Oculoplastic Surgery

Editors

JOHN B. HOLDS

GUY G. MASSRY

FACIAL PLASTIC SURGERY CLINICS OF NORTH AMERICA

www.facialplastic.theclinics.com

Consulting Editor

J. REGAN THOMAS

May 2021 • Volume 29 • Number 2

ELSEVIER

1600 John F. Kennedy Boulevard • Suite 1800 • Philadelphia, Pennsylvania, 19103-2899

http://www.theclinics.com

**FACIAL PLASTIC SURGERY CLINICS OF NORTH AMERICA Volume 29, Number 2
May 2021 ISSN 1064-7406, ISBN-13: 978-0-323-75641-9**

Editor: Stacy Eastman
Developmental Editor: Ann Gielou M. Posedio

Facial Plastic Surgery Clinics of North America (ISSN 1064-7406) is published quarterly by Elsevier Inc., 360 Park Avenue South, New York, NY 10010-1710. Months of issue are February, May, August, and November. Business and Editorial Offices: 1600 John F. Kennedy Blvd., Suite 1800, Philadelphia, PA 19103-2899. Periodicals postage paid at New York, NY, and additional mailing offices. Subscription prices are $412.00 per year (US individuals), $895.00 per year (US institutions), $459.00 per year (Canadian individuals), $944.00 per year (Canadian institutions), $546.00 per year (foreign individuals), $944.00 per year (foreign institutions), $100.00 per year (US students), $100.00 per year (Canadian students), and $255.00 per year (foreign students). Foreign air speed delivery is included in all *Clinics* subscription prices. All prices are subject to change without notice. POSTMASTER: Send address changes to *Facial Plastic Surgery Clinics*, Elsevier Health Sciences Division, Subscription Customer Service, 3251 Riverport Lane, Maryland Heights, MO 63043. **Customer service: 1-800-654-2452 (US and Canada); 1-314-447-8871 (outside US and Canada); Fax: 314-447-8029; E-mail: journalscustomerservice-usa@elsevier.com (for print support); journalsonlinesupport-usa@elsevier.com (for online support).**

Reprints. For copies of 100 or more of articles in this publication, please contact the Commercial Reprints Department, Elsevier Inc., 360 Park Avenue South, New York, NY 10010-1710. Tel.: 212-633-3874; Fax: 212-633-3820; E-mail: reprints@elsevier.com.

Facial Plastic Surgery Clinics of North America is covered in *MEDLINE/PubMed* (*Index Medicus*).

Contributors

CONSULTING EDITOR

J. REGAN THOMAS, MD
Professor, Facial Plastic and Reconstructive
Surgery, Department of Otolaryngology–Head
and Neck Surgery, Northwestern University
School of Medicine, Chicago, Illinois, USA

EDITORS

JOHN B. HOLDS, MD, FACS
Clinical Professor, Departments of
Ophthalmology and Otolaryngology–Head and
Neck Surgery, Saint Louis University School of
Medicine, Ophthalmic Plastic and Cosmetic
Surgery, Inc, St Louis, Missouri, USA

GUY G. MASSRY, MD
Beverly Hills Ophthalmic Plastic and
Reconstructive Surgery, Beverly Hills,
California, USA; Division of Oculoplastic
Surgery, Department of Plastic Surgery,
Cedars-Sinai Medical Center, Division of
Oculoplastic Surgery, Department of
Ophthalmology, Keck School of Medicine of
USC, University of Southern California, Los
Angeles, California, USA

AUTHORS

CLAUDIA AMARAL, BS
University of Puerto Rico School of Medicine,
San Juan, Puerto Rico

BRIAN BIESMAN, MD, FACS
Assistant Clinical Professor, Ophthalmology,
Dermatology, Otolaryngology, Vanderbilt
University Medical Center, Nashville,
Tennessee, USA

BRIAN H. CHON, MD
Oculofacial Plastic Surgery, Department of
Ophthalmology, Cole Eye Institute, Cleveland
Clinic Foundation, Cleveland, Ohio, USA

LIZA M. COHEN, MD
Division of Orbital and Ophthalmic Plastic
Surgery, Doheny and Stein Eye Institutes,
University of California, Los Angeles, Los
Angeles, California, USA

RAYMOND S. DOUGLAS, MD PhD
Department of Surgery, Division of
Ophthalmology, Cedars-Sinai Medical Center,
Los Angeles, California, USA; Beverly Hills
Ophthalmic Plastic and Reconstructive
Surgery, Beverly Hills, California, USA; State
Key Laboratory of Ophthalmology, Zhongshan
Ophthalmic Center, Sun Yat-sen University,
Guangzhou, China

DINO ELYASSNIA, MD
Marten Clinic of Plastic Surgery, San
Francisco, California, USA

KERRY HEITMILLER, MD
Department of Dermatology and Cutaneous
Biology, Thomas Jefferson University,
Philadelphia, Pennsylvania, USA

JOHN B. HOLDS, MD, FACS
Clinical Professor, Departments of
Ophthalmology and Otolaryngology–Head and
Neck Surgery, Saint Louis University School of

Medicine, Ophthalmic Plastic and Cosmetic Surgery, Inc, St Louis, Missouri, USA

CATHERINE J. HWANG, MD, FACS
Oculofacial Plastic Surgery, Department of Ophthalmology, Cole Eye Institute, Cleveland Clinic Foundation, Cleveland, Ohio, USA

ANDREW A. JACONO, MD, FACS
Associate Clinical Professor, Department of Otolaryngology–Head and Neck Surgery, Division of Facial Plastic Surgery, Albert Einstein College of Medicine, New York, New York, USA; Chief, Department of Facial Plastic and Reconstructive Surgery, Northwell Health (North Shore LIJ), Manhasset, New York, USA

HANNAH LANDSBERGER
Nova Southeastern University Dr. Kiran C. Patel College of Allopathic Medicine, Davie, Florida, USA

ALYSSA LOLOFIE, BS
Medical Student, University of Utah School of Medicine, Salt Lake City, Utah, USA

TIMOTHY MARTEN, MD
Founder and Director, Marten Clinic of Plastic Surgery, San Francisco, California, USA

GUY G. MASSRY, MD
Beverly Hills Ophthalmic Plastic and Reconstructive Surgery, Beverly Hills, California, USA; Division of Oculoplastic Surgery, Department of Plastic Surgery, Cedars-Sinai Medical Center, Division of Oculoplastic Surgery, Department of Ophthalmology, Keck School of Medicine of USC, University of Southern California, Los Angeles, California, USA

BRYAN C. MENDELSON, FRCS (Ed), FRACS, FACS
The Centre for Facial Plastic Surgery, Toorak, Victoria, Australia

JOSÉ RAÚL MONTES, MD, FACS, FACCS
Department of Ophthalmology, University of Puerto Rico School of Medicine, José Raúl Montes Eyes and Facial Rejuvenation, San Juan, Puerto Rico

FARZAD R. NAHAI, MD
Private Practice, The Center for Plastic Surgery at Metroderm, Assistant Clinical Professor of Plastic and Reconstructive Surgery, Atlanta, Georgia, USA

FOAD NAHAI, MD
Private Practice, The Center for Plastic Surgery at Metroderm, Adjunct Professor of Plastic and Reconstructive Surgery, Atlanta, Georgia, USA

CRISTEN OLDS, MD
Roxbury Institute, Beverly Hills, California, USA; Roseville Facial Plastic Surgery, Roseville, California, USA

JULIAN D. PERRY, MD
Oculofacial Plastic Surgery, Department of Ophthalmology, Cole Eye Institute, Cleveland Clinic Foundation, Cleveland, Ohio, USA

CHRISTINA RING, MD
Department of Dermatology and Cutaneous Biology, Thomas Jefferson University, Philadelphia, Pennsylvania, USA

DANIEL B. ROOTMAN, MD, MS
Division of Orbital and Ophthalmic Plastic Surgery, Doheny and Stein Eye Institutes, University of California, Los Angeles, Los Angeles, California, USA

NAZANIN SAEDI, MD
Department of Dermatology and Cutaneous Biology, Thomas Jefferson University, Philadelphia, Pennsylvania, USA

RENATO SALTZ, MD, FACS
Adjunct Professor, University of Utah, Salt Lake City, Utah, USA; Past President, ISAPS; Past President, ASAPS; Owner of Saltz Plastic Surgery & Saltz Spa Vitoria, Salt Lake City, Utah, USA

ELIZABETH SANTOS, MPH-A, DrPH
José Raúl Montes Eyes and Facial Rejuvenation, San Juan, Puerto Rico

DENIZ SARHADDI, MD
Private Practice, Saint Louis Cosmetic Surgery, Inc, Chesterfield, Missouri, USA

KENNETH D. STEINSAPIR, MD
Orbital and Ophthalmic Plastic Surgery Division, Stein Eye Institute, David Geffen School of Medicine at UCLA, Los Angeles, California, USA

SAMANTHA STEINSAPIR
Orbital and Ophthalmic Plastic Surgery Division, Stein Eye Institute, David Geffen School of Medicine at UCLA, Los Angeles, California, USA

JONATHAN SYKES, MD
Professor Emeritus, Facial Plastic and Reconstructive Surgery, UC Davis Medical Center, Sacramento, California, USA; Roxbury Institute, Beverly Hills, California, USA

YAO WANG, MD
Fellow, Department of Plastic Surgery, Division of Oculoplastic Surgery, Cedars-Sinai Medical Center, Los Angeles, California, USA; Beverly Hills Ophthalmic Plastic and Reconstructive Surgery, Beverly Hills, California, USA

CHIN-HO WONG, MMed (Surg), FAMS (Plast Surg)
W Aesthetic Plastic Surgery, Singapore, Singapore

Contents

The anatomy of the eyelids and periorbital region is delicate. The individual anatomic variations determine each person's eyelid appearance and function. It is essential that every surgeon that evaluates and treats the aesthetic conditions of patients desiring periorbital enhancement understands the association of anatomy and diagnosis. Each periorbital aesthetic diagnosis has an anatomic basis, and knowledge of the applied anatomy allows a targeted treatment plan. This article outlines the layered anatomy with its clinical significance for the eyelids and periorbital region. Specific examples are used to illustrate the applied anatomy. A contemporary treatment plan for each anatomic problem is given.

The endoscopic approach for forehead rejuvenation and brow lift has many advantages. It provided excellent exposure for release of periorbital soft tissues combined with endoscopic magnification, shorter scars, and reduced risk of alopecia and scalp sensory changes compared with the traditional open coronal brow lift. The technique has improved over the last 15 years with better fixation devices, a better understanding of the longevity, and decreased complications of the procedure. The endoscopic brow lift offers the patient a much easier and safer solution for the aging forehead, active wrinkles from corrugator and frontalis hyperactivity, and the ptotic, asymmetric brow.

 Video content accompanies this article at http://www.facialplastic.theclinics.com.

Given the central importance of the "eyes," meaning the periorbital region, to facial appearance, the motivated blepharoplasty patient has the opportunity to improve appearance significantly beyond the minimum of age reversal, to reveal inner beauty or add attractiveness. Bright and beautiful eyes have good three-dimensional contouring. The benefits of a quality eyelid crease enable the surgical focus to be on lid contouring with a reduced requirement for lid skin and fat excision. A durable crease maintains fixation of both the tarsal and infrabrow segments. The softness of youthful eyes can be regained by precise, but cautious, use of lipofilling.

Ptosis surgery is performed via an anterior/external or posterior/internal approach, primarily defined by the eyelid elevator muscle surgically addressed: the levator complex anteriorly or Muller muscle posteriorly. Posterior ptosis surgery via Muller muscle conjunctival resection is an excellent first choice for cases of mild to moderate ptosis with good levator function, as it is predictable, provides a reliable cosmetic outcome, requires no patient cooperation during surgery, portends a lower rate of reoperation, and rarely leads to lagophthalmos and/or eyelid retraction postoperatively. External levator resection is preferred in patients with severe ocular surface/cicatricial conjunctival disease, shortened fornices, and lesser levator function.

The aging appearance of the lower eyelids is multifactorial, involving changes in the skin, orbital fat, orbicularis muscle, soft tissue of the midface, and tear trough. The extent of these changes differs in each case and happens in a background of volume loss that occurs with facial aging. We present the indications, advantages, and technique for volumizing transcutaneous lower blepharoplasty with fat transposition. The absolute and relative contraindications to transcutaneous surgery are discussed, and surgical details of transconjunctival blepharoplasty with fat repositioning and autologous fat grafting as alternative approaches are included.

Transconjunctival lower lid blepharoplasty is a safe and effective procedure with a low complication rate. Success with this procedure depends on proper patient analysis and selection. The lower lid periorbital fat can be resected, or preserved, and draped over the orbital rim or used as free fat grafts, depending on the clinical presentation. The lower lid skin can be resurfaced with a peel, with a laser, or by skin pinch depending on surgeon preference.

Fat grafting represents the most important new addition to surgical procedures to rejuvenate the orbit since the inception of the "blepharoplasty" technique. Traditional blepharoplasty procedures do not always address the changes that occur with age in the orbital area and can actually degrade the appearance of the eye. Fat grafting allows treatment of age-associated loss of periorbital volume not addressed by traditional blepharoplasty procedures. Fat grafting is an artistically powerful method to rejuvenate the periorbital orbital area that often provides a more healthy, fit, youthful, and sensual appearance than traditional blepharoplasty procedures.

Aesthetic canthal suspension can be an effective adjunct to lower eyelid blepharoplasty. Understanding the anatomy and function of the lateral canthal tendon is critical for preoperative evaluation and surgical decision making. In this article, the authors discuss the lateral canthal terminology, anatomy, and aging changes. Various canthal suspension procedures, including open and closed canthal suspension, commissure sparing open canthoplasty, and canthopexy, are described. Finally, the preoperative evaluation, postoperative course, and complications of surgery are reviewed.

 Video content accompanies this article at http://www.facialplastic.theclinics.com.

Numerous solutions for post-blepharoplasty lower eyelid retraction are reviewed. Patients require permanent recruitment of skin and soft tissue to lengthen the lower eyelid and control of the lower eyelid shape. The authors use a hand-carved expanded polytetrafluoroethylene (ePTFE) implant held with microscrews to provide volume and felting material at the orbital rim and to permanently fix vertically lifted cheek soft tissue into the lower eyelid. The eyelid margin is also controlled with a hard palate graft inset into the conjunctival surface below the tarsus. This eyelid reconstruction avoids tension on the lateral canthoplasty, a point of failure in other solutions.

Festoons represent a combination of fluid accumulation and soft tissue laxity in the superolateral cheek. They remain a difficult entity to treat. The ideal treatment for festoons would possess minimal invasiveness and recovery time, and predictably improve the condition. No nonsurgical treatment currently meets these criteria, and surgical treatments have significant limitations. Fortunately, a variety of treatment options exist that can benefit each patient and be tailored to their specific needs. Knowledge of the underlying anatomy, clinical characteristics, and clinical evaluation will better equip the treating physician to manage festoons.

Globe prominence (proptosis) may be caused by a variety of congenital or acquired conditions and poses unique challenges to aesthetic and reconstructive surgery. Once the underlying cause of proptosis is determined, a treatment plan consisting of surgical and medical procedures can be formed. Thyroid eye disease is the most common cause of proptosis and helps guide treatment options for proptosis. Although common eyelid and orbital procedures are used for proptosis correction, special care must be taken due to the unique difficulties of the distorted anatomy. Various surgical procedures and less invasive treatments can be combined to provide optimal aesthetic and functional results.

Periorbital rejuvenation is a common reason for patients to seek cosmetic treatment. There are several nonsurgical light and energy–based devices available to treat various aspects of periorbital rejuvenation without risks of an invasive, surgical procedure. Although ablative laser resurfacing appears to offer the most impressive clinical improvements, nonablative devices result in noticeable cosmetic improvement with more favorable side-effect profiles and shorter recovery times. The specific modality selected for periorbital rejuvenation should be tailored to patients' individual characteristics, preferences, and aesthetic goals. With continued advancements, additional nonsurgical light and energy–based devices will become available in the future for periorbital rejuvenation.

 Video content accompanies this article at http://www.facialplastic.theclinics.com.

A retrospective observational case study and a literature review were conducted to evaluate how anatomic findings, especially those related to the periorbital zone, serve as a guiding compass for injectable implants. Treatment techniques and product selection will be discussed for patients with negative vector, shallow orbit, and deep set eyes. Versatility of injectables will be demonstrated on patients with peanut face, iatrogenically altered anatomy (after surgery), and trauma.

 Video content accompanies this article at http://www.facialplastic.theclinics.com.

Dermal fillers, in particular hyaluronic acid gel (HAG) fillers, are used in the treatment of aging changes in the periocular area. Filler treatment requires in-depth knowledge of specific issues relating to product performance and administration, safety protocols, and recognition and treatment of complications. There are different approaches to treatment of the tear trough. Prior filler treatment must be suspected in patients presenting for aesthetic evaluation, and the possibility of migration with a dysmorphic appearance and/or Tyndall effect appearance always is kept in mind. Treatment with hyaluronidase injection generally is effective in reducing overcorrection or migration of HAG in this area.

Dermal fillers remain popular for facial rejuvenation but with its increasing use, the potential for more complications including blindness is present. This article focuses on the mechanism of filler-associated blindness, possible treatments, and future directions. Unfortunately, to date there is no proven treatment to reverse filler-induced blindness or visual compromise. It is essential for all injectors to discuss the potential ocular risks including blindness with their patients and obtain informed consent before filler injection.

FACIAL PLASTIC SURGERY CLINICS OF NORTH AMERICA

Foreword
Oculoplastic Surgery

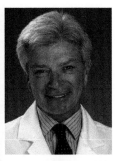

J. Regan Thomas, MD
Consulting Editor

The appearance of the eyelids and periocular area of the face is an important component of an individual's overall appearance. Changes of the skin and anatomy related to aging represent a frequent request by the patient population for correction and improvement in the eyelid and periorbital region. Surgery and other treatments of eyelids, brows, and periorbital areas have been incorporated into the expertise of several specialties, including facial plastic surgery and otolaryngology–head and neck surgery, ophthalmology, and plastic surgery. Based on the patient's needs and desires in addition to their anatomic presentation and aesthetic appearance, there are multiple techniques and rejuvenation procedures available to be utilized by the physician. Dr Holds and Dr Massry, as Guest Editors of this issue, titled Oculoplastic Surgery, have assembled an outstanding group of experienced physician authors who cover the broad array of treatment alternatives related to the eyelid and periorbital regions.

The contributing authors represent a variety of the above-noted specialties and provide key insights of various treatment techniques and modalities. All of the selected contributing authors, while representing a variety of specialties, are experienced and well-recognized experts in the treatment approaches that they describe. In addition to surgical procedures, a variety of useful treatments, including periocular dermal fillers and light and energy-based modalities, are described. There is important attention to preventing as well as correcting complications from treatment of this challenging and sensitive anatomic region.

Blepharoplasty and related procedures are frequent and popular treatments for a growing patient population. Possessing appropriate approaches and techniques through expertise in these areas is valuable to the treating physicians and their respective patients. This issue of *Facial Plastic Surgery Clinics of North America* as organized by Dr Holds and Dr Massry offers salient and valuable insights and is a useful reference for our readership in this important component of our represented specialties.

I am particularly pleased to provide this issue of *Facial Plastic Clinics of North America* to our readership as a valuable resource based on the insights, experience, and expertise of our multispecialty contributors.

J. Regan Thomas, MD
Facial Plastic and Reconstructive Surgery
Department of Otolaryngology
– Head and Neck Surgery
Northwestern University School of Medicine
60 East Delaware Place
Chicago, IL 60611, USA

E-mail address:
regan.thomas@nm.org

Facial Plast Surg Clin N Am 29 (2021) xiii
https://doi.org/10.1016/j.fsc.2021.02.009
1064-7406/21/© 2021 Published by Elsevier Inc.

Preface

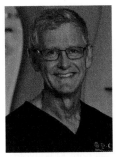 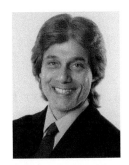

John B. Holds, MD, FACS   Guy G. Massry, MD

Editors

This text, which will update the reader regarding key issues in Oculofacial Surgery, was developed in the year no one will forget: 2020. The chaos, uncertainty, death, and destruction of the first global pandemic in over a century affected us all and created unique challenges, but also unique opportunities to observe, reflect, grow, and refine our practices, friendships, and world view.

The authors included are seminal contributors in their fields and were selected based on relationships fostered through years of fruitful interaction, collaboration, and shared learning. Many more topics and worthy authors could have been included, but, unfortunately, space limitations often control these decisions. For anyone omitted, we apologize in advance for the oversight. We are proud of this issue of *Facial Plastic Surgery Clinics of North America*, and of the broad range of subjects reviewed. We feel it provides a contemporary overview of the essential surgical and nonsurgical procedures and concepts relevant to all who perform eyelid and periorbital rejuvenation. We are especially excited that the authorship is multidisciplinary in nature, which provides the most well-rounded view of the topics discussed.

We would like to individually thank all our authors. This includes Drs Sykes and Olds for their thought-provoking introductory article on anatomy and how it applies to surgery; Dr. Saltz and Ms. Lolofie for their personal and historical perspective on endoscopic brow lifting; Dr Mendelson and Wong for their insights of platform upper

blepharoplasty; Drs Rootman and Cohen for tackling the always vexing problem of blepharoptosis; and Drs Jacono, Nahai, Nahai, and Sarhaddi for sharing their experience on the open approach and transconjunctival lower blepharoplasty. Dr Massry and I (with Drs. Wang and Douglas) were honored to add our insights on the various options of canthal suspension, while Drs Chon, Hwang, Perry, and Steinspair have provided concise and detailed pearls and approaches to the most challenging of eyelid and periorbital deficits, the management of festoons and postblepharoplasty lower-eyelid retraction.

The final surgical procedures covered are from surgeons who have been leaders, and generationally innovative, on our understanding of these topics. Drs. Biesman, Heitmiller, Ring and Saedi contribute their encyclopedic knowledge regarding the utility of light and energy-based devices. Drs Douglas and Wang, along with Ms Landsberger, present relevant issues and approaches integral to our treating the patient with the prominent eye, while Drs. Maarten and Elyassnia has provided a treatise describing his masterful and artistic approach to facial fat transfer.

Regarding nonsurgical interventions, Drs. Montes and Santos with Ms. Amaral beautifully and artistically cover the appropriate use of periocular dermal fillers, while Drs Hwang, Chon, and Perry cover the important issues relating to vascular embolization of dermal fillers, a topic every injector needs intimate knowledge of. We are joined by Dr Wang in discussing a frequent

Facial Plast Surg Clin N Am 29 (2021) xv–xvi
https://doi.org/10.1016/j.fsc.2021.02.008
1064-7406/21/© 2021 Published by Elsevier Inc.

facialplastic.theclinics.com

situation in the periorbital cosmetic surgeon's office, managing periorbital filler.

We cannot thank our colleagues who authored this text enough for their hard work and perseverance. It was difficult to focus during this year, when each turn raised questions regarding our health, financial stability, and happiness. Editorship of this issue provided a unique opportunity to stay in touch with the authors during a year with no in-person meetings, during which we would normally be able to share scientific knowledge, share surgical observations, and socialize with friends and colleagues. In that regard, we grew as friends during this year, and our friendship and professional regards with our authors grew as well, despite lockdowns, financial stresses, and personal and generalized anxiety. Kudos to all who helped make this issue of *Facial Plastic Surgery Clinics of North America* a reality.

John B. Holds, MD, FACS
Ophthalmic Plastic and Cosmetic Surgery, Inc
St. Louis, MO, 63131, USA

Guy G. Massry, MD
Beverly Hills Ophthalmic Plastic Surgery
150 North Robertson Boulevard, #314
Beverly Hills, CA 90211, USA

E-mail addresses:
jholds@gmail.com (J.B. Holds)
gmassry@drmassry.com (G.G. Massry)

Website:
http://Drmassry.com

Anatomic Trends and Directions in Periorbital Aesthetic Surgery

Jonathan Sykes, MD[a,b,*], Cristen Olds, MD[b,c]

KEYWORDS

- Periorbital aesthetic surgery • Eyelid appearance • Brow

KEY POINTS

- The orbit and periorbital region is anatomically complex and contains crucial muscular, neurovascular structural components.
- A thorough understanding of periorbital anatomy is crucial to safely and effectively addressing periorbital pathology and aging.
- The eyelid and eyebrow should be considered in tandem when assessing periorbital pathology.

PERIORBITAL TOPOGRAPHY

The eyelids and brows have a variable surface covering that differs from the covering in all other parts of the body. The thin eyelid skin is in stark contrast to the skin adjacent to the eyelids (brow, temple, and cheek), all of which have much thicker skin cover and underlying superficial fat. The skin of the eyebrow is thick, having a variable amount and density of eyebrow hairs.

The vertical distance between the upper eyelid margin and the eyebrow is variable and is related to the eyebrow height. The upper eyelid crease is an infolding of upper eyelid skin and is variable in height and depth. This gently curved upper eyelid crease is formed by the insertion of fibers of the levator aponeurosis into the orbicularis muscle and the eyelid skin (**Fig. 1**). In whites, the height of the upper lid crease at the midpupillary line is usually between 6 and 10 mm and tapers to 3 to 4 mm medially and laterally. In Asians, the height of the supratarsal fold is usually lower (and sometimes absent) than is the crease in most whites and is approximately 3 to 6 mm in the midpupillary line[1] (**Fig. 2**). An elevated supratarsal crease can be associated with upper eyelid ptosis, as disinsertion of the levator aponeurosis can cause both malposition of the eyelid margin (ptosis) and elevation of the supratarsal fold.

The lower eyelid skin fold is located approximately 3 mm from the lower eyelid margin.[2] This fold is related to the position and contraction of the orbicularis oculi muscle (OOM) and is more commonly seen in children, descending and becoming more irregular with age.

The palpebral fissure is approximately 10 mm in height and 30 mm in width. The aperture can be decreased from eyelid ptosis (weakening or dehiscence of the levator complex) or from hypertrophy of the OOMs. The level of the upper eyelid margin is usually 1 to 2 mm below the superior limbus, and the lower eyelid margin is usually at the inferior limbus.

THE BROWS

The eyebrows are not a part of the forehead or the eyelids but are an important portion of the periorbital complex, as they form the superior frame of the region. For this reason, eyebrow height, orientation, thickness, and general appearance get the attention of patients, surgeons, and cosmetic brow specialists.[3,4] The skin of the eyebrow is thick, and it contains dermal appendages that produce short, course hairs. The brow hairs emerge

[a] Facial Plastic & Reconstructive Surgery, UC Davis Medical Center, Sacramento, CA, USA; [b] Roxbury Institute, Beverly Hills, CA, USA; [c] Roseville Facial Plastic Surgery, Roseville, CA, USA
* Corresponding author.
E-mail addresses: dr.jonathan.m.sykes@gmail.com; jmsykes@ucdavis.edu

Facial Plast Surg Clin N Am 29 (2021) 155–162
https://doi.org/10.1016/j.fsc.2021.02.006

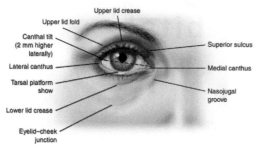

Upper lid crease

Upper lid fold

Canthal tilt
(2 mm higher
laterally)

Superior sulcus

Lateral canthus

Medial canthus

Tarsal platform
show

Nasojugal
groove

Lower lid crease

Eyelid–cheek
junction

Fig. 1. External topography of the upper and lower eyelid. (*Reproduced from*: Patel AD, Massry GG. Eyelid and Periorbital Anatomy. In: Nahai F, Nahai F, eds. *The Art of Aesthetic Surgery: Principles and Techniques* Vol 1. 3 ed.: Thieme 2020. (Figure 31.7 in original).)

from the skin surface at markedly oblique angles. The shape, thickness, and orientation of the brow hairs vary with personal style and preference and fashion trends.

The height of the brow is based on the movements and relative contraction of the muscles that move the brows (**Fig. 3**). The only elevators of the eyebrows are the paired frontalis muscles, which form the anterior belly of the occipitofrontalis musculofascial muscle complex. The frontalis muscle is enveloped by the galea aponeurosis. Contraction of this muscle creates horizontal rhytids of the forehead skin and produces brow elevation and scalp tightening. The frontalis muscle has no bony attachments. Superiorly, it thins into an aponeurosis, and inferiorly, its medial attachments are continuous with the procerus muscle and the orbital portion of the orbicularis muscles.[5]

Depression of the eyebrows is accomplished with several muscle groups. The midline procerus muscle arises from the fascia covering the lower portion of the nasal bones and the upper lateral cartilages and inserts into the skin of the central lower forehead. Contraction of the procerus muscle produces a transverse fold at the nasal root and central brow depression. The paired corrugator supercilii muscles are obliquely oriented muscles that originate from medial frontal bone at the superomedial orbit. The muscle passes obliquely in a superolateral direction and inserts into the skin of the eyebrow and deep fascia of the inferior frontalis muscle.[6] Contraction of the corrugator muscle produces vertical glabellar folds and pulls the brow inferiorly and medially. Contraction of this muscle also creates a frowned appearance.

The OOM has pretarsal and preseptal components that act as the protractors of the eyelids (**Fig. 4**). The more peripheral orbital portion of the OOM interdigitates with the inferior frontalis muscle fibers. These orbital fibers contribute to depression of the eyebrows.

The height and position of the eyebrows are related to the relative contraction of the brow elevators (frontalis muscle) versus the contraction of the brow depressors (corrugator supercilii, depressor supercilii, procerus, and orbicularis oculi).[7] Excessive brow elevation can confer a surprised expression, whereas excess brow

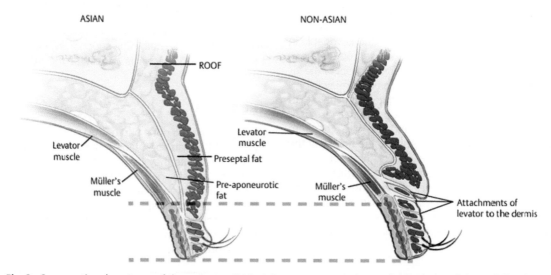

Fig. 2. Cross-sectional anatomy of the upper eyelid in Asian versus non-Asian eyelids. Asian eyelids are fuller than those of non-Asians, as preaponeurotic fat rides lower in the lid and there is a preseptal fat layer, which is continuous with the brow fat pad. Also, note potentially blunted attachments of the levator to the dermis, which can lead to an incomplete or absent crease in many patients. (*Reproduced from*: Patel AD, Massry GG. Eyelid and Periorbital Anatomy. In: Nahai F, Nahai F, eds. *The Art of Aesthetic Surgery: Principles and Techniques* Vol 1. 3 ed.: Thieme 2020. (Figure 31.12 in original).)

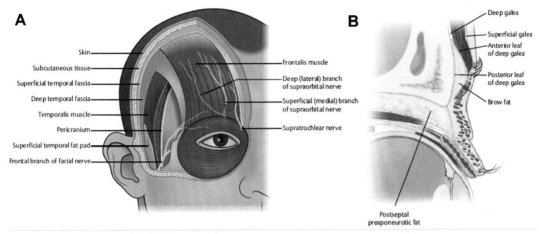

Fig. 3. Layers of the forehead. (*A*) Frontal view. (*B*) Parasagittal section through eyeball. ([*A*] *Reproduced from* Sokoya M, Inman J, Ducic Y. Scalp and forehead reconstruction. Semin Plast Surg 2018;32(02):90–94; and [*B*] Codner M, McCord C, eds. Eyelid & Periorbital Surgery, 2nd ed. New York, NY: Thieme; 2016. (Figure 31.6 in original.).)

depression can depict anger, consternation, or worry. Brow elevation also has a functional purpose, as contraction of the frontalis muscle may compensate for primary eyelid ptosis.[8–10]

LAYERS OF THE EYELID, UPPER LID

The upper eyelid is composed of very thin skin, structurally dense fibrous tissue (tarsal plate), and muscles that close (protractors) and open (retractors) the eyelids (**Fig. 5**). The upper eyelid crease is a horizontal indentation formed by the attachment of the superficial levator aponeurosis fibers into the orbicularis oris intermuscular septa and subcutaneous tissue. The crease is located approximately 6 to 10 mm above the eyelid margin centrally in most whites. When present, the upper lid crease in Asians is located at 3 to 6 mm.[11] In patients with dehiscence of the levator aponeurosis,

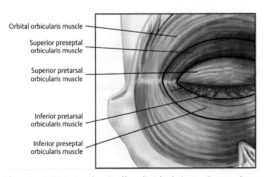

Fig. 4. OOM is classically divided into 3 portions: orbital, preseptal, and pretarsal. (*Reproduced from*: Patel AD, Massry GG. Eyelid and Periorbital Anatomy. In: Nahai F, Nahai F, eds. *The Art of Aesthetic Surgery: Principles and Techniques* Vol 1. 3 ed.: Thieme 2020.)

the eyelid crease is usually elevated, and the eyelid is thin.[12,13]

The eyelid is covered by very thin skin, usually only 400 to 500 μm in thickness.[14,15] There is almost no subcutaneous tissue in the eyelids. The OOM (protractors of the eyelids) are located just deep to the skin. The orbital septum is located just deep to the OOM. The septum is a thin, multilayered connective tissue beginning at the arcus marginalis along the orbital rim. The septum is a continuation of the periorbita within the orbit and contains the eyelid fat pads, which lie just deep to the septum. The upper eyelid has 2 fat pads: a nasal (medial) fat pad and a central (preaponeurotic) fat pad (**Fig. 6**). In the lateral portion of the upper eyelid is the lacrimal gland. The medial and central fat pads are separated by the superior oblique muscle and its associated trochlea. The nasal fat pad is whiter and contains more fibrotic fat than does the central pad.[16]

The central eyelid fat pad is termed preaponeurotic because it is located just superficial to the levator aponeurosis (upper eyelid retractor) (see **Fig. 6**). The levator palpebrae superioris (LPS) muscle originates from the lesser wing of the sphenoid bone just above the annulus of Zinn and superolateral to the optic canal (**Fig. 7**). The muscle travels within the orbit in a relatively horizontal orientation in close approximation to the superior rectus muscle. At a point just posterior to the superior orbital rim, the LPS widens and changes to a vertical orientation at a fascial condensation. This fascial thickening is termed the Whitnall ligament (superior transverse ligament). The fascia attaches medially to the fascia around the trochlea and laterally to the capsule of the lacrimal gland and the frontal bone periosteum. As the upper

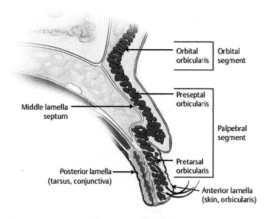

Fig. 5. Upper eyelid cross-section. (*Reproduced from*: Patel AD, Massry GG. Eyelid and Periorbital Anatomy. In: Nahai F, Nahai F, eds. *The Art of Aesthetic Surgery: Principles and Techniques* Vol 1. 3 ed.: Thieme 2020. (Figure 31.8a in original).)

eyelid retracts, the fascial sheet helps elevate the upper eyelid fat pockets, preventing unsightly eyelid bulging.[17]

At the level of Whitnall ligament, the levator muscle separates into anterior (superficial) aponeurosis and a posterior (deep) component (see **Fig. 7**). The retractor complex also changes from a horizontal orientation to a vertical one. The deep muscle is termed the Muller muscle and is innervated by sympathetic (autonomic) nerve fibers. These fibers course with the third (oculomotor) cranial nerve. Muller muscle attaches to the superior border of the tarsal plate, while most of the more anterior aponeurotic fibers insert onto

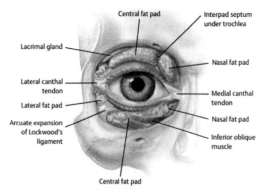

Fig. 6. Fat pads of the upper and lower eyelids. The trochlea separates the upper nasal and preaponeurotic fat pad. The inferior oblique separates the nasal and central fat pad of the lower eyelid. The arcuate expansion separates the lateral fat pad of the lower eyelid. (*Reproduced from*: Patel AD, Massry GG. Eyelid and Periorbital Anatomy. In: Nahai F, Nahai F, eds. *The Art of Aesthetic Surgery: Principles and Techniques* Vol 1. 3 ed.: Thieme 2020. (Figure 31.13 in original).)

the lower one-third of the anterior surface of the tarsal plate.

The tarsal plates are dense fibrous tissue that gives structural integrity and form to the upper eyelid. The upper lid tarsal plate measures 8 to 12 mm centrally and tapers medially and laterally to 2 to 3 mm as the plate inserts into the canthal tendons.[18,19] The levator apparatus attaches to the tarsal plate on its superficial and superior surfaces (see **Fig. 4**). The palpebral conjunctiva is densely attached and bound to the undersurface of the tarsal plate.

LOWER EYELIDS

The lower eyelid is composed of very thin skin, a small tarsal plate, and muscles that close (protractors) and open (retractors) the lid (**Fig. 8**). The shape of the lower eyelid is determined by the attachment of the medial and lateral canthal tendons, the tone, and contraction of the lower eyelid OOM (**Fig. 9**). The lateral canthal angle is usually positioned 1 to 2 mm above the medial canthal angle. The infratarsal crease of the lower eyelid is variable but is often most noticeable at the inferior border of the short lower eyelid tarsal plate.

The lower eyelid is also covered by very thin skin with almost no subcutaneous tissue being present. The OOM is located just deep to the skin, with the pretarsal OOM contributing to the tone and shape of the lower eyelid. The septum orbitale of the lower eyelid is located just deep to the lower OOM. This septum covers and contains the 3 fat pads of the lower eyelid (see **Fig. 6**). Herniation of these fat pads is associated with unsightly bulges of the lower eyelid. The medial (nasal) and central lower lid fat pads are separated by the inferior oblique muscle. The central and lateral (temporal) fat pads are separated by the arcuate extension of the oblique muscle.[20] The inferior oblique muscle is the most superficial extraocular muscle, and injury to this should be avoided during lower blepharoplasty.

The retractors of the lower eyelid arise from fibers of the inferior rectus and inferior oblique muscles (see **Fig. 8**). The retractors begin as a fibrous sheet and emanate from the suspensory ligament of the eye (Lockwood ligament) and fuse with fibers from the orbital septum approximately 5 mm below the inferior border of the tarsal plate.[1] These conjoined fibers insert onto the inferior border of the tarsal plate.[21]

The lower lid tarsal plate is shorter than the upper tarsal plate and measures approximately 4 mm centrally and tapers medially and laterally to 2 mm as the plate inserts into the canthal tendons. Again, the palpebral conjunctiva of the lower eyelid

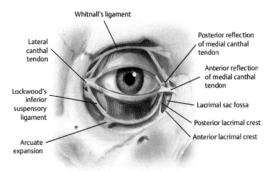

Fig. 7. Relevant anatomic structures for upper and lower lid anatomy. ROOF, retroorbicularis oculi fat; SOOF, suborbicularis oculi fat. (*Reproduced from*: Patel AD, Massry GG. Eyelid and Periorbital Anatomy. In: Nahai F, Nahai F, eds. *The Art of Aesthetic Surgery: Principles and Techniques* Vol 1. 3 ed.: Thieme 2020. (Figure 31.11 in original).)

is densely adherent to the deep surface of the lower eyelid tarsal plate.

PERIOCULAR AESTHETIC CONDITIONS
Skin

The skin of the eyelids is the thinnest in the body. In addition, there is no subcutaneous (superficial) fat supporting the eyelid skin from the eyelid margin to near the brow. Early periorbital aging changes are often seen in the eyelids because of the thin skin and lack of superficial fat.[22,23] This condition, known as dermatochalasis, is treated with an upper blepharoplasty, during which excess skin above the supratarsal fold is removed.

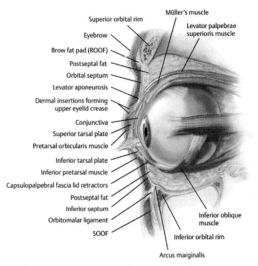

Fig. 8. Lower lid cross-section. (*Reproduced from*: Patel AD, Massry GG. Eyelid and Periorbital Anatomy. In: Nahai F, Nahai F, eds. *The Art of Aesthetic Surgery: Principles and Techniques* Vol 1. 3 ed.: Thieme 2020. (Figure 31.8b in original).)

Orbicularis Oculi Muscle

The OOM is an oval sheet of concentric muscle fibers that cover the upper and lower eyelids, parts of the forehead, and the upper portion of the midface. This muscle is the main protractor of the eye. Its contraction leads to a narrowing of the palpebral aperture and contributes to tear drainage.[24] The muscle can be divided anatomically into 2 parts: the orbital and palpebral portions. The pars palpebralis can be further divided into the preseptal and pretarsal regions.[25]

The muscle is located just deep to the skin and is supplied by divisions of cranial nerve VII (facial nerve). This muscle is responsible for eyelid closure (protractor), performing both involuntary (blinking) and voluntary (squinting) muscle activity. The origin of the palpebral portion of the OOM is the medial palpebral ligament, with the insertion of the muscle being the lateral palpebral raphe.

The OOM receives its motor innervation through branches of the facial nerve. The temporal branch courses superomedially to innervate the upper half of the orbicularis, frontalis, and corrugator supercilii muscles. The lower half of the orbicularis is supplied by the zygomatic branches of the facial nerve. Sensory input to the skin above the OOM is provided through branches of the infraorbital and zygomaticofacial nerves that travel through the muscle terminating in the pretarsal region.[26]

The Orbital Septum

The orbital septum is a thin fibrous membrane that begins at the orbital rim at the arcus marginalis. The septum is fused to the arcus marginalis along most of the bony orbital rim. Within the eyelid, the septum forms a layer that separates the anterior and posterior eyelid lamellae, and the eyelids from the orbit proper. In the upper eyelid, fibers of the septum merge with those of the anterior portion of the levator aponeurosis. In the lower eyelid, the orbital septum fuses with the capsulopalpebral fascia below the tarsus, and this fused fascial sheet inserts into the inferior border of the tarsus.[27]

The septum is variable in thickness and strength. The septum is usually thicker in younger individuals and thins with aging.[28] In both the upper and the lower eyelids, the septum is the immediate cover and restrains the preaponeurotic fat (deep eyelid fat). When the septum thins, the preaponeurotic fat just deep to it may bulge forward.[29]

Fat Pads

The nasal fat pad of the upper eyelid is in continuity with the extraconal orbital fat.[30] The preaponeurotic

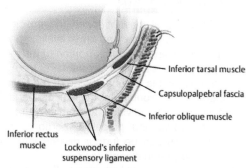

Inferior tarsal muscle

Capsulopalpebral fascia

Inferior oblique muscle

Inferior rectus muscle

Lockwood's inferior suspensory ligament

Fig. 9. Critical structures and landmarks in canthal anatomy. (*Reproduced from*: Patel AD, Massry GG. Eyelid and Periorbital Anatomy. In: Nahai F, Nahai F, eds. *The Art of Aesthetic Surgery: Principles and Techniques* Vol 1. 3 ed.: Thieme 2020. (Figure 31.10 in original).)

fat of the upper eyelid is separated from deep orbital fat by the LPS. All fat pads, except the nasal upper eyelid fat, of both eyelids overlie the eyelid retractors and are important surgical landmarks to identify the retractors.[31] In the upper eyelids, the 2 fat pads (compartments), medial (or nasal) and central, are separated by a facial layer, which connects with the trochlea. This facial condensation designates the position of the superior oblique muscle. There is no fat pad laterally in the upper eyelid; rather, the lacrimal gland is located in this region.

In the lower eyelid, there are 3 fat pads: nasal (medial), central, and lateral (temporal). These fat pads are separated by connective tissue fibrous septae. The arcuate expansion is a connective tissue extension that spans from Lockwood ligament to the orbital rim and separates the central and lateral lower lid fat compartments. The nasal and central fat pads are separated by the inferior oblique muscle.

When the orbital septum thins and weakens with age, the septum is no longer able to contain the orbital fat. The fat then bulges forward, creating a convexity on the eyelid surface. In the lower eyelid, the fat prominence can be continuous or appear as 2 or 3 separate convex bulges. The convex highlight of the fat bulge is often worsened by a strong orbicularis retaining ligament (ORL). This ligament attaches the posterior aspect of the OOM to the underlying maxilla and zygoma. The medial portion of the ORL (from the midpupillary line medially) is euphemistically termed the "tear trough ligament."

Improving the lower eyelid bags or circles can be performed in several ways. The lower eyelid fat pads can be partially resected to remove the bulge. The fat pads can also be repositioned (transposed) onto and over the orbital rim. The fat transposition procedure has the advantage of

decreasing the convexity caused by the fat herniation and augmenting the convexity caused by the adherence of the tear trough ligament just inferior to the bulge. Lower eyelid bags can also be improved by adding to the concavity inferior to the fat herniation with either injectable "off-the-shelf" fillers or with injectable fat.

Eyelid Retractors

The upper eyelid retractor begins as a muscle, the LPS, which originates from the lesser wing of the sphenoid just above the annulus of Zinn. The muscle travels in a mostly horizontal orientation in close approximation to the superior rectus muscle. The LPS widens into a fascial band, which forms the superior tarsal ligament (ligament of Whitnall). This fascial condensation inserts medially into the trochlear fascia and laterally into the capsule of the lacrimal gland.

At the superior tarsal ligament, the levator complex begins more vertically, splitting into an aponeurotic portion anteriorly (levator aponeurosis) and a muscular portion posteriorly (Muller muscle). The aponeurosis travels inferiorly in the eyelid to insert both onto the anterior surface of the tarsus and into the interfascicular septa of the pretarsal OOM. The levator aponeurosis is supplied by a branch of CN III (oculomotor).

Muller muscle underlies the levator aponeurosis. The aponeurosis and muscle are adherent by a small fascial plane that attaches the 2 structures. Muller muscle is supplied by branches of the sympathetic nervous system and inserts into the superior border of the tarsus. The muscle and aponeurosis work in tandem to elevate the upper eyelid. Contraction of the horizontally oriented LPS muscle transmits a posterior and vertical action on the upper eyelid, which is transmitted through a pulley system via the levator aponeurosis and Muller muscle.

PALPEBRAL APERTURE

The palpebral aperture consists of the space between the upper and lower eyelid margins. The shape of the eyelid aperture is created by the underlying tarsoligamentous sling. The fissure height (eyelid aperture) is normally 26 to 30 mm in width and 8 to 10 mm in height. The palpebral fissure height is related to the relative contraction of the eyelid protractors (OOMs) versus the contraction of the eyelid retractors (levator complex). The palpebral fissure height is shortened in patients with ptosis and increased in patients with Graves ophthalmopathy and congenital conditions, such as cri-du-chat syndrome.

A narrow palpebral aperture is seen in patients with a hyperdynamic OOM (eyelid protractor);

this occurs in patients with blepharospasm. Overactive orbicularis contraction can occur with facial rest or be associated with facial synkinesis (narrowed aperture when smiling). Ptosis of the upper eyelid can also cause a narrowed eyelid aperture. Ptosis is caused by a dehiscence of the eyelid retractors or a weakened contraction of the retractor musculature.

SUMMARY

The periorbital region is an anatomically complex region with a myriad of structures that support the eyelid, globe, lacrimal system, and surrounding neurovascular structures. In order to fully address periorbital aging, the brow should be considered part of the aesthetic unit when this area is being evaluated. A thorough knowledge of this anatomy is required to evaluate and treat aesthetic and reconstructive issues in this region to avoid injury to critical structures of the orbit and surrounding region.

CLINICS CARE POINTS

- The brow's position is determined by the relative activity of muscular brow elevators and depressors.
- Upper eyelid ptosis is characterized by brow elevation, a deep, elevated upper eyelid crease, and malposition of the upper eyelid margin.
- Thinning of the orbital septum leads to pseudoherniation of the underlying fat pads which is characteristic of periorbital aging.

DISCLOSURE

The authors have nothing to disclose.

REFERENCES

1. Goold LA, Casson RJ, Selva D, et al. Tarsal height. Ophthalmology 2009;116(9):19.
2. Sykes JM, Suarez GA, Trevidic P, et al. Applied facial anatomy. In: Azizzadeh B, Murphy MR, Johnson CM, et al, editors. Master Techniques in facial rejuvenation. (Second Edition). Edinburgh: Elsevier; 2018. p. 6–14.
3. Lam VB, Czyz CN, Wulc AE. The brow-eyelid continuum: an anatomic perspective. Clin Plast Surg 2013; 40(1):1–19.
4. Clevens RA. Rejuvenation of the male brow. Facial Plast Surg Clin North Am 2008;16(3):299–312.
5. Sykes JM. Applied anatomy of the temporal region and forehead for injectable fillers. J Drugs Dermatol 2009;8(10):24–7.
6. Park JI, Hoagland TM, Park MS. Anatomy of the corrugator supercilii muscle. Arch Facial Plast Surg 2003;5(5):412–5.
7. Sykes JM, Trevidic P, Suárez GA, et al. Newer understanding of specific anatomic targets in the aging face as applied to injectables: facial muscles-identifying optimal targets for neuromodulators. Plast Reconstr Surg 2015;136(5):56S–61S.
8. Beaulieu R, Andre K, Mancini R. Frontalis muscle contraction and the role of visual deprivation and eyelid proprioception. Ophthal Plast Reconstr Surg 2018;34(6):552–6.
9. Ben Simon GJ, Blaydon SM, Schwarcz RM, et al. Paradoxical use of frontalis muscle and the possible role of botulinum A toxin in permanent motor relearning. Ophthalmology 2005;112(5):918–22.
10. Knize DM. An anatomically based study of the mechanism of eyebrow ptosis. Plast Reconstr Surg 1996;97(7):1321–33.
11. Jeong S, Lemke BN, Dortzbach RK, et al. The Asian upper eyelid. Arch Ophthalmol 1999;117(July): 907–12.
12. Alkeswani A, Hataway F, Westbrook B, et al. Changes in lid crease measurements in levator advancement for ptosis. Ann Plast Surg 2020; 84(6S Suppl 5):S358–60.
13. Martin JJ. Ptosis repair in aesthetic blepharoplasty. Clin Plast Surg 2013;40(1):201–12.
14. Chopra K, Calva D, Sosin M, et al. A comprehensive examination of topographic thickness of skin in the human face. Aesthet Surg J 2015;35(8):1007–13.
15. Hwang K, Kim DJ, Kim SK. Does the upper eyelid skin become thinner with age? J Craniofac Surg 2006;17(3):474–6.
16. Sires BS, Saari JC, Garwin BS, et al. The color difference in orbital fat. Arch Ophthalmol 2001;119(6):868–71.
17. Kakizaki H, Takahashi Y, Nakano T, et al. Whitnall ligament anatomy revisited. Clin Exp Ophthalmol 2011; 39(2):152–5.
18. Kim YS, Hwang K. Shape and height of tarsal plates. J Craniofac Surg 2016;27(2):496–7.
19. Coban I, Sirinturk S, Unat F, et al. Anatomical description of the upper tarsal plate for reconstruction. Surg Radiol Anat 2018;40(10):1105–10.
20. Rohrich RJ, Arbique GM, Wong C, et al. The anatomy of suborbicularis fat: implications for periorbital rejuvenation. Plast Reconstr Surg 2009;124(3):946–51.
21. Kakizaki H, Zako M, Nakano T, et al. Three ligaments reinforce the lower eyelid. Okajimas Folia Anat Jpn 2004;81(5):97–100.
22. Bravo BSF, Da Rocha CRM, De Bastos JT, et al. Comprehensive treatment of periorbital region with hyaluronic acid. J Clin Aesthet Dermatol 2015;8(6):30–5.
23. Kashkouli MB, Abdolalizadeh P, Abolfathzadeh N, et al. Periorbital facial rejuvenation; applied anatomy and pre-operative assessment. J Curr Ophthalmol 2017;29(3):154–68.

24. Pottier F, El-Shazly NZ, El-Shazly AE. Aging of orbicularis oculi. Anatomophysiologic consideration in upper blepharoplasty. Arch Facial Plast Surg 2008;10(5):346–9.

25. Hoorntje LE, van der Lei B, Stollenwerck GA, et al. Resecting orbicularis oculi muscle in upper eyelid blepharoplasty - a review of the literature. J Plast Reconstr Aesthet Surg 2010;63(5):787–92.

26. Choi Y, Kang HG, Nam YS, et al. Facial nerve supply to the orbicularis oculi around the lower eyelid: anatomy and its clinical implications. Plast Reconstr Surg 2017;140(2):261–71.

27. Casabona G, Bernardini FP, Skippen B, et al. How to best utilize the line of ligaments and the surface volume coefficient in facial soft tissue filler injections. J Cosmet Dermatol 2020;19(2):303–11.

28. Sykes J, Cotofana S, Trevedic P, et al. Upper face: clinical anatomy and regional approaches with injectable fillers. Plast Reconstr Surg 2015;136(5):204S–18S.

29. Mendelson BC. Herniated fat and the orbital septum of the lower lid. Clin Plast Surg 1993;20(2):323–30.

30. Rohrich RJ, Ahmad J, Hamawy AH, et al. Is intraorbital fat extraorbital? Results of cross-sectional anatomy of the lower eyelid fat pads. Aesthet Surg J 2009;29(3):189–93.

31. Ferneini EM, Halepas S, Aronin SI. Antibiotic prophylaxis in blepharoplasty: review of the current literature. J Oral Maxillofac Surg 2017;75(7):1477–81.

My Evolution with Endoscopic Brow-Lift Surgery

Renato Saltz, MD, FACS[a,b,c,]*, Alyssa Lolofie, BS[d]

KEYWORDS

- Facial rejuvenation • Endoscopic facial rejuvenation • Endoscopic brow lift

KEY POINTS

- Brow aesthetics and surgical options for brow lift and forehead rejuvenation.
- Ideal candidates for the endoscopic brow-lift technique.
- Forehead and periocular anatomy.
- Surgical technique and the 4 key steps for endoscopic brow rejuvenation.
- Long term results and complications.

INTRODUCTION

The endoscopic approach for forehead rejuvenation and brow lift has many advantages.[1–19] It provided excellent exposure for release of periorbital soft tissues combined with endoscopic magnification, shorter scars, and reduced risk of alopecia and scalp sensory changes compared with the traditional open coronal brow lift. The technique has improved over the last 15 years with better fixation devices, a better understanding of the longevity, and decreased complications of the procedure. The endoscopic brow lift offers the patient a much easier and safer solution for the aging forehead, active wrinkles from corrugator and frontalis hyperactivity, and the ptotic, asymmetric brow.

CONTENT
Indications

The generally accepted ideal for the shape and position of the brow has been changing over the years and through different cultures; therefore, brow aesthetics cannot be generalized and must be evaluated in relation to gender, ethnicity, orbital shape, culture, and overall facial aging and proportions. Currently, we consider the "ideal aesthetic brow" with the medial brow at or below the level of the orbital rim, above the medial canthus, and with a gentle peak on the last two-thirds toward the lateral end with the lateral tail higher than the medial (**Fig. 1**). Men's brows should be straight and located at the level of the supraorbital rim with no lateral temporal elevation, which is a characteristic of the female brow. With facial aging, the eyebrows gradually fall and lose volume, encroach on the orbit, and bunch the skin over the lateral orbital rim, creating what is known as "temporal hooding." Anatomically, there is no levator mechanism on the lateral brow allowing tissue ptosis and loss of volume for causing the lateral or temporal brow ptosis. Eyebrow ptosis, eyebrow asymmetry, temporal hooding, and forehead wrinkles are all indications for forehead rejuvenation and a brow lift (**Fig. 2**).

Patient Selection

Techniques for forehead rejuvenation include open coronal, lateral temporal brow lift, direct

[a] University of Utah, 5445 South Highland Drive, Salt Lake City, UT 84117, USA; [b] ISAPS; [c] ASAPS; [d] University of Utah School of Medicine, 5445 South Highland Drive, Salt Lake City, UT 84117, USA
* Corresponding author. Saltz Plastic Surgery, 5445 South Highland Drive, Salt Lake City, UT 84117.
E-mail address: rsaltz@saltzplasticsurgery.com

Facial Plast Surg Clin N Am 29 (2021) 163–178
https://doi.org/10.1016/j.fsc.2021.02.007

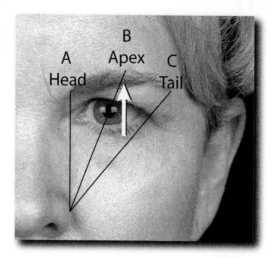

Fig. 1. Brow aesthetics. *Arrows* show the ideal brow position.

approach through the brow, transpalpebral brow lift with direct excision of the corrugator muscles, endoscopic brow lift, and neurotoxin injections. Since the introduction of the endoscopic approach to brow lift in 1993 by Vasconez and Core, I have not performed an open coronal brow lift. Almost all of my facial rejuvenation cases today include forehead and brow rejuvenation through an endoscopic technique. The best candidates for endoscopic forehead rejuvenation and brow lifts are patients with flat foreheads (flat frontal bone), no receding hairline (low hairline), and minimal redundant forehead skin. High hairlines and male-pattern baldness add to the challenge of being able to see and remove the glabellar muscles and achieve fixation. In patient selection, the key problems to be addressed are eyebrow ptosis, eyebrow position, brow asymmetry, hyperactive frontalis and corrugator muscles, and frontal and glabellar frown lines.

Anatomy (Brief Review)

The anatomy of the forehead and periorbital regions should be appreciated by the surgeon. The temporal ridge is bound by the temporal line of fusion, which is a deep bony point of fixation of the overlying soft tissue. The junction of the facial bone periosteum with the deep temporal fascia is what is known as the temporal fusion line. It is most caudal extension named fusion ligament. In order to adequately release and mobilize the lateral brow and temporal region, the temporal line of fusion should be released to the level of the supraorbital rim. There are also supraorbital ligamentous attachments that require release in

order to elevate the brow and forehead soft tissues **(Fig. 3)**.

The nerves that are encountered and preserved during endoscopic brow lift include the supratrochlear and supraorbital nerves, the 2 main sensory nerves, and the frontal nerve, the main motor branch of the facial nerve. Care is taken to appreciate and preserve these nerves during dissection. Subgaleal dissection (below superficial temporal fascia) lateral to the temporal line of fusion will maintain the plane of dissection deep to the frontal branch. Inferior dissection to the level of the sentinel vein while remaining the dissection superficial to the deep temporal fascia protects the frontal branch from direct division or traction neuropraxia (injury). Appreciation that the neurovascular bundles for the supratrochlear and supraorbital nerves exit the orbit 1.5 and 2.5 cm from midline, respectively, allows gentle division of the periosteum at that location to avoid division of the associated vascular bundles or damage to the nerves **(Fig. 4)**.

The sentinel vein is inferior to the inferior temporal septum and approximates the level of the frontal branch for the facial nerve.

The muscles of the forehead include the frontalis, procerus, corrugator supercilii (with oblique and transverse heads), the depressor supercilii, and the orbicularis muscles. The brow elevator is the frontalis muscle, whereas the other muscles all act in various fashions as brow depressors. Although release and physical repositioning of the brow and forehead elevate the brow, division and weakening of the brow depressors also correct dynamic brow ptosis and glabellar frown lines **(Fig. 5)**.

Preoperative Preparation

Assessment of the patient includes evaluation of both the medial and the lateral brow position, the ratio from brow to upper eyelid, glabella and forehead lines, forehead shape and height, and the hairline shape and position. To assess the strength of the muscle action, movement, and depth of soft tissue folds, the patient should be asked to frown as well as to raise the eyebrows. The eyebrows should also be assessed for the thickness, shape, position, and symmetry. In preoperative consultation, the doctor should advise as to the number of incisions and type of fixations. Based on the patient assessment, the operation can be planned. Patient inclusion is important in that brow lifts are individualized. The preoperative evaluation in front of a mirror with input from the patient is key for a successful outcome and reasonable expectations. The discussion and markings should focus on

A

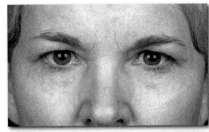

- *Soft Tissue descent*

- *Soft Tissue deflation*

- *Loss of lid crease*

- *No frontalis muscle lateral to the temporal crest*

  - *25-30% of the tail of the brow has no levator*

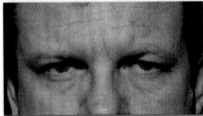

B

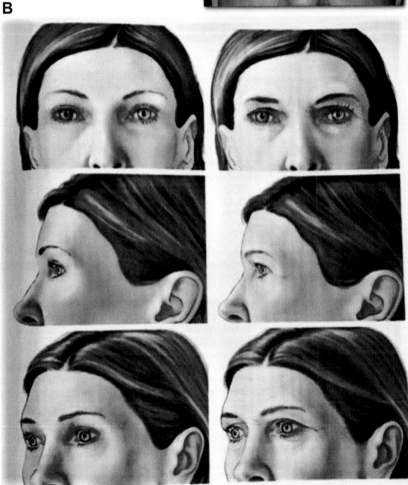

Fig. 2. Brow aging. (*A*) Age-related changes of the brow involve brow descent, furrowing, vertical and transverse frown lines, and crow's-feet. (*B*) Early signs of brow and periorbital aging include deflation and brow ptosis with a lowering of the medial and lateral hair-bearing brown and development of vertical glabellar and horizontal forehead lines. These changes often result in alterations to facial expression producing a tired, concerned, or even angry look. There is also real or apparent excess skin on the upper eyelid. (*From* Foad N., et al. Endoscopic Plastic Surgery. QMP (Thieme NY). 2008; with permission.)

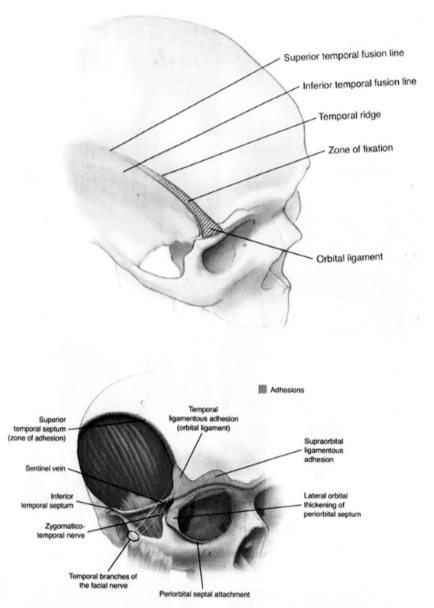

Fig. 3. Structural landmarks in the brow. The temporal fusion line lies at the junction of the periosteum and the deep temporal fascia. It must be released to achieve brow mobility. The orbital retaining ligament, situated at the lateral supraorbital rim, must also be released. (*From* Foad N., et al. Endoscopic Plastic Surgery. QMP (Thieme NY). 2008; with permission.)

possible elevation of the anterior hairline; medial brow elevation; position, shape, and elevation of the lateral brow; softening and spreading of the intermedial brow space after corrugator resection (**Fig. 6**).

The endoscopic technique is based on the use of modern technology whereby the traditional eye-hand surgical coordination is done through a video-endoscopic system. Additional extensive training is necessary not only for the surgeon but also for all medical and nursing personnel involved in the surgical case. The novice should take his or her first assistant to cadaver workshops and/or courses to learn together. The equipment, from endoscope to camera and monitors, is usually standard in centers where aesthetic surgeries are performed. It has become important to test each system, inspect each instrument, and check for a backup system as a safeguard. The surgeon must have knowledge of the principles extending

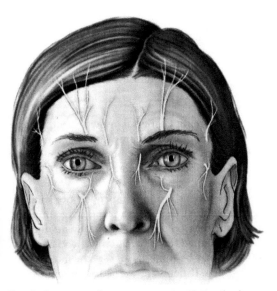

Fig. 4. Sensory and motor nerve supply to the brow. The supraorbital and supratrochlear nerves are protected during dissection. The frontal branches of the facial nerve lie anterior to the deep temporal fascia. (*From* Foad N., et al. Endoscopic Plastic Surgery. QMP (Thieme NY). 2008; with permission.)

from training, equipment needs and operation, and technical skills.

Equipment

Although use of the endoscopic brow lift has nearly eliminated the need for open coronal brow lifts, there are additional equipment requirements. Equipment should be tested before induction of anesthesia, and backup equipment should be available. The endoscopic equipment on the cart for visualization includes a monitor (preferably high definition), a 3-chip camera with the ability to record the procedure digitally and take still photographs, light source, electrocautery base unit, and suction. The additional equipment on the field should include an endoscope (most commonly a 4- to 5-mm 30-degree Hopkins rod with an endoscopic sheath), camera connector, light source connector, endoscopic dissectors, endoscopic forceps, endoscopic scissors, endoscopic graspers, and a malleable Durden suction cautery. The devices used for fixation can include a drill for a cortical tunnel, a drill for temporary screw fixation, a drill for use of the Endotine device (MicroAire, Charlottesville, Virginia, USA), or a variety of other fixation methods preferred by the surgeon. The endoscopic cart should be positioned at the foot of the bed with the surgeon positioned at the head of the bed (**Fig. 7**).

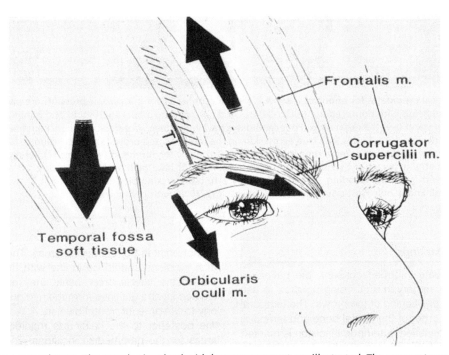

Fig. 5. Brow musculature. The muscles involved with brow movement are illustrated. The corrugators and procerus contribute to vertical and transverse brow furrows, respectively. (*From* Knize DM. An anatomically based study of the mechanism of eyebrow ptosis. Plast Reconstr Surg. 1996 Jun;97(7):1321-33. https://doi.org/10.1097/00006534-199606000-00001. PMID: 8643714; with permission. (Figure 9 in original).)

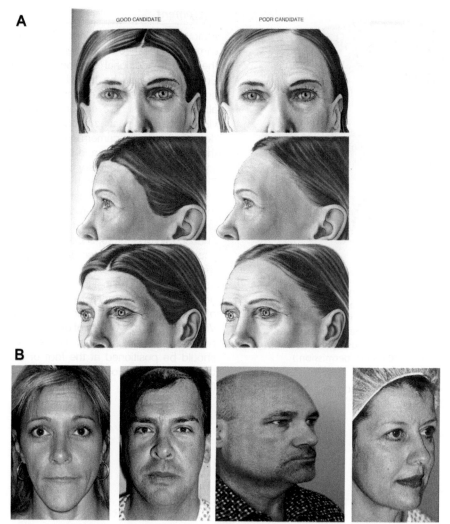

Fig. 6. (A) Ideal candidates for endoscopic brow lift. Ideal candidates for endoscopic brow lift are patients with short flat foreheads with nonreceding, thick hairlines and normal skin, moderate rhytids, and minimal true skin excess laterally and over the nasal radix. Poor candidates have high convex forehead, high receding hairline with thin hair, thick skin, deep rhytids, and true excess skin on the forehead and brow. (B) Clinical candidates for endoscopic brow lift: (1) young woman, repeated user of neurotoxins for foreheads wrinkles; (2) young man with brow asymmetry, hyperactive corrugator, and high forehead; (3) bald man with brow ptosis; (4) aging forehead/brow with temporal hooding "camouflaged" by artificially waxing/plucking the lateral brow. ([A] *From* Foad N., et al. Endoscopic Plastic Surgery. QMP (Thieme NY). 2008; with permission.)

Position/Markings

After adequate informed consent, the patient is marked for surgery in a standing position to use the natural positioning of the brows. The temporal crest and border of the frontal bone and temporal fossa are identified; a temporal incision is marked along a superior lateral vector line from the nasal ala crossing the lateral canthus and continues to a point approximately 2 cm behind the temporal hairline. A 2-cm curved line is then marked medial to that point in both temporal areas. The paramedian incisions should be in line with the desired pull of the lateral brow peak; they are usually located as straight lines from the mid pupil superiorly to the anterior frontal hairline. A 1-cm vertical line posterior to the hairline is marked in those areas for the paramedian incisions. The location of the supratrochlear and supraorbital nerves is also identified and marked. The location of the deep branch of the supraorbital nerve when it reaches the hairline is also marked at approximately

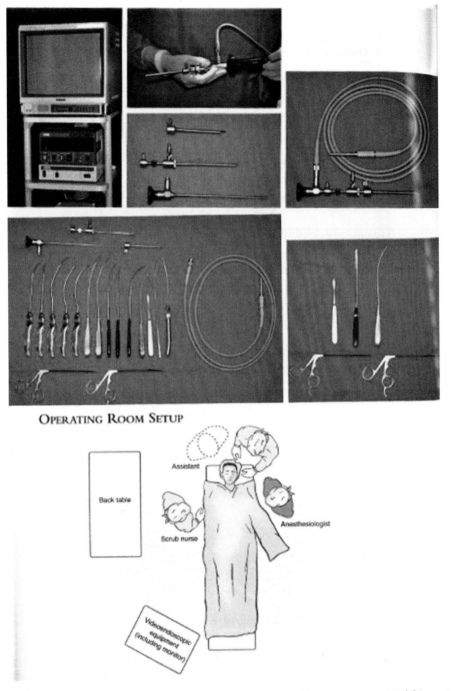

Fig. 7. Surgical table and equipment. (*From* Foad N., et al. Endoscopic Plastic Surgery. QMP (Thieme NY). 2008; with permission.)

1 cm medial to the temporal crest line. In addition, the desired vector of brow elevation is also mapped (**Fig. 8**).[20]

If the patient is found to have brow asymmetry on preoperative evaluation, careful examination should be performed for true brow asymmetry or for underlying unilateral upper lid ptosis, which causes ipsilateral elevation of the brow to compensate for upper lid ptosis. In the latter clinical setting, repair of eyelid ptosis often equalizes brow position, avoiding overcorrection of 1 brow compared with the other.

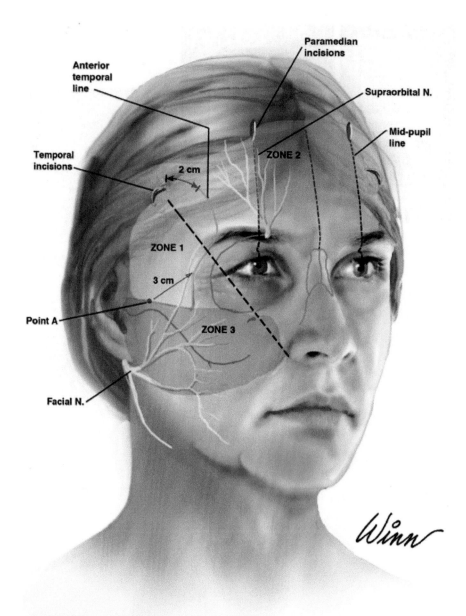

Fig. 8. Preoperative markings. I prefer the 4-port approach with 2 temporal and 2 paramedian incisions. The temporal incisions are placed on a straight line from the nasal ala in the direction of the lateral canthus, usually 2 cm behind the temporal hairline. The paramedian incisions are at mid pupil line and start at the hairline. (*From* Saltz R, Ohana B. Thirteen Years of Experience With the Endoscopic Midface Lift, *Aesthetic Surgery Journal*, Volume 32, Issue 8, November 2012, Pages 927–936, https://doi.org/10.1177/1090820X12462714; with permission. (Figure 3 in original).)

Anesthesia

Most commonly, the patient is placed under general anesthesia using an endotracheal tube secured to the upper teeth with dental floss. Infiltration is achieved using a mixture of 20 mL of 2% lidocaine, 20 mL of 0.25% Marcaine, 1 mL of epinephrine solution in 140 mL of normal saline. Infiltration is done using a 20-gauge spinal needle in a tumescent fashion. The patient is prepared and draped in a sterile fashion. The endotracheal tube is wrapped with sterile plastic drape, so it is inside the sterile field and easily manipulated when the head is turned to either side.

Surgical Technique

The brow-lift procedure is divided into the following 4 key steps:

1. Blunt subperiosteal dissection over the frontal bone down to the supraorbital rim
2. Meticulous division and spreading of the supraorbital rim periosteum under endoscopic visualization
3. Muscle resection under endoscopic visualization
4. Fixation in the temporal and paramedian wounds

The procedure starts approximately 20 minutes after infiltration is completed to obtain maximum vascular constriction. The temporal incision allows visualization and dissection on top of the deep temporal fascia. Periosteal dissectors are used on the surface of the deep temporal fascia in the lateral area and on the periosteum in the medial area. After these pockets are completed, the temporal line of fusion is released in a lateral-to-medial direction, and subperiosteal dissection is completed over the frontal bone. At this point, a 4-mm 30-degree scope is introduced to continue the dissection (**Fig. 9**).

The sentinel veins are identified and preserved (**Fig. 10**). The "fusion ligament," characterized by the junction of the forehead periosteum with the deep temporal fascia at the level of the lateral supraorbital rim, is identified and divided using the endoscopic scissors; it is a key component to allow full elevation of the lateral brow. The lack of proper identification and division of the fusion ligament can cause suboptimal elevation of the lateral brow and early relapse of the brow-lift result (**Fig. 11**).

The dissection continues medially where the supraorbital nerve is identified and preserved. I do not transect the periosteal attachments in between the corrugator muscles to minimize the medial brow elevation and the so-called surprised look. At this point, the corrugator muscles are identified and completely excised (**Fig. 12**). Manual palpation and gentle pressure over the skin avoid trauma to the dermis and possible indentations during endoscopic corrugator resection. In the case of very thin skin and possible indentation, I recommend immediate placement of fat grafts with suture fixation. At this point, the surgeon should feel how mobile the lateral brow is and be sure that both are equally mobile and symmetric in preparation for fixation.

Experimental work from Boutros and Romo in guinea pigs and rabbit periosteum demonstrated that periosteal partial adherence can take up to 6 weeks, with permanent adherence requiring up to 12 weeks. This work adds convincing support to the anecdotal observation that short-term fixation often causes surgical relapse.

The temporal fixation is best achieved by using interrupted 3-0 PDS sutures from the superficial temporal fascia (and galea) into a superior lateral direction to the deep temporal fascia. The central portion of the inferior scalp flap may be excised in triangular wedges in order to prevent redundancy at the lateral brow. My experience on brow fixation at paramedian incisions has evolved since 1994 from simple compressing dressings, tissue glues, plain sutures, cortical tunnels, external screws, and absorbable screws that did not offer always adequate fixation and consistent long-term results. Since 2002, fixation of brow elevation at the paramedian areas is best achieved with the Endotine device (**Fig. 13**). At this point, still under general anesthesia, the patient is examined in a sitting position for brow position and brow symmetry; measurements for comparison include the mid pupil to top of the middle brow and the lateral cantus to the tail of the brow. The 4 scalp incisions are then approximated with the 4-0 plain gut. The hair is washed, and the patient is taken to the recovery room. No dressings are applied.

Postoperative Care

In the recovery room, the position of the patient's head is maintained as elevated to 30° to avoid airway obstruction and excessive facial edema. The patient's blood pressure must be carefully monitored to avoid bleeding and hematomas, usually maintaining it at less than 120/80 mm Hg. Bags of crushed ice can be used over the eyes and forehead. The patient is allowed to shower on the first postoperative day. Oral analgesia is given, and antibiotics are used for up to 24 hours. Lymphatic drainage massage, starting at 48 to 72 hours postoperatively, can help with initial swelling improvement in the initial postoperative period and improve discomfort, bruising, and appearance in the early postoperative period.

Pitfalls and How to Correct

Despite the advantages, the endoscopic approach for forehead rejuvenation and brow lift is not without complications. Relapse has declined over the years because of increased use of longer-term fixation. The "surprised look" has been eliminated by preserving a bridge of periosteum at the midline and by avoiding fixation in the para median incisions in patients that have very mobile medial brows or a hyperactive medial frontalis muscle. Alopecia has been eliminated in

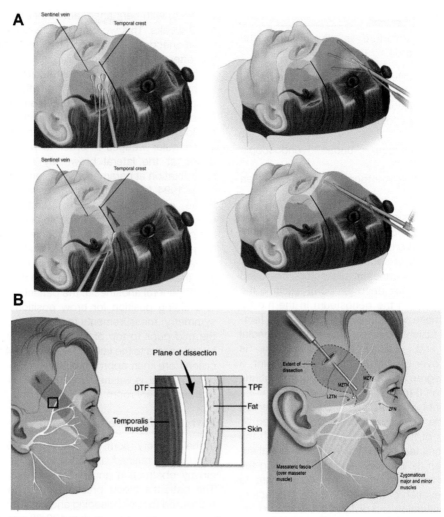

Fig. 9. (*A, B*) Forehead dissection. Dissection starts at the temporal region using periosteal dissectors on the surface of the deep temporal fascia in the lateral area and on the periosteum in the medial area. After these pockets are completed, the temporal line of fusion is released in a lateral-to-medial direction. This "blind dissection" is kept above the supraorbital rim by approximately 1 cm. The index finger of the contralateral hand stays on top of the supraorbital rim to protect the orbit and its contents. The 30-degree-angle 4-mm endoscope is only introduced after the temporal and forehead regions are completely undermined. The temporal pocket is developed easily and safely by smooth dissection on top of the deep temporal, above the temporalis muscle and below the superficial temporal fascia, protecting the intermediate fat pad and the frontal branch of the facial nerve. DTF, deep temporal fascia; LZTN, lateral zygomatic temporal nerve; MZTN, medial zygomatic temporal nerve; TPF, temporal parietal fascia also known as superfical temporal fascia; ZFN, zygomatic facial nerve. (*From* Foad N., et al. Endoscopic Plastic Surgery. QMP (Thieme NY). 2008; with permission.)

my practice after I abandoned percutaneous screw fixation and changed to the completely buried Endotine device. The alopecia was caused by improper local pressure in the surrounding scalp skin with the screw fixation technique. Anecdotal reports have blamed the cortical tunnel technique for fixation as the cause of an intracranial bleeding during an endoscopic brow-lift procedure. Injury to the supratrochlear and supraorbital nerves causing temporary paresthesia is another

potential complication. It can be minimized by adequate scalp incision placement, avoiding trauma to the deep branch of the supraorbital nerve as well as gentle tissue manipulation and careful soft tissue retraction using the endoscope. The subperiosteal dissection plane retains the vascular blood supply within the forehead flap; therefore, subperiosteal dissection maximizes flap blood supply and minimizes trauma to the deep branch of supraorbital nerve. Temporary

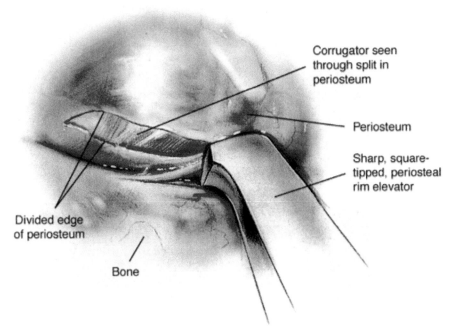

Corrugator seen through split in periosteum

Periosteum

Sharp, square-tipped, periosteal rim elevator

Divided edge of periosteum

Bone

Fig. 10. Division of supraorbital periosteum, starting from lateral to medial with full release of the "fusion liga-ment" and stopping short of the midline, which is the key to avoiding complete release from side to side and to avoiding migration of the medial brow and the "surprised look." (*From* Foad N., et al. Endoscopic Plastic Surgery. QMP (Thieme NY). 2008; with permission.)

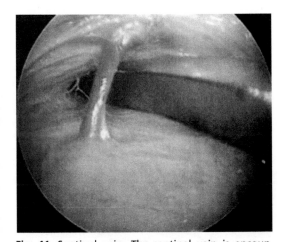

Fig. 11. Sentinel vein. The sentinel vein is encoun-tered during endoscopic dissection. The identification of the sentinel vein identifies a standard landmark for the frontal branch of the facial nerve. Dissection should not proceed beyond this. (*Reproduced from* Saltz R, Codner M. Endoscopic brow lift. In: Nahai FR, Nahai F, Codner M (eds). Techniques in Aesthetic Plastic Surgery: Minimally Invasive Facial Rejuvena-tion. Philadelphia, PA: Saunders Elsevier; 2009; with permission. (Figure 3.23 in original).)

paresthesia and some irregularities of the frontalis muscle are occasionally seen but usually improve within 2 to 3 weeks. Correction of eyelid ptosis with levator aponeurotic advancement corrects lid malposition and brow asymmetry from compensatory brow elevation. Early detection of postoperative brow asymmetry (within 24–48 hours) can be improved by repositioning the paramedian fixation through reelevation and pos-terior displacement of galea/skin from the Endo-tine. Delayed temporary brow asymmetry can be improved with Botox injections. If the brow asym-metry persists and there is obvious recurrence of brow ptosis, reintervention is advised.

Blind Brow Lifts

Nonendoscopic procedures for forehead rejuve-nation are now very popular; I call them "blind brow lifts" because the better one can see, the more precise and safer the technique can be. Su-praorbital neve variations are common (**Fig. 14**). The operative time for blind brow lifts is no better than endoscopic; one would have to dissect widely around all potential anomalous variations of the supraorbital nerve to avoid injuries and per-manent paresthesia in the forehead and anterior scalp. They require larger incisions with potential

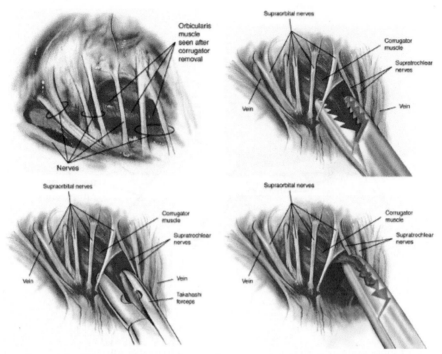

Fig. 12. Corrugator muscle. The corrugator muscles may be resected endoscopically with grasping forceps, taking care not to injure the supraorbital or supratrochlear nerves. (*From* Foad N., et al. Endoscopic Plastic Surgery. QMP (Thieme NY). 2008; with permission.)

damage to the deep branch of the supraorbital nerve with permanent sensory loss and alopecia. Nonendoscopic "blind brow lifts" are applicable in selected patients in whom only lateral lift is needed and no forehead wrinkles and no corrugator release is indicated or required.

Pearls

- Endoscopic brow lifts are dependent on technology and dissociation of eye-hand

coordination. The ability to master both skills will affect the safety and quality of the results. It involves significant learning curve for the surgeon and staff.
- Surgeon and operating room personnel should be familiar with the endoscopic equipment and advanced technology and be able to troubleshoot problems.
- The procedure has basically 4 steps: (1) dissection of temporal and forehead soft tissues, (2) release of supraorbital rim

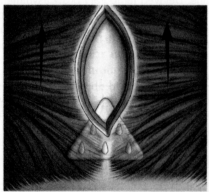
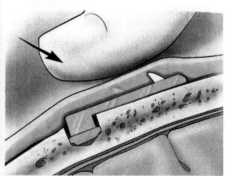

Fig. 13. Endotine fixation. The Endotine divot hole is drilled through the first layer of skull bone and situated at the caudal extent of the incision. The Endotine is snapped into place. The scalp can then be repositioned vertically and held into place by fixation tines. *Arrow* demonstrates applying pressure of skin over the endotine. (*From* Foad N., et al. Endoscopic Plastic Surgery. QMP (Thieme NY). 2008; with permission.)

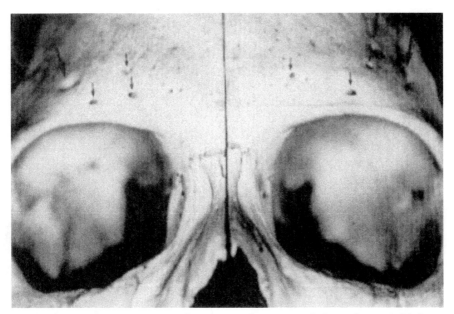

Fig. 14. Supraorbital nerve variations. *Arrows* demonstrate the many variations of supra orbital nerve position.

periosteum, (3) corrugator removal, and (4) forehead and temporal fixation.

- Keeping the dissector close to the deep temporal fascia is much safer and avoids any trauma to the frontal branch of the facial nerve.
- Knowledge of the anatomy of motor and sensory nerves and careful dissection during brow-lift surgery are essential to prevent complications.
- Keeping the assistant's fingers palpating the skin while avulsing the corrugators may prevent overresection of subcutaneous fat with resulting depression.
- Avoid dividing periosteum from side to side. Preserving the periosteum intact at midline will prevent elevation of the medial brow and the "surprised look."
- In most cases, in women, the lateral brow needs to be elevated higher than the central and medial brow. In men, the elevation should be equal to avoid feminization of the male brow.
- Early failure is caused by inadequate release of periosteal septa and adhesions. Late failure is caused by inadequate fixation.

SUMMARY

Our experience from 1994 to 2020 includes more than 2000 cases with 80% of the endoscopic brow lifts combined with facelifts. The longest well-documented follow-up is 15 years with overall good long-term results and no visible scars. In our series, 20% of patients report Endotine sensitivity for approximately 1 month and a weak frontalis muscle (unilateral or bilateral) for 2 to 4 weeks with all recovering full muscle function without requiring any additional treatment besides reassurance and occasional neurotoxin injections to soften the temporary brow asymmetry. Endoscopic forehead rejuvenation is a safe and reproducible technique that requires proper endoscopic training and learning curve with proper informed consent.

The endoscopic approach for brow lift has many advantages and is the gold standard in forehead rejuvenation. It has many advantages: it provides excellent exposure for safe release of periorbital tissues combined with endoscopic magnification; it is performed through small scalp incisions with reduced risk of alopecia and scalp sensory changes compared with traditional open coronal brow lift; and it can be combined with blepharoplasty when indicated and safe resurfacing techniques (CO_2 laser, trichloroacetic acid peels) to forehead and periocular areas. The technique has improved over the years with a better understanding of the periosteal adherence and consequently better fixation devices, a better understanding of the long-term results, and decreased complications. It offers the patient a much easier and safer solution for the aging forehead and the ptotic, asymmetric brow. The endoscopic brow lift is a time-tested method of providing highly accurate, precise, safe, long-lasting, and aesthetically focused rejuvenation of the entire forehead, brow, and periocular region in a reasonable amount of time when done properly by a trained surgeon. It is also the safest and easiest "gate" to the midface. (**Figs. 15-19**).[20-22]

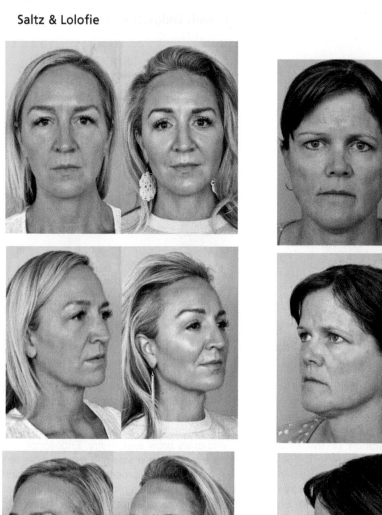

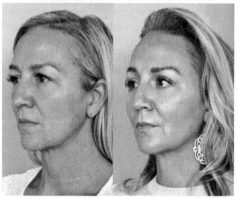

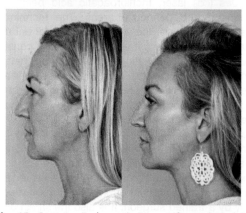

Fig. 16. Case 2 - Endoscopic Brow Lift combined with Endoscopic Midface Lift using 2 temporal and 2 paramedian scalp 1cm incisions. Fixation of the brow with ultratines and fixation of the midface with the endomidface device. Follow up at 1 year

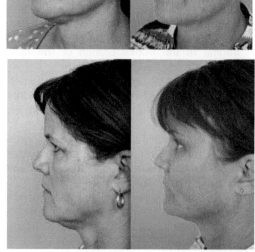

Fig. 15. Case 1 - Endoscopic Brow Lift combined to Transconjuntival Blepharoplasty. Ultratines used for paramedian fixation and 3-0 PDS for temporal fixation. Follow up at 1 year.

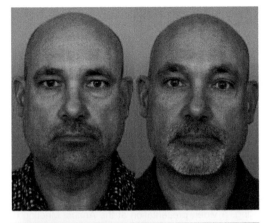

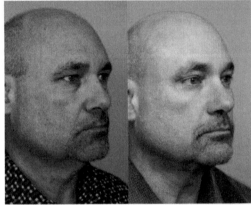

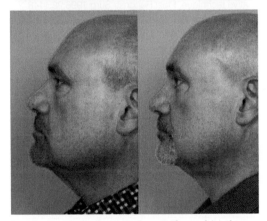

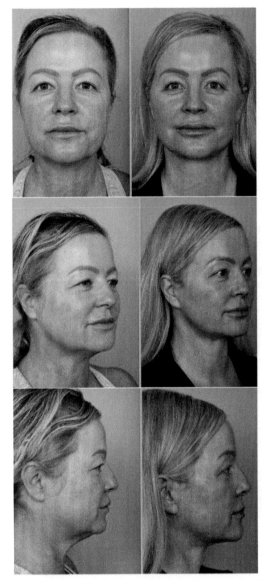

Fig. 18. Case 4 - Endoscopic Brow Lift 2 temporal and 2 paramedian scalp 1cm incisions combined to Facelift and Necklift. Endotines used for paramedian fixation and 3-0 PDS for temporal fixation. Follow up at 1 year.

Fig. 17. Case 3- Endoscopic Brow Lift combined to upper and lower blepharoplasty (transconjuntival) and neck liposuction. Emdotines used for paramedian fixation and 3-0 PDS for temporal fixation. Follow up at 2 years.

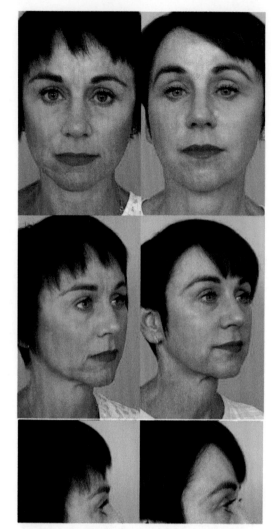

Fig. 19. Case 5 - Endoscopic Brow Lift 2 temporal and 2 paramedian scalp 1cm incisions combined to Facelift and Necklift. Endotines used for paramedian fixation and 3-0 PDS for temporal fixation. Follow up at 10 years.

REFERENCES

1. Isse NG. Endoscopic forehead lift: evolution and update. Clin Plast Surg 1995;22:661.
2. Knize DM. Limited-incision forehead lift for eyebrow elevation to enhance upper blepharoplasty. Plast Reconstr Surg 1996;97:1334.
3. Mackay GJ, Nahai F. The endoscopic forehead lift. Operative techniques in plastic and re-constructive surgery. Operative Techniques in Plastic and Reconstructive Surgery 1995;2:137.
4. Matarasso A, Matarasso SL. Endoscopic surgical correction of glabellar creases. Dermatol Surg 1995;21:695.
5. Paul MD. Subperiosteal transblepharoplasty forehead lift. Aesthet Plast Surg 1996;20:129.
6. Ramirez OM. The anchor subperiosteal forehead lift. Plast Reconstr Surg 1995;95:993.
7. Ramirez OM. Endoscopically assisted biplanar forehead lift. Plast Reconstr Surg 1995;96:323.
8. Rohrich RJ, Beran SJ. Evolving fixation methods in endoscopically assisted forehead rejuvenation: controversies and rationale. Plast Reconstr Surg 1997; 100:1575.
9. Vasconez LO. The use of the endoscope in brow lifting. A video presentation at the Annual Meeting of the American Society of Plastic and Reconstructive Surgeons. Washington, DC, 1992.
10. Core GB, Vasconez LO, Askren C, et al. Coronal face lift with endoscopic techniques. Plast Surg Forum 1992;25:227.
11. Isse NG. Endoscopic facial rejuvenation: endoforehead, the functional lift. Case reports. Aesthetic Plast Surg 1994;18:21.
12. Trinei FA, Januszkiewicz J, Nahai E. The sentinel vein: an important reference point for surgery in the temporal region. Plast Reconstr Surg 1998;101:27.
13. Chajchir A. Endoscopic subperiosteal forehead lift. Aesthet Plast Surg 1994;18:269.
14. Daniel RK, Tirkanits B. Endoscopic forehead lift: an operative technique. Plast Reconstr Surg 1996;98:1148.
15. Del Campo AF, Lucchesi R, Cedillo Ley MP. The endo-facelift: basics and options. Clin Plast Surg 1997;24:309.
16. Isse NG. Endoscopic forehead lift. Presented at the Annual Meeting of the Los Angeles County Society of Plastic Surgeons, Los Angeles, Sept 12, 1992.
17. Bostwick J III, Nahai F, Eaves F III. Endoscopic brow lift in endoscopic plastic surgery. St Louis (MO): Quality Medical Publishing; 1996.
18. Paul M. The evolution of the brow lift in aesthetic plastic surgery. Plast Reconstr Surg 2001;108:1409–24.
19. Casagrande C, Saltz R, Chem R, et al. Direct needle fixation in endoscopic facial rejuvenation. Aesthet Surg J 2000;20(5):361–7.
20. Foad N, Saltz R. Endoscopic plastic surgery qmp. New York: Thieme; 2008.
21. Saltz R, Ohana B. Thirteen years of experience with the endoscopic midface lift. Aesthetic Surgery 2012; 32(8):927–36.
22. Saltz R, Casagrande C, Saciloto A, et al. Rejuvenation of the midface. In: Foad N, Saltz R, editors. Endoscopic plastic surgery qmp. New York: Thieme; 2008. p. 237–70.

Upper Blepharoplasty – Nuances for Success

Bryan C. Mendelson, FRCS (Ed), FRACS, FACS[a],*, Chin-Ho Wong, MMed (Surg), FAMS (Plast Surg)[b]

KEYWORDS

- Upper eyelid • Tarsal fixation blepharoplasty • Postblepharoplasty look • Brow ptosis
- Dermatochalasis • Orbital rim augmentation • Hydroxyapatite

KEY POINTS

- Because the "eyes" are of the highest importance in facial appearance and identity, it behooves the surgeon of the motivated patient to go beyond simple age reversal, to reveal inner beauty or add attractiveness.
- A nuanced understanding of facial aesthetics is required of the surgeon, along with refined surgical technique, which includes detailed intraoperative recognition of lid anatomy.
- A blepharoplasty technique based on a lid crease that is stable and lasting provides independent control of both lid segments. A major skin resection is avoided as is unnatural skin tension, visible scars, and the subsequent postblepharoplasty "look."
- Simultaneous correction of the age-related diminution of the orbital rim fat volume adds a level of aesthetic refinement, while avoiding the "operated eye look." Simultaneous correction of a deficient supraorbital rim projection enhances the result in those patients.

 Video content accompanies this article at http://www.facialplastic.theclinics.com

---

Good is the enemy of best.
—Mark Twain

This article represents the personal understanding of an individual plastic surgeon that evolved with a broad experience over the course of his career in aesthetic surgery of the face. It does not replace the "how to guide" for the learning surgeon, for whom much is well presented elsewhere. Rather the concepts may appeal to some individual surgeons, who find satisfaction in the possibilities of aesthetic surgery. All surgery requires quality of practice, but when a person's face is involved, quality has a different significance. This is because of the personal and social impact that surgery of facial appearance has on that person's identity and self-esteem, reflecting how other people are influenced by, and respond to the appearance, usually at a subconscious level.

This significance was succinctly described last century by Egon Brunswick (1934), a psychologist: "*a small change in facial proportion, changes our perception of a person's personality*".

This article is based around a refinement in perceptual understanding, then of the relevant anatomy, leading to the surgery required to obtain the intended result. There are several aspects involved in the aesthetics of the "eye" including illusion, something women know from their experience of using cosmetic eye makeup. Even the term "makeup" tells a story!

Upper lid blepharoplasty is the centerpiece in rejuvenation of the periorbital region and also in glamorization of the eyes. However, a blepharoplasty is part of a larger story. This is because attractive eyes have a strong 3-dimensional aspect to them. Beautiful eyes are in a "picture

---

[a] The Centre for Facial Plastic Surgery, 109 Mathoura Road, Toorak, Victoria 3142, Australia; [b] W Aesthetic Plastic Surgery, 06 – 28/29, Mount Elizabeth Novena Specialist Center, 38 Irrawaddy Road, Singapore 329563, Singapore
* Corresponding author.
E-mail address: drbryan@bmendelson.com.au

Facial Plast Surg Clin N Am 29 (2021) 179–193
https://doi.org/10.1016/j.fsc.2021.01.001
1064-7406/21/© 2021 Elsevier Inc. All rights reserved.

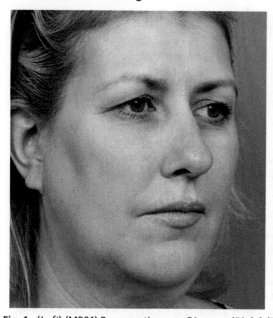 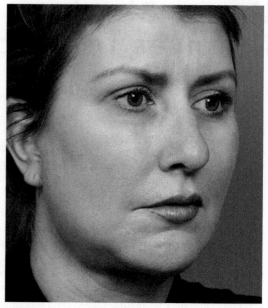

Fig. 1. (*Left*) (MB01) Preoperative, age 51 years. (*Right*) (B02) One year postop tarsal fixation blepharoplasty, with a temporal lift and face/necklift. Tarsal plate 10.0 mm height, 5 mm skin excision only. The visual impact of the eyes on overall facial appearance is so significant that the benefit to her overall appearance from having a quality contouring of the lid from the upper blepharoplasty compares strongly with the impact of her facelift.

frame" formed by the bony orbital rim, which is highlighted by the brows (**Fig. 1**).

The 3-dimensional contour begins with the relationship between the picture frame, the superior orbital rim, and the globe and continues with the relationship between the 2 parts of the lid (**Fig. 2**). The upper part of the lid is the connection between the brow and the globe. Eye shadow is traditionally applied to glamourize the eyes by creating the illusion of a greater depth of the lid recess, which indicates its importance in Society.

Although the lid is considered a single entity, it is structured of 2 segments that are anatomically separated by the *lid crease* (**Fig. 3**). These are the lid proper, the lower part, the *tarsal segment*, and above that, the *infrabrow segment*.[1] The *lid fold* is the lower part of the infrabrow segment that tends to hang over and conceal the lid crease to a varying degree. The lid fold varies considerably according to race, it may even be absent, and its variation over time is such that it ages a person. Hence, management of an excess lid fold is the usual surgery of upper lid blepharoplasty. Although interrelated, the 2 segments are visually and functionally separate. The hidden crease, with its function of internal fixation influences the appearance of the lid by balancing the 2 lid segments. Unfortunately, there is some confused terminology in some quarters; the terms "crease" and "fold" are confused as if they are the same thing. The crease is an inversion, which cannot be filled, and the fold is the opposite.

The *tarsal segment* moves across the upper globe as a unit, based on the fixed tarsal plate dimensions. Its moves as a unit. In contrast, the *infrabrow segment* is constantly changing its shape and dimensions, as it bridges the gap between the brow above and the mobile tarsal segment. The "look" of the eyes is most strongly determined by *the lid show*, the amount of the tarsal segment visible below the lid fold. Clearly the fold is under the influence of the infrabrow segment. It varies not only in its position but also in its quality. The well-defined surface appearance of an attractive lid reflects the internal anatomy (**Fig. 4**).

UPPER LID BLEPHAROPLASTY

For more than 30 years the senior author has used, and refined, a tarsal fixation technique of upper lid blepharoplasty, first learnt from Dr Robert Flowers.[2–4] This technique progressively replaced the use of the previously used standard excision technique because it provides the surgeon with precise control and predictable and extraordinarily lasting results. These benefits come at the price of a longer operating time and increased risk, both of which are reduced with experience involving a learning curve. The aesthetic, anatomic, and technical considerations are shared later, and the role of the brow is integral in the result.

Surgical control, paramount for quality surgery, is obtained in the technique by considering the 2 interconnected segments of the lid as separate and distinct. Each lid segment is appropriately corrected, independent of the other. The procedure is not difficult to master once the surgical steps are understood, although, the surgeon's ability to recognize the internal anatomy is more critical than in traditional blepharoplasty.

Planning the tarsal segment is the first priority. The location of the marking for the lower incision (lower marking) is traditionally placed at a predetermined distance from the lid margin, correlating with the lowest skin crease. A logical alternative is to precisely locate the lower incision, whichis determined by the patient's tarsal plate.

Surgical Technique

Preliminary markings

These are performed with the patient relaxed but cooperative. Three cardinal reference points are first marked on the lashline, with the patient looking at the same distant object. These are the medial limbus, medial pupil, and lateral limbus. Then the provisional lower marking is lightly placed.

The upper marking is made from the brow down, with the brow gently pushed down or naturally relaxed with the patient sitting.

The upper marking of the excision is challenging, as it requires judgment. It is located in reference to the patient's brow position, being placed lower (less skin excision) if more skin needs to be retained due to inherently high and/or forward projecting brows. The usual distance is within the range, 17 to 21 mm, which according to standard excisional only blepharoplasty is not removing sufficient skin. More skin must be retained for the skin inversion of the tarsal fixation. This skin is "released" during lid closure, which prevents lagophthalmos.

Final markings

When the patient is deeply sedated or asleep, the lid is readily everted. Now, the shape of the patient's tarsal plate is clearly seen and noted, then using the caliper, the maximum height of the tarsal plate (distance X) is measured (**Fig. 5**).

The position for the lower skin incision is calculated (X plus 1 mm) and this skin marking now

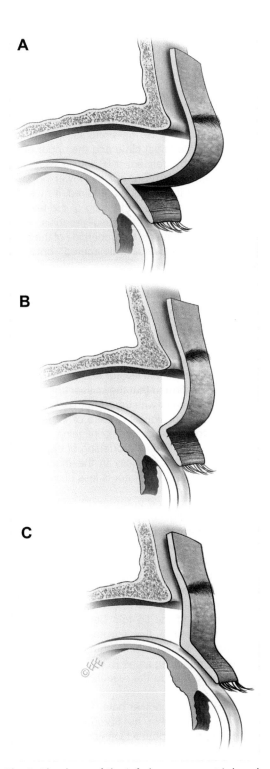

A

B

C

Fig. 2. The shape of the infrabrow segment is largely determined by the skeleton, specifically the amount of superior orbital rim projection relative to the position of the globe. (*A*) The most aesthetically pleasing relationship is where the superior orbital rim projects well forward of the anterior surface of the globe.

Accordingly, as the infrabrow segment descends from the brow, it curves inward (recedes). (*B*) An intermediate situation, not as aesthetically pleasing, where the amount of forward projection of the rim is small, leading to less receding (curvature) of the descending upper lid. (*C*) An aesthetically difficult relationship is the prominent eye. In this configuration there cannot be an attractive, receding lid fold. Pseudoptosis may result in the absence of a lid fold. (*Courtesy of* Dr. Levent Efe, CMI, Australia.)

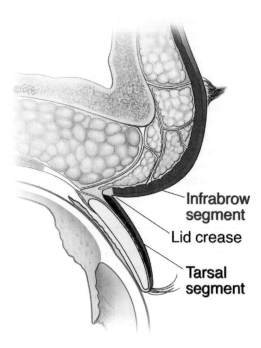

Infrabrow segment

Lid crease

Tarsal segment

Fig. 3. The 2 segments of the upper lid are anatomically separated by the lid crease. (*Courtesy of* Dr. Levent Efe, CMI, Australia.)

made at the 3 cardinal points. As the marking is being performed, the skin should be placed under the natural tension intended for the final result.

Medial to the medial limbus up to the punctum, the marked distance is reduced to 7 to 8 mm. Similarly, over the lateral canthus the marking is about 8 mm, extending laterally as far as required to excise any moderate temporal hooding but significantly less than with a standard blepharoplasty due to the skin inversion inherent in the technique. The planned skin excision is confirmed by a pinch test and adjusted accordingly.

Excision of skin and muscle

Compared with a traditional blepharoplasty a considerably smaller amount of skin is resected as skin tension is to be avoided.

The skin only is incised, first along the lower incision, then the upper incision, and then carefully removed off the outer surface of the orbicularis with meticulous hemostasis on the muscle surface.

The orbicularis is then incised along the lower incision (*cutting diathermy or scalpel*), bevelling down slightly toward the upper border of the tarsal plate. Lateral to the lateral canthus a small strip of orbicularis is removed to avoid a dog ear at closure.

Defining the tarsal plate

The filmy areola tissue (the pretarsal extension of the levator) is then removed off the tarsal plate. To do this, the orbicularis is first elevated, then the areolar tissue carefully released from the underside of the orbicularis muscle fascia, continuing this dissection as far down toward the lashes as required, according to the pretarsal skin laxity. Both ends of the tarsal plate and the upper edge should be clearly defined. It is not necessary to routinely clean soft tissue off the lower edge of the levator, but if trimming is required, it must be done carefully to avoid shortening of the levator. The removal of the areolar tissue enables, what Dr Flowers described as, the underside of the orbicularis (its fascia) being "wallpapered" onto the tarsal plate surface.

Defining the Levator Edge

The septum orbitale is incised just above the *sling*, where it joins the levator. Identification of the levator is commenced at the lateral extent where it is safer from unintentional levator shortening.

Once it is confirmed that the scissor tip is on the surface of the levator with the septum orbitale, just superficial, a meticulously release of the septum off the levator is performed, continuing medially (**Fig. 6** C,D). Unintended shortening of the levator must be avoided, especially in the medial third where the edge of the levator is less distinct.

Adjusting the fat pad volumes

The lateral prolongation of the central fat pad just above the lateral canthus is reviewed. It is often considerable, especially when there is fullness over the lateral lid. The prolongation is mobilized, from lateral to medial, at times to the lateral limbus, to be folded over later as a fat flap.

If enhancement of the lateral extension of the inferior border of the lid fold beyond the lateral orbital rim is desired, this is obtained by removal of preaponeurotic fat here, with more contouring obtained by removing some ROOF fat here, being mindful not to overdo the resection, especially in men.[5]

Medially, the distinctive pale, nasal fat pad is mobilized from within its fibrous capsule and managed in the standard technique (**Fig. 6**E). As this is Y shaped, the second limb of the Y should be sought.[6]

Reconstruction using Flowers sutures

Reconstruction is performed using a series of standard 3-point fixation sutures (tarsus, levator, pretarsal orbicularis) (**Fig. 6** F,G). The 6/0 Vicryl Rapide suture used is fine, yet provides sufficient

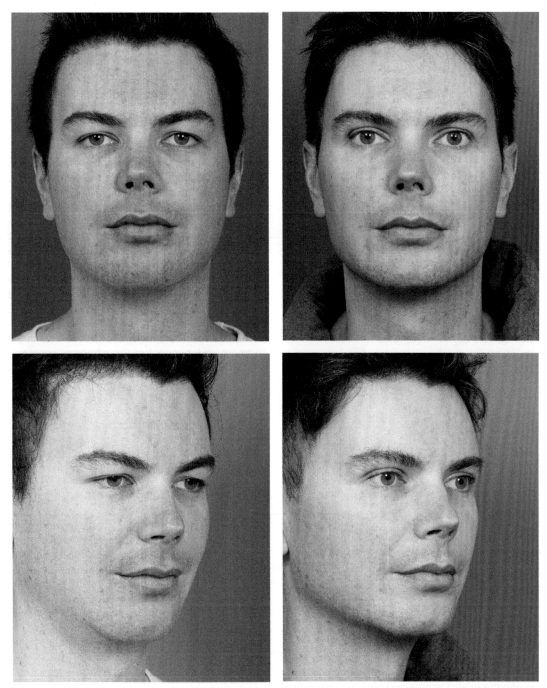

Fig. 4. (*Left above*) (LH01) and (*left below*) (LH02) Preoperative, 36-year-old man, tired eyes, in someone with a favorable skeletal configuration having a broad flat forehead with inherently good projection of his superolateral orbital rims. Highlighting the principle that attractive eyes have a strong 3-dimensional configuration. (*Right above*) (LH04) and (*Right below*) (LH06) Eighteen months postoperative following tarsal fixation blepharoplasty (only 3 mm maximum skin removal). Lipofill performed for subtle contour enhancement, using Lipogems via a Maft gun. 2 mL infrabrow mainly medial. 1.0 mL brows, 1.0 mL superior temple. Also 1.0 mL upper maxilla, 1.0 mL zygoma. Vividly demonstrating that "a small change in facial proportion changes our perception of a person's personality."

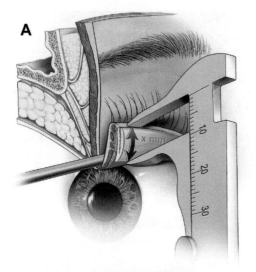

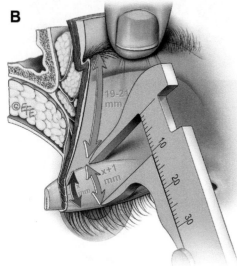

Fig. 5. Lid marking using the tarsal plate. (*A*) The height of the tarsal plate, distance x, measured in the midpupil position. (*B*) Transposed to the skin as x plus 1 mm for the lower incision. (*Courtesy of* Dr. Levent Efe, CMI, Australia.)

strength and durability, without causing tissue reaction.

The first suture at the medial end is placed between the medial (first and second) cardinal points, between the medial limbus and medial pupil. With the upper edge of the tarsal plate stabilized with fine forceps the needle enters the outer surface of the tarsus just below the upper edge and exits the upper edge of the tarsal plate. Note that the needle must not go through to the conjunctival surface.

The second bite of the suture is to the levator, taking a secure bite near the free edge.

The third bite of the suture picks up the orbicularis, more specifically the fascia on its underside.

Rather than tightening the pretarsal skin directly, it is indirectly toned by this suture placement here.

With the suture tied, the levator functions, whereas the incision is fixed in the lid crease.

The second suture is the most important, being in line with the medial pupil, the usual high point for the lid margin. It is placed in the same standard technique, as is the third suture, placed at the marking for the lateral limbus.

A fourth suture, not as important as the others, bisects the distance between the lateral limbus and the lateral canthus where the tarsal plate is beginning to reduce in height.

The fifth suture at the lateral canthus is different from the others, because the tarsal plate is so narrow here. This suture has a different objective, that of reducing the temporal hooding lateral to the lateral canthus. The suture ignores the narrow tarsus and picks up the orbicularis first, which is then sutured up and medial to the levator, several mms above its free edge to shape the lateral tarsal contour.

This completes the correction of the tarsal segment, independent of the infrabrow segment. It has been achieved with natural skin tension, yet the lashes are everted.

Fat flap Lateral fat, if mobilized, is translocated medially to restore central infrabrow volume and stabilized by a suture to the septum orbitale beneath the area of peaking in the medial third of the lid.

Skin closure As the lateral skin closure must be meticulous, interrupted sutures are used here for precision. These sutures include the underlying orbicularis, whereas the most medial suture incorporates a bite of the underlying levator edge, at its lateral horn.

A continuous monofilament suture (5/0 pronova) is mainly used for lid closure, commencing at the medial end. As the closure continues across the lid, the suture picks up the edge of the levator, which becomes fixed to the incision.

Summary

The blepharoplasty is completed with natural tension of both the pretarsal and infrabrow skin, yet with eversion of the lashes.

Minimal skin is excised when using the tarsal fixation technique.

The orbicularis is preserved, being incised only at the level of the upper border of the tarsal plate for safe access to its anterior surface.

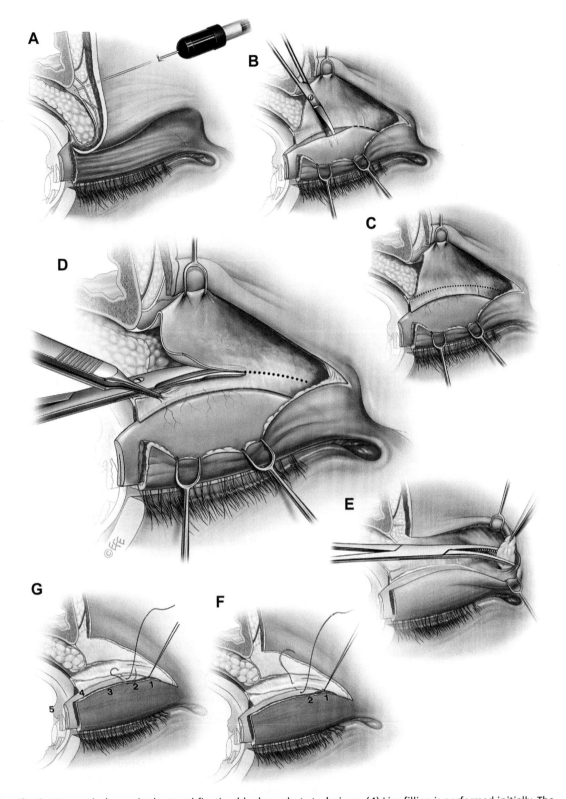

Fig. 6. Key surgical steps in the tarsal fixation blepharoplasty technique. (*A*) Lipofilling is performed initially. The fine cannula is directed vertically through entry points in the brow to the periosteum of the superior orbital rim. Volume is placed deep in the triangular recess formed by the attachment of the septum to the posterior border of the rim and continued up on the rim. (*B*) Following the incision through skin and orbicularis, the pretarsal areolar-like tissue is removed off the tarsal plate. (*C, D*) Following definition of the sling, the septum orbitale is released from the levator, with care to avoid shortening the levator. (*E*) Excess deep medial fat is adjusted. (*F, G*) Series of "Flowers" 3-point fixation sutures placed, each commencing at the upper border of the tarsal plate, then to the levator edge, and finally to the pretarsal orbicularis. (*Courtesy of* Dr. Levent Efe, CMI, Australia.)

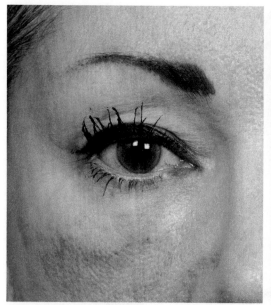 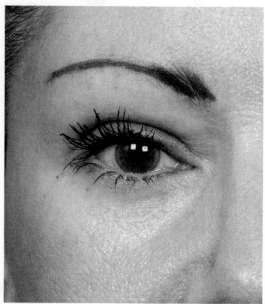

Fig. 7. (*Left*) (RG03) Preoperative, age 48 years. (*Right*) (RG04) One year postoperative tarsal fixation upper blepharoplasty. Markings: tarsal plate 9.5 mm height, lower incisional line at 10 mm, upper incision at 22 mm from midbrow (maximum skin removal 3 mm). Medial translocation of excess lateral fat and reduction of moderately large excess deep medial fat. Superolateral orbital rim projection contour enhanced with 1.0 mL hydroxyapatite rim augmentation and lipofilling with Maft gun of 2.0 mL, to medial lid and 1.0 mL beneath the brow. (Associated, lower lid cheek refinement, with hydroxyapatite augmentation medial orbital rim, 0.4 mL, maxillary concavity I.6 mL, and zygoma1.0 mL). Demonstrating that control of the shape of the infrabrow segment is not limited to the lid fold. Attention to the deficient volume high in the segment is required, in addition to the reduction of low medial fullness from medial brow fat pad excess.

The removal of the areolar tissue on the tarsal plate minimizes long-term recurrence of crepey pretarsal skin.

The exposure of the levator aponeurosis and tarsus and the internal suture repair integral with the procedure most likely prevents the subsequent development of involutional ptosis and allows the simultaneous correction of previously diagnosed clinical ptosis.

The absence of skin tension allows early suture removal. This Video 1 illustrates the technique.

Discussion

Importance of the shape of the lid fold

Most attractive lids have a lid fold that is soft, rounded, and definitely not flaccid as it descends from the brow. It curves around and inward into the crease in the depth of the lid, at the top of the tarsal plate (**Fig. 7**). The crease itself, although concealed by some overhang of the fold at rest, fulfills its second function, to maintain the pretarsal segment smooth with an even tone, without being taut.

When it has been brought to one's attention, it becomes quite obvious that the curvature of the

lid fold has a real but subliminal visual impact. The curvature gives the illusion of the eye appearing more attractively open and brighter, than 2-dimensional measurements reflect (**Fig. 8**).

This focus on shape of the lid fold is not generally appreciated but is of such aesthetic significance as to be a priority in upper lid surgery. Because fixation at the lower edge of the infrabrow segment is a key controller of the shape of the lid fold, there is strong reason for using a technique that provides a secure lid crease. People who attend a plastic surgeon for improvement of their tired eyes appearance are not aware of the importance of the lid crease, especially when not having been blessed by nature with this anatomic attribute.

The benefits of tarsal fixation

Analysis of the lid presentation of patients leading them to secondary upper lid blepharoplasty has only recently received attention. The presentation is different from that of patients presenting for primary upper lid blepharoplasty (lid fullness and excessive hanging of the lid fold). It has acquired a specific term, a "*post blepharoplasty look*."[7,8] This "look" is essentially one of pretarsal skin laxity

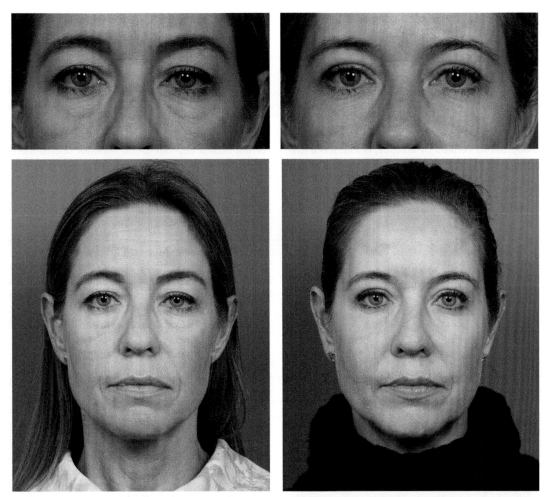

Fig. 8. (*Left*) (RS04) A 43-year-old, showing tired eyes. (*Right*) (RS05) Postoperative at 1 year, looking fresher after tarsal fixation blepharoplasty (3 mm maximum skin resection). Also, enhancing of the lid contour with supero-lateral orbital rim projection increased by 1.0 mL hydroxyapatite orbital rim augmentation. (Associated lower lid-cheek refinement from hydroxyapatite augmentation of the inferior orbital rim, maxilla, and zygoma, along with transconjunctival lid fat adjustment). Demonstrating that the brighter, more open eyes look is partly an illusion that the lid fold is higher due to the round shape of the fold with more incurving of the infrabrow segment.

(dermatochalasis with pleated horizontal skin folds), in the absence of a lid fold. As would be expected for this amount of laxity or if present, the fold tends to be high and flaccid (due to previous fat removal). The lid is hollowed due to the absence of infrabrow fat volume, yet a medial fat bulge is common (persistent or recurrent).

In the sample of 100 secondary upper blepharoplasty patients, who subsequently underwent tarsal fixation blepharoplasty a median 8.7 years following their initial blepharoplasty, nearly 40% did not require further skin resection with the median amount of only 2.0 mm for the others. Medial fat pad correction was required in 90% and lid ptosis correction in 12%. When a lid fixation technique is used, the emphasis is on contouring the

shape of the lid, not on skin tension. Similar to other facial rejuvenation surgery, the skin is only a covering, not a support.

The likelihood of a postblepharoplasty look developing, even in small degrees, is inherently reduced, whereas the results are more pleasing and more lasting (**Fig. 9**).

The internal lid tightening results in a youthful restoration of the lash tone, that lasts, while incipient or mild lid ptosis is corrected.

PART 2: PERIORBITAL LIPOFILLING

The advent of lipofilling has provided a quantum advance in the quality of rejuvenation possible around the eyes. The restoration of soft tissue volume directly improves the contour of the infrabrow segment of the lid.[9–11] A further effect of infrabrow lipofilling is the indirect improvement of the pretarsal segment tissue tone and smoothness, which is possible when the pretarsal tissues are not exceptionally loose. In some cases, lipofilling alone is all that is required to obtain a blepharoplasty effect, without surgery.[12]

An important observation about lid aging (yet to be objectively verified by a study) is that there is a progressive diminution of the preperiosteal fat of the superior orbital rim. This results in a loss of youthful fullness of the upper part of the infrabrow segment, which over time leads to flaccidity and

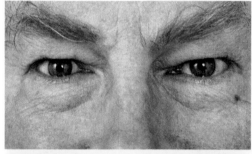

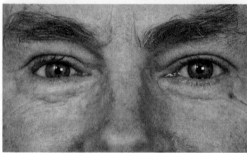

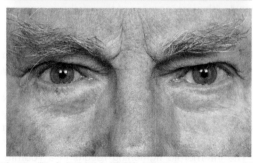

Fig. 9. (*Top*) (*Middle*) (JR02) (JR02) Preoperative, 53-year-old, man. One year following tarsal fixation blepharoplasty. (*Bottom*) (JR04) Twenty-four years postop. No further surgery. Observe the maintenance of the shape and smooth quality of the pretarsal skin, reflecting the durable fixation of the surgically created but unseen lid crease. Subsequent aging is limited to the infrabrow segment, secondary to forehead, brow descent.

sagging in the lower part, the lid fold. Ultimately, a gaunt hollowing of the upper lid occurs, whereas earlier in this process the reduction of youthful freshness is subliminal but evident.

This aging change is readily improved using a fine lipofilling cannula. Importantly, the focus of the lipofilling is to place the fat volume deep on the periosteum.

It is not widely appreciated that the attachment of the orbital septum to the superior orbital rim is not where you would assume it to be, at the center of the rim. It was demonstrated early on, to be at the posterior edge of the rim.[13] This leaves a triangular recess in the angle between the bony rim above and the septum behind and below. This is not usually clinically apparent, as the recess is filled in youth with fat (see **Fig. 5**A, **Fig. 10**).

The early and significant concerns about lipofilling leaving visible lumps no longer remain an impediment to its use in practice; this is due to improved understanding and the improvements in technology. Practically speaking, lipofilling of the periorbital area provides unique challenges, even for a surgeon experienced in lipofilling elsewhere in the body, due to the unusual characteristics of the lid, it's exceptional amount of active mobility, and the exceptional thinness of the eyelid skin that allows even minor imperfections to be revealed. In addition, the reduction of the lid soft tissue volume with age is profound. Although the classic Coleman technique is modified by using smaller fat parcels with finer aspiration and infiltration cannulas, the few difficulties experienced by the author caused a rethink.

In practice, patients are extraordinarily intolerant of even the most minor imperfection with lid lipofilling, which reflects the importance of their eyes to them. Patients may obsess with a corrosive concern about even a microlump that can scarcely be seen! This effect can be most damaging, as the concern does not necessarily abate, even after the imperfection has been objectively improved. This is an intolerable situation for the patient and surgeon to go through, for surgery of such importance to the patient, and must be avoided at all costs.

For grafted fat to take and survive requires certain conditions. The focus has correctly been on the graft size, but the substrate is of importance, even in well-vascularized eyelid tissue. In significantly depleted lids very little remaining fat is present to act as a substrate into which a graft can be placed, that inherently only a small amount of take can occur. It may require repeated grafting, to progressively build the substrate volume for improved take of the subsequently grafted fat. It is much simpler to predictably augment a smaller volume deficiency with adequate substrate, than

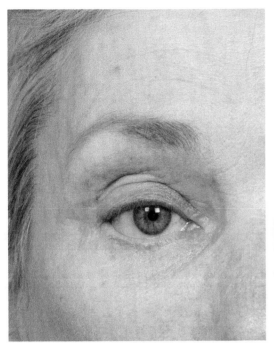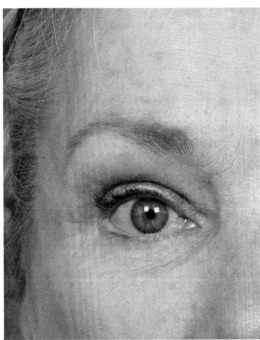

Fig. 10. (*Left*) (JE01) A 65-year-old woman with past history of conventional blepharoplasty 8 years before, with full facial rejuvenation surgery. (*Right*) (JE02) Postoperative. One year following secondary blepharoplasty (tarsal fixation technique) with only 2 mm skin excision. Also, lipogems performed using the Maft gun. A secondary lipogems was performed 4 months later, mainly to the infrabrow orbital rim, temple, and forehead.

a depleted lid. In such a situation, it is important to explain this to the patient as the rationale for the plan of a staged series of lipofilling. It is always safer to slightly underfill, avoiding the risk of even a slight unintended excess. There is more precision control with a smaller final increment, as the second putt in golf.

Preparing the injected fat by washing and diluting with saline or Ringer solution is beneficial for ease of injection and dispersing the injected volume. The author has found that the Llpogems closed system of washing with some microfracturing of the fat has avoided lumps, although it is not inexpensive. Precision control of the injection process is fundamental to safety and the avoidance of irregularities. The precision of use with the MAFT (Micro Autologous Fat Transfer) gun[14] provides a new dimension of risk prevention obtained by mechanical trigger control of calibrated microquantities of injected fat. With this degree of control comes the confidence to inject in areas not previously considered for correction. Now subliminal volume correction is performed along the superomedial orbital rim inferior to the brow, often extending down to the medial canthus and sometimes extending to a dark hollow just inferior to the canthus. This thin preperiosteal lipofilling may be extended medially to where it is blended into the side of the nose.

Although transposition of medial orbital fat can be used to correct superomedial orbital deficiency, controlled lipofilling is more versatile, not limited in volume and with the ability to taper volume at the edge.

Subsequent lipofilling, although an inconvenience for the patient, is often required in some areas to obtain the optimum youthful look without risk. Fortunately, this can be performed using local anesthesia in most instances.

PART 3: SUPERIOR ORBITAL RIM AUGMENTATION

Because of their visual importance, the brows hold a major place in the cosmetics world, where eyebrow thickness, shape, and color are regularly attended to by most adults. Nonsurgical cosmetic procedures benefit eyebrow height and shape to a degree, whereas surgery is required to obtain more significant and permanent improvements.

The intrinsic position and shape of the brow is an external manifestation of the shape of the underlying skeleton, specifically, projection of the superior orbital rim and the superolateral part of the rim formed by the zygomatic process of the frontal bone, on which the brow rests (**Fig. 11**). There is no evidence that this bone changes with aging as there is for some other orbital rim bone.[15,16]

Endeavors to surgically impose a certain shape to the brow unrelated to the skeleton may not necessarily convey an aesthetically balanced look. To a certain extent, the brow and the related infrabrow segment of the lid can be positioned indirectly by surgically enhancing the underlying skeleton. This is a relatively simple procedure with low risk and permanent benefit. The author has performed surgical augmentation of the superolateral orbital rim in more than 150 patients, specifically enhancing the projection of the zygomatic process of the frontal bone, lateral to the supraorbital nerve foramen[17] Ref (**Fig. 12**).

Although a gentle enhancement can be achieved with filler or lipofilling, a definitive contour improvement is obtained by performing a bony augmentation using subperiosteal hydroxyapatite. This increases projection of the superolateral orbital rim, relative to the globe, lateral to the supraorbital nerve[18] (**Fig. 13**).

Markings 1: Incision

With the patient awake, the vertically oriented bony superior temporal line is palpated and marked. Then with the patient raising their brow maximally, mark a prominent frontalis crease immediately medial to the superior temporal line on both sides, between 35 and 50 mm above the brow. This incision line in the crease can be as short as 12 mm in length.

Markings 2

A pair of markings from the planned incision is extended down to the brow. The lateral line

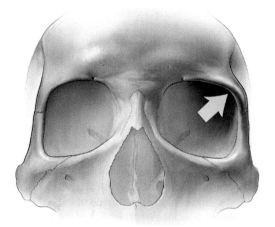

Fig. 11. A well-shaped zygomatic process of the frontal bone provides strong visual emphasis. Projection of the superolateral orbital rim is enhanced while the outer brow is supported over the lid. (*Courtesy of* Dr. Levent Efe, CMI, Australia.)

extends to the palpable lateral prominence of the superior orbital rim, the zygomatic process of the frontal bone.

The medial line extends inferomedially to the orbital rim at about the location of the supraorbital nerve. Within the area for augmentation indicate the volumes to be placed, increasing from medial to lateral and then tapering along the superior temporal line.

Preparation

Local anesthetic/adrenaline solution is injected into the incision and subperiosteally within the demarcated area. The periosteum readily hydrodissects here, as it is loosely attached. Given sufficient time for the adrenaline effect, there is virtually no bleeding with the procedure.

Incision and Subperiosteal Pocket Dissection

First incise the dermis only. Then vertically spread to open between the neurovascular structures. The periosteum is then easily entered and partially opened, without bleeding.

Use a narrow periosteal dissector to dissect medially first, which is not at all difficult, extending the dissection to the orbital rim, but not beyond (Fig. 15A). Continue the dissection laterally right up to the periosteal attachment at the lateral extent of the frontal bone, preserving its lateral periosteal boundary. Change the periosteal elevator to one that the tip curves inward, to enable dissection part way around the orbital rim to allow the granules to be placed on the lowest part of the anterior surface of the bone, better supporting the brow. Avoid overdissection, as the shape of the periosteal pocket defines the basic shape of the implant (Fig. 15B).

Placement of the Hydroxyapatite

Using a narrow retractor, the first of the loaded syringes is inserted into the pocket (recommended 1.0 mL syringe, with the hub amputated and loaded with 0.2 mL of the hydroxyapatite mixture). The tip of the syringe is directed to the most medial extent. The tip is felt through the skin to be just above the rim. With a finger protecting the inferior edge of the rim, the content is progressively added while the finger feels the granules emerging onto the bony rim. The plunger is further used to position the granules.

Then the next syringe volume is placed immediately lateral to the first and so on, and the granules are shaped using a small periosteal dissector until the volume along the rim is complete. Additional hydroxyapatite extends along the periosteal edge, tapering up along the superior temporal

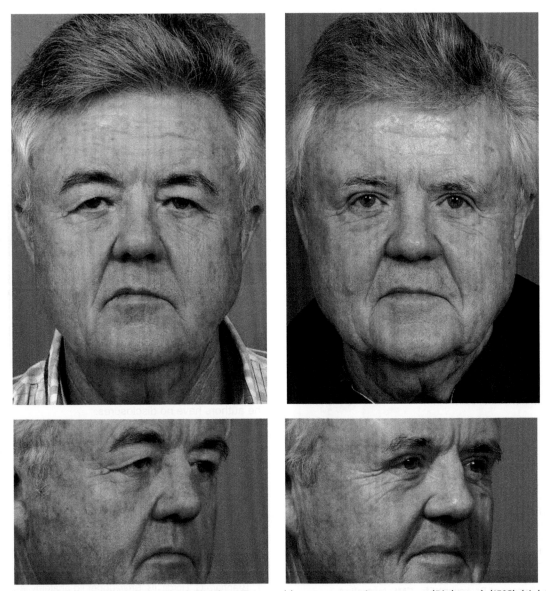

Fig. 12. (*Left top*) (JF01) (*left below*) (JF03) A 67-year-old man, no previous surgery. (*Right top*) (JF03) (*right below*) (JF04) Seven years after tarsal fixation blepharoplasty (only 5 mm maximum skin removal), a small reduction of central fat and large reduction of medial fat. Also, lateral brow contour projection was enhanced by a hydroxyapatite augmentation (1.2 mL) of the superolateral orbital rim to enhance 3D contouring. No further surgery since the original. This case impressively demonstrates that less excision of lid skin than expected results from the deeper invagination of the lid skin into the lid crease. The maintenance of pretarsal smoothness and the lid fold shape highlights the long-term benefits of having the lid crease and provides secure and durable fixation.

line. The feathering, shaping process is completed using a finger externally and the dissector internally.

Closure

A simple closure using 3 to 5 everting dermal sutures of 5/0 monofilament is all that is required. The periosteum does not require closure, only a broad Steri-Strip across the upper edge of the granule-based implant.

AFTERCARE: there is minimal need for postop analgesia. With proper wound care the incision is inconspicuous by 8 weeks. The subtle, but permanent, benefit is seen in the "look of the eyes" of the patients (**Figs. 7, 8** and **12**). It is not detectable that surgery has been done to the brows from this essentially risk-free procedure.

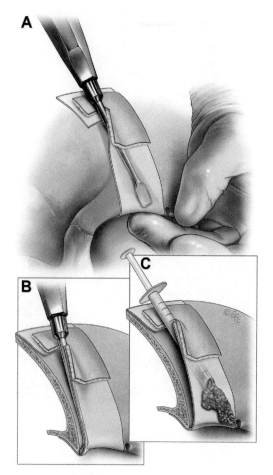

Fig. 13. Surgical steps in augmentation of the supero-lateral orbital rim using hydroxyapatite granules. (*A*) Through a forehead skin crease incision medial to the superior temporal line a precise subperiosteal dissection is performed down to the orbital rim. (*B*) The pocket extends not further than the lower edge of the rim. (*C*) The hydroxyapatite granule mixture is introduced into the pocket in 0.2 mL increments. (*Courtesy of* Dr. Levent Efe, CMI, Australia.)

SUMMARY

Given the central importance of the "eyes," meaning the periorbital region, to facial appearance, the motivated blepharoplasty patient has the opportunity to improve appearance significantly beyond the minimum of age reversal, to reveal inner beauty or add attractiveness. Bright and beautiful eyes have good 3-dimensional contouring.

The benefits of a quality eyelid crease enable the surgical focus to be on lid contouring with a reduced requirement for lid skin and fat excision. A durable crease maintains fixation of both the tarsal and infrabrow segments, providing lasting benefits while reducing the possibility of a postblepharoplasty look.

The softness of youthful eyes is regained by precise but cautious use of lipofilling. The shape of the lid fold, is important, adding in the concepts of cosmetic makeup illusion.

CLINICS CARE POINTS

- The key to attractive 'eyes' is in the appearance of the infrabrow segment of the lid.
- A rounded and full lid fold that recedes as it descends, suggests a fresh and youthful look.
- The shape of the skeletal orbital frame intrinsically determines the infrabrow segment shape.
- A lid crease that is precise and secure is essential to maintain tone of both the infrabrow and pretarsal skin.
- The 'post blepharoplasty look' is explained by the failure of lid crease fixation.

DISCLOSURE

The authors have no disclosures.

SUPPLEMENTARY DATA

Supplementary data related to this article can be found online at https://doi.org/10.1016/j.fsc.2021.01.001.

REFERENCES

1. Branham G, Holds JB. Brow/upper lid anatomy, aging and aesthetic analysis. Facial Plast.Clin N Am 2015;23(2):117–27.
2. Flowers RS. Blepharoplasty. Chapter 21. In: Courtiss EH, editor. Male aesthetic surgery. C.V. St Louis (MO): Mosby; 1982. p. 207–37.
3. Flowers R. Upper blepharoplasty by eyelid invagination - Anchor blepharoplasty. Clin Plast Surg 1993; 20(2):193–207.
4. Siegal R. Surgical anatomy of the upper eyelid fascia. Ann Plast Surg 1984;13(4):263–73.
5. May J, Fearon J, Zingarelli P. Retro-orbicularis oculus fat (ROOF) resection in aesthetic blepharoplasty: A 6 year study in 63 patients. Plast Reconstr Surg 1990;86(4):682–9.
6. Ullmann Y, Levi Y, Ben-Izhak O, et al. The surgical anatomy of the fat in the upper eyelid medial compartment. Plast Reconstr Surg 1997;99:658–61.

7. Mendelson BC, Luo D. Secondary Upper Lid Blepharoplasty: A Clinical Series Using the Tarsal Fixation Technique. Plast Reconstr Surg 2015;135:508e.

8. Steinsapir KD, Yoon-Duck K. Pathology of "Post- Upper Blepharoplasty Syndrome" Implications for Upper Eyelid Reconstruction. Clin Opthalmol 2019;13: 2035–42.

9. Fagien S. Advanced rejuvenative upper blepharoplasty: enhancing aesthetics of the upper periorbita. Plast Reconstr Surg 2002;110:278–91.

10. Trepsat F. Periorbital rejuvenation combining fat grafting and blepharoplasties. Aesthet Plast Surg 2003;27:243–53.

11. Massry GP, Azizzadeh B. Periorbital fat grafting. Facial Plast Surg 2013;29:46–57.

12. Tonnard PL, Verpaele AM, Zeltzer AA. Augmentation blepharoplasty: a review of 500 consecutive patients. Aesthet Surg J 2013;33:341–52.

13. Meyer D, Linberg J, Wobig J, et al. Anatomy of the Orbital Septum and Associated Eyelid Connective Tissues - Implications for Ptosis Surgery. Opthalmic Plast Reconstr Surg 1991;7(2):104–13.

14. Lin TM, Lin TY, Chou CK, et al. Application of micro-autologous fat transplantation in the correction of sunken upper eyelid. Plast Reconstr Surg Glob Open 2014;2:e259.

15. Pessa JE, Chen Y. Curve analysis of the aging orbital aperture. Plast Reconstr Surg 2002;109(2):751–5.

16. Mendelson B, Wong C. Changes in the facial skeleton with aging: implications and clinical applications in facial rejuvenation. Aesth.Plast.Surg. 2012;36:753–60.

17. Minelli L, Richa De Arco J, Mendelson B C. Hydroxyapatite augmentation of the superolateral orbital rim. Aesth Plast Surg, in press.

18. QMP stream Rhytidectomy. Hydroxyapatite Facial Augmentation, Bryan Mendelson. Available at: https://www.qmp.com/login.

Blepharoptosis Repair: External Versus Posterior Approach Surgery: Why I Select One over the Other

Liza M. Cohen, MD, Daniel B. Rootman, MD, MS*

KEYWORDS

- Eyelid • Blepharoptosis • Ptosis surgery • External levator resection
- Muller's muscle conjunctival resection

KEY POINTS

- There are 2 major approaches to ptosis surgery, anterior/external and posterior/internal, primarily defined by the respective eyelid elevators surgically addressed: the levator complex anteriorly and Muller muscle posteriorly.
- Posterior approach Muller muscle conjunctival resection (MMCR) surgery is an excellent first choice for most cases of mild to moderate ptosis with good levator function because it is predictable, provides a reliable cosmetic outcome, requires no patient cooperation during surgery, is associated with a lower rate of reoperation, and rarely leads to lagophthalmos and/or eyelid retraction.
- There are cases in which an anterior approach external levator resection (ELR) is preferred, including severe ocular surface/cicatricial conjunctival disease, shortened fornices, and in patients with poor levator function.
- There are circumstances in which the authors prefer MMCR and others may traditionally favor ELR. These include patients with mild congenital ptosis and good levator function, contact lens–associated ptosis, glaucoma with superior filtering blebs, and myasthenia gravis.

INTRODUCTION

Blepharoptosis is one of the most common problems presenting to the ophthalmic plastic surgeon. Most ptosis surgery involves some combination of resecting and advancing or plicating the eyelid retractors (the levator muscle/aponeurosis or Mueller muscle) with the intention of elevating the upper eyelid margin. Excluded from this paradigm are bypass procedures, such as frontalis suspension, which is not a focal topic of this discussion. Although ptosis surgery may conceptually appear straightforward, it requires a detailed knowledge of relevant eyelid anatomy, understanding of the pathophysiology of the cause of ptosis, and careful surgical planning to execute effectively. Even with these considerations, ptosis surgery can be frustratingly unpredictable, signifying that major gaps exist in our knowledge as it relates to ptosis physiology, mechanisms of repair, and the biological healing process.

Current surgical management of ptosis is typically by 1 of 2 approaches, anterior and posterior, mostly defined by the respective eyelid elevators surgically addressed: the levator anteriorly and Muller muscle posteriorly. The anterior/external approach involves advancement or resection of the levator aponeurosis, and for consistency in this discussion this will be referred to as an

Division of Orbital and Ophthalmic Plastic Surgery, Doheny and Stein Eye Institutes, University of California Los Angeles, Los Angeles, 300 Stein Plaza, Los Angeles, CA 90095, USA
* Corresponding author.
E-mail address: rootman@jsei.ucla.edu

Facial Plast Surg Clin N Am 29 (2021) 195–208
https://doi.org/10.1016/j.fsc.2021.01.002
1064-7406/21/© 2021 Elsevier Inc. All rights reserved.

external levator resection (ELR). Posterior/internal approach ptosis surgery involves resection of the Muller muscle and conjunctiva, and for consistency this will be referred to as Muller muscle conjunctival resection (MMCR). It should be noted that neither of these surgeries is likely pure, and in each case some manipulation of the other elevator is expected. It is also important to differentiate the conceptual approach from surgical access. The incision does not define the approach. Techniques in which a posterior incision is used to plicate the levator are considered anterior approaches. Vice versa, methods in which an anterior incision is used to plicate the Muller muscle would be considered posterior approaches. We refer to anterior and posterior as they relate to the elevators primarily involved in the surgery, not the position of the incision or surgical access. Thus, whether the skin or conjunctiva is incised is not particularly relevant for this discussion of anterior and posterior ptosis surgery.

The decision of whether to perform anterior or posterior ptosis surgery in many ways ultimately depends on surgeon preference, although there are circumstances in which one approach may be preferred over the other. In this article, we discuss relevant anatomy, pathophysiology, surgical techniques, and our decision-making process for selecting the appropriate ptosis surgery.

ANATOMIC CONSIDERATIONS

The 2 primary retractors of the upper eyelid are the levator palpebrae superioris (LPS) muscle and Muller muscle. The frontalis muscle is often considered a secondary retractor of the eyelid; however, recent investigations suggest that the mechanical action of the frontalis (elevating the brow) does not transmit to the eyelid under normal circumstances.[1] The frontalis is thus not considered an eyelid elevator for this discussion.

The LPS is a skeletal muscle, originating from the lesser wing of the sphenoid bone superolateral to the optic canal.[2,3] Its muscular portion is approximately 36 mm long and fans out as it courses anteriorly from a width of 4 mm posteriorly to 18 mm at the level of the superior transverse (Whitnall) ligament.[3] The Whitnall ligament consists of a band of fibrous tissue extending from the lacrimal gland fossa laterally to the trochlea medially. Whitnall's ligament is believed to function as a pulley for the LPS, allowing the muscle to change direction.[4]

Anterior to the Whitnall ligament, the LPS courses inferiorly as a fibrous aponeurosis. Microscopically, the transition from LPS to aponeurosis is gradual with muscular fibers present in diminishing amounts as it travels distally into the eyelid.[5–8] The levator aponeurosis expands medially to form the medial horn, which coalesces with the posterior portion of the medial canthal tendon and inserts onto the posterior lacrimal crest.[5] Similarly, a lateral horn is formed laterally, which divides the lacrimal gland into orbital and palpebral lobes and attaches to the lateral orbital (Whitnall) tubercle.[2,3,5]

The levator aponeurosis has been classically thought to insert inferiorly onto the lower half of the anterior surface of the tarsus in white eyelids. Histopathological evidence suggests though that this insertion may be more diffuse and variable, effectively anywhere along the tarsus.[9] This is particularly evident in Asian eyelid configurations. Fibers of the aponeurosis additionally extend anteriorly through the orbicularis oculi muscle and insert onto the skin, which is believed to form the eyelid crease.[5,10]

The Muller muscle is a smooth muscle. Its origin is found within the Whitnall ligament, where the LPS undergoes muscle-aponeurosis transition. Histologic studies demonstrate interweaving smooth and striated muscle fibers at this position.[11,12] The Muller muscle is approximately 8 to 12 mm in length and courses deep to the levator aponeurosis, in what some consider to be a potential "postaponeurotic" space.[13] Distally, there is some controversy regarding the insertion of the Muller muscle. Classically it is described as inserting onto the superior border of the tarsus.[6] Other investigations have suggested that it may insert more inferiorly onto the anterior surface of the tarsus.[14] Some have further proposed that the Muller muscle terminates above the tarsus[15] within a complex network of elastic and collagen fibers involving the levator aponeurosis, Muller muscle, and orbicularis.[16,17] It is likely that this insertion is variable across populations, and may even change over time. Interestingly, the LPS-Muller configuration is somewhat unique in the body, with the skeletal LPS and smooth Muller muscle being arranged in series without a fixed anchor point.

The Muller muscle receives sympathetic innervation, a finding that has been confirmed clinically by its involvement in Horner syndrome, experimentally by immunostaining of sympathetic receptors,[18] and pharmacologically by using sympathetic agonists and antagonists.[19] Although it is known to be sympathetically innervated, the precise nervous pathway within the orbit is poorly understood. It is likely that innervation is derived from multiple sympathetic roots.[20] The Muller muscle is responsible for approximately 3 mm of upper eyelid excursion. This has been confirmed experimentally in healthy subjects where from a neutral position, the eyelid can be lowered

1.5 mm with sympathetic antagonists and raised 1.5 mm with agonists.[19]

There is some controversy regarding the function of the Muller muscle. Some suggest it is a transmitter of the levator aponeurosis action,[16] whereas others propose it is a stretch receptor for the LPS,[21] providing a primarily proprioceptive role. The most widely accepted hypotheses suggest that it functions to maintain tonic eyelid position, allowing for responses based on sympathetic stimulation,[22] or that it maintains a 3 mm "fine tuning" role in upper eyelid position. It is additionally possible (and plausible) that the Muller muscle is multifunctional.

PATHOPHYSIOLOGY

The determination of eyelid position likely involves a comprehensive maintenance system with afferent inputs, central processing, and efferent outputs.[23] Dysfunction anywhere in this system may lead to ptosis, and ptosis surgery is theorized to modify this system, leading to a re-setting of static eyelid position.

Potential afferent inputs to this system include vision, touch sensation, and proprioception. Although it is well-documented that functional visual field impairment due to ptosis can be reversible with surgery,[24–26] visual stimuli may not be a critical component in the development of ptosis, as patients with anophthalmic sockets can demonstrate ptosis and respond to both anterior and posterior ptosis surgery.[27] Simple touch sensation also may be a less relevant input, as it is well known that an anesthetic eye, for instance after topical proparacaine use, is not reliably associated with ptosis. Proprioceptive stimuli are of keen interest as potential vital inputs[28–32]; however, much of the evidence for this pathway is speculative at this point. Further research is needed to determine the influence of these various afferent factors.

The flow of afferent information is also incompletely understood. Presumably these signals follow the trigeminal system. The trigeminal sensory pathway passes through the trigeminal ganglion, synapses in the main sensory trigeminal nucleus, decussates, and travels along the contralateral ventral trigeminal lemniscus before synapsing in the ventral posteromedial (VPM) nucleus of the thalamus. The proprioceptive signals from the extraocular muscles and eyelid elevators presumably follow this pathway; however, animal data suggest that at least some of the extraocular muscle proprioceptive input travels directly to the lateral geniculate nucleus with retinal ganglion cells[33] and even with motor nerves, including the oculomotor nerve.[34] From the thalamus, these signals travel diffusely throughout the brain to visual, sensory, and balance centers. Indirect evidence of eyelid position signals traveling through the thalamus can be drawn from studies in which thalamic injury (infarct, hemorrhage) can be associated with ptosis.[35] These afferent systems are relatively poorly understood; however, they clearly play a role in eyelid position homeostasis.

Output systems are more completely characterized. Motor innervation to the LPS via the superior division of the third cranial nerve is well-established.[36,37] Muller muscle innervation is part of the sympathetic system. There is some controversy as to the precise anatomic projection of efferent intraorbital pathways to the Muller muscle, and the motor control could perhaps have input from other related extraorbital systems.[18] However anatomically transmitted, much evidence of sympathetic innervation exists.[18–20]

The integration and coordination of the afferent and efferent signals is the most sparsely investigated and consequently most poorly understood aspect of eyelid position physiology. Some have proposed a reflex arc involving afferent stretch receptors in the Muller muscle and efferent output via the LPS and frontalis muscles.[21,38] This work is theoretic, yet perhaps it does provide some framework for conversion of afferent to efferent signals, though without central processing.

There is, however, much emerging evidence of integration capacity, and thus central processing, in the eyelid position maintenance system. For instance, eyelid position is relatively preserved when gravitational forces are altered. We examined photographs of astronauts both on Earth and in space and found zero gravity does not significantly change marginal reflex distance 1 (MRD1). We have also shown that in healthy individuals, changing postural position was also associated with relative preservation of eyelid position.[39] In addition, reducing protracting forces in facial palsy is in most cases associated with maintenance of normal eyelid position, although it should be noted that more severe facial weakness is associated with a breakdown in this system and eyelid position abnormalities.[40,41] These results together suggest there is adaptive capacity within the eyelid position maintenance system. However, at present the capacity, functionality, and neural basis for this system are each very poorly characterized. Clearly, more research in this area is needed to more accurately understand the determinants of eyelid position, particularly as it relates to central processing and proprioception.

MECHANISMS OF REPAIR
External Levator Resection

ELR surgery was developed based on the principle that the primary defect in ptosis is a disinsertion or lengthening (thinning) of the levator aponeurosis. Surgery is directed at the presumed root cause of the disorder and involves reinserting (with or without shortening) the levator aponeurosis to the tarsus. This is supported histopathologically, as one study demonstrated aponeurotic defects in most patients with involutional ptosis.[42]

However, various pieces of information have challenged this assertion over time. Some believe the high incidence of levator aponeurosis disinsertion is iatrogenic, and with careful dissection its incidence can be decreased dramatically.[43] Others have demonstrated fatty infiltration of the LPS with an attenuated aponeurosis but no disinsertion or dehiscence in patients with ptosis, suggesting again that the incidence of disinsertion is lower than originally suspected.[44,45] Additional studies noting decreased levator function in patients affected by involutional ptosis suggest an alternative myogenic rather than aponeurotic etiology for involutional ptosis.[46] Further, as described in the preceding sections, it is quite likely that there are more complicated pathophysiologic processes involved in at least some proportion of patients with ptosis. Simple mechanical theories appear to incompletely explain the pathophysiology of ptosis generally and the mechanisms of ELR efficacy specifically.

Overall, although it is widely believed that mechanical advancement/reinsertion of the levator aponeurosis onto the tarsus is the mechanism of eyelid elevation in ELR,[47] the system may in fact be more complicated. There is emerging evidence that the surgery may have more nuanced effects on eyelid position.

Muller Muscle Conjunctival Resection

The mechanism for MMCR surgery is even less clear. It was originally proposed that resection/plication of the Muller muscle would raise the eyelid an equal amount as would phenylephrine applied in the preoperative setting.[48] However, phenylephrine response is not entirely predictive of surgical change. This suggests that the mechanism is more complicated than mechanically replicating the configuration of a contracted muscle. Further supporting this notion, histologic studies have demonstrated little association between the amount of Muller muscle resected[49–51] or the quantity of adrenergic receptors[18] and degree of eyelid elevation.

In response to this unequal relationship between Muller muscle resection and eyelid elevation, some have proposed that plication of the levator aponeurosis is an essential aspect of the mechanism for MMCR surgery. This is supported by histologic identification of levator fibers in MMCR specimens.[50,52] However, there are observations that challenge this explanation as well. Mechanical levator plication does not explain the variability in response to similar tissue resection lengths. For instance, the standard deviation of change in MRD1 for 1 mm of resection length is close to 1.0 mm, indicating high variability.[53] In addition, there is little empiric evidence of a relationship between resection length and change in MRD1 when preoperative MRD1 is taken into account.[54,55] Further, MMCR surgery appears to have less effect on eyelid contour compared with ELR,[56] and with similar levator-related mechanisms, one would expect the contour effects to be the same.

Finally, the progression of MRD1 change after ELR and MMCR surgery is also different, suggesting alternative mechanisms. In patients who undergo ELR, change in MRD1 evident by 1 week postoperatively is stable at 3 months,[57] and this is independent of the degree of swelling.[58] However, patients who undergo MMCR experience an increase in MRD1 from 1-week to 3-month follow-up, although there is no difference in final MRD1 result between the groups.[57] These studies suggest that the 2 surgeries work by different mechanisms, albeit with some overlap.

Although there is ample evidence as to the deficiencies of mechanical Muller or levator-specific mechanisms, there is unfortunately little evidence for alternative theories. The unequal evidence for any one theory can suggest 2 overlapping possibilities. The first is that multiple pathophysiologic processes are at play, and thus in some but not all cases mechanical mechanisms are managed appropriately and primarily responsible for efficacy. Alternatively, mechanical processes may be only marginally involved, in so much as they stimulate more adaptive neural processing mechanisms that reset eyelid position. These systems may be functional or dysfunctional, creating variability in the response. This dichotomy would be akin to the mechanical and sensory theories of strabismus. Emerging research will ideally provide better answers for this question in the future. Presently, we can use practical experience to guide best practices, accepting some variability in outcome.

SURGICAL TECHNIQUE
External Levator Resection

Anterior ptosis surgery was first described by Everbusch in 1883,[59] but gained popularity after Jones and colleagues[13] demonstrated disinsertion of the levator aponeurosis in 1975. The surgery involves advancement/reattachment of the levator aponeurosis onto the tarsus, typically via an external upper eyelid skin incision.

Steps of procedure

1. Mark the upper eyelid crease.
2. Local anesthesia with or without conscious sedation. Conservative use of local anesthesia may preserve levator function and allow for accurate assessment of eyelid position intraoperatively.
3. Incise skin.
4. Traverse orbicularis muscle (**Fig. 1**A) and identify levator aponeurosis (**Fig. 1**B) and tarsus.
5. Dissect the levator free from the superior border of the tarsus.
6. At this point, many dissect the levator free of the Muller muscle below and/or the septum (**Fig. 1**C) and pre-aponeurotic fat pads (**Fig. 1**D) above.
7. Determine point of maximal eyelid elevation and pass a double-armed suture partial thickness through the tarsus at this location (**Fig. 1**E), then through the posterior surface of the levator (**Fig. 1**F) and tie on a slip knot.
8. Sit the patient up vertically and assess eyelid position and contour. Suture may need to be adjusted. A second suture may need to be placed to attain optimal lid height and contour.
9. Tie suture ends permanently and cut.
10. Close skin (**Fig. 1**G,H).

Variations in technique

It should be noted that huge variability in the steps of this procedure exist in the community. A wide range of modifications have been proposed from changing the size and location of the skin incision,[60,61] to the order of dissection along the anterior or posterior portions of the levator (or both), even including whether to disinsert the levator at all or to include the horns in a wide dissection. The number, placement, and configuration of sutures have also been varied in as many ways as would be conceptually possible.[62] There is no standard procedure for ELR surgery and no convincing evidence that one incision, dissection, or suture technique is better (or worse) than another.

More significant procedural modifications also have been described. Intraoperative evaluation of the eyelid in the sitting position with patient cooperation has been shown to more accurately predict postoperative eyelid position,[63] supporting the use of upright patient positioning and suture adjustment intraoperatively. The use of adjustable

sutures has been reported to decrease the reoperation rate to 5% to 18%.[64–66]

To predict surgical outcome and decrease reoperation rates, there have been attempts to modify the amount of aponeurosis advancement via the creation of nomograms. Various approaches have been described. The levator function technique assumes that the eyelid height set during surgery will elevate or fall a predictable amount after surgery based on preoperative levator function.[67] In the MRD technique, the preoperative MRD1 dictates the amount the levator is advanced.[67] This approach has been refined to a 2:1 aponeurosis resection to expected eyelid elevation algorithm, suggesting that for every 2 mm of resection, 1 mm of eyelid elevation is to be expected.[68] This has been further modified by using a spring scale to apply a constant force on the aponeurosis to account for its expansile nature.[69,70] None of these nomograms have gained wide popularity for a number of reasons, including the variability in defining the "end of the levator" and empiric experience revealing extensive variability in the response. These nomograms simply do not demonstrate the type of consistency required for practical utility and have thus not been widely adopted.

Muller Muscle Conjunctival Resection

Since it was originally described by Putterman and Urist in 1975,[48] MMCR surgery has gained acceptance and popularity, particularly among younger surgeons in the United States,[71] although less so internationally.[72,73] The basic premise of the surgery involves excision of a tissue flap containing the Muller muscle, conjunctiva, and some levator aponeurosis fibers.

Steps of procedure

1. Local anesthesia with or without conscious sedation. The posterior eyelid can be anesthetized by everting the eyelid and injecting directly into the Muller muscle plane (**Fig. 2**A).
2. Evert the eyelid over a Desmarres retractor to expose the conjunctiva and tarsus.
3. Mark the conjunctiva at 2 positions (medial and lateral one-third) across the tarsus at half of the total distance to be resected from the upper margin of the tarsus.
4. Grasp the medial and lateral positions with a locking forceps or sutures, taking care to involve conjunctiva, Muller muscle, and likely some posterior levator aponeurosis (**Fig. 2**B). Classically, a suture is passed for this purpose.

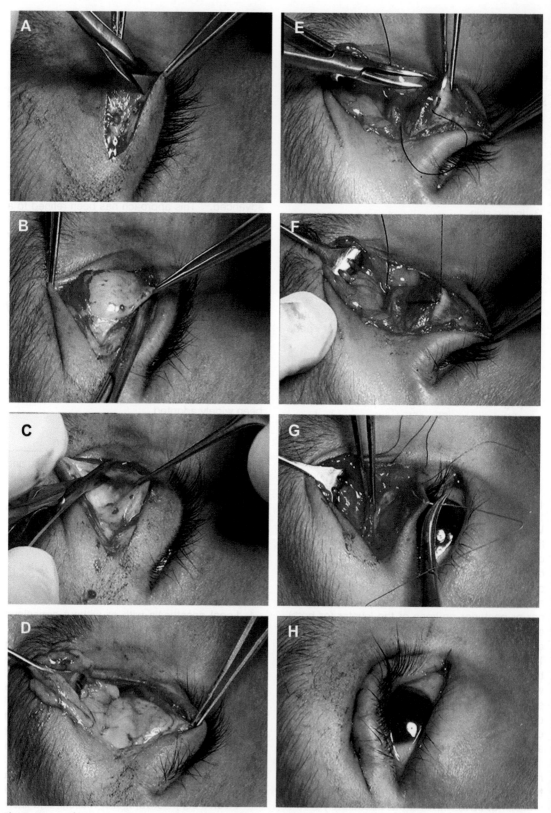

Fig. 1. Steps of ELR procedure. (*A*) The orbicularis oculi muscle is incised, and (*B*) levator aponeurosis identified. The levator is dissected free from the septum (*C*) and pre-aponeurotic fat pads (*D*) above. (*E*) A suture is passed partial thickness through the tarsus at the desired point of maximal elevation, then through the posterior surface of the levator (*F*). (*G, H*) The skin is closed, with incorporation of levator aponeurosis if eyelid-crease formation is desired.

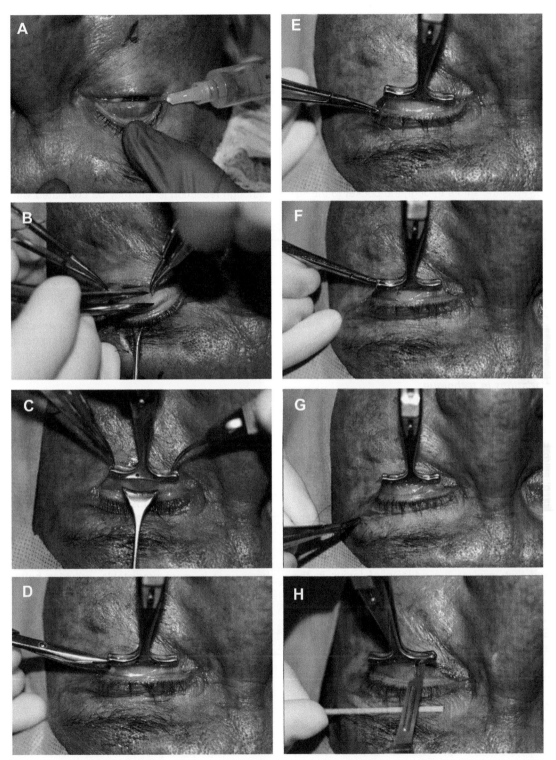

Fig. 2. Steps of MMCR procedure. (*A*) The eyelid is everted and local anesthesia injected directly into the Muller muscle plane. (*B*) The conjunctiva/Muller muscle is grasped with locking forceps at 2 positions (medial and lateral one-third) across the tarsus at half of the total distance to be resected from the upper margin of the tarsus (3.5 mm in this case). (*C*) The tissue is elevated on tension and superior traction applied to the eyelid margin with a Desmarres retractor, while the ptosis clamp is applied. (*D*) A conjunctival pocket is created using Westcott scissors above the tarsus laterally to bury the suture. (*E*) A suture is passed through the pocket to the inferior or

5. Elevate these positions on tension and apply superior traction to the eyelid margin, stretching the elevated positions from the tarsus to full extension.
6. Apply ptosis clamp (**Fig. 2**C). Tarsus can be incorporated into the clamp if tarsectomy is desired.
7. Create conjunctival pocket using Westcott scissors above the tarsus laterally to bury the suture (**Fig. 2**D). Alternatively, the suture can be passed to and from the skin surface to externalize the knot.
8. Pass the suture through the pocket to the superior conjunctival position (**Fig. 2**E), then underneath the clamp in a serpentine fashion to the medial side (**Fig. 2**F), where the direction is reversed. Suture is passed in the intervening spaces to the lateral side and externalized to the conjunctival pocket or through the eyelid.
9. Suture is tied and ends cut (**Fig. 2**G).
10. Pass a blade at a 45-degree angle away from the tarsus underneath the clamp, along the length of the resection (**Fig. 2**H).
11. Reposition eyelid.

Variations in technique

Most of the technical literature regarding MMCR has focused on development of a tissue resection length algorithm[48,74–79] and only slight modifications to the technique have been proposed.[80–83] Such modifications in operative technique, including excising and closing the tissue under direct visualization,[80] by using a single horizontal mattress suture,[81] no suture,[82] or tissue glue[83] have all demonstrated efficacy. Although many variations in surgical technique for MMCR exist, they all appear to result in similar outcomes.

One modification, however, may be different, and that involves the addition of tarsus in the MMCR resection. This technique blurs the lines between the Fasanella Servat procedure and MMCR and can be effective in certain patients.[78] Some would consider this a separate procedure and thus may not be described by the bulk of MMCR experience. The use of tarsectomy is beyond the present discussion.

The original conceptualization of the procedure presumed that excision of most of the Muller muscle would re-create the effect of maximal muscle contraction under phenylephrine stimulation.[48] However, this simple relationship did not hold,

leading to variations in the amount of tissue resected intended to improve predictability of the surgical outcome. The most commonly cited nomogram for resection length to elevation is the "4:1 rule."[76,79] This algorithm suggests that for every 4 mm of resection, 1 mm of eyelid elevation is to be expected. This was developed based on data that found on average 8 mm of tissue is resected, and the MRD1 response to this is 2 mm of elevation.[76,77,79,84,85] Simple division is then used to create the 4:1 nomogram. However, more recent literature has demonstrated that although resection length may be correlated with MRD1 elevation, so is preoperative MRD1. Essentially, lower eyelids always receive longer resection lengths. In multivariate modeling, it has been shown that preoperative MRD1 is the more critical factor in determining response, resection length being only secondary.[55] When directly compared, a standard resection length of 7 mm performs approximately the same as a variable 4:1 rule, with no difference in final outcome.[54] Despite this evidence, a variable 4:1 algorithm persists in being almost universally used clinically, though this may change over time.

CHOICE OF APPROACH FOR PTOSIS SURGERY

The decision of whether to perform anterior or posterior ptosis surgery is largely based on surgeon preference, as in most cases, either technique is appropriate. Our preference is for MMCR as a primary intervention in most cases.

Most patients with ptosis present with mild to moderate involutional ptosis. MRD1 is typically in the range of 0 to 3 mm with good levator function (>12 mm excursion). In such cases, we consider MMCR to be a good first choice for surgery because it is more predictable, provides better cosmetic outcome in terms of eyelid contour and symmetry, has a lower rate of reoperation for undercorrection or overcorrection, and very rarely leads to lagophthalmos and/or eyelid retraction above the limbus.[56,86] Furthermore, should a second surgery be required, it is less complicated to perform this surgery (ie, MMCR, tarsectomy, or ELR), due to less scarring and disruption of tissue planes in the eyelid. Empirically, a second procedure after MMCR appears to be effective if needed, with similar complication profiles to primary ELR or MMCR surgery (Karlin JN, Katsev B, Kapelushnik

---

superior conjunctival position. (*F*) The suture is passed underneath the clamp in serpentine fashion from lateral to medial and then medial to lateral and externalized through the conjunctival pocket. (*G*) Suture is tied within the pocket and ends cut. (*H*) The tissue is excised by passing a blade at a 45-degree angle away from the tarsus underneath the clamp, along the length of the resection.

N, Simon GB, Rootman DB. Revision ptosis surgery for undercorrected Müller muscle conjunctival resection. Unpublished data, 2020.).

A positive response to phenylephrine (>2 mm change) is considered by many to be a necessary criterion to pursue MMCR surgery. This may not be the case. We have demonstrated that even patients with a moderate phenylephrine response can achieve good outcomes with MMCR. These patients often present with less severe ptosis (higher MRD1) and achieve less change in MRD1; however, final outcomes are typically similar to those with larger phenylephrine responses. The phenylephrine response is thus again related to the preoperative MRD1 and larger responses are seen in lower cases; both strong and weak responders at any preoperative MRD1 can benefit from MMCR surgery. We do not routinely use phenylephrine response as a criterion for patient selection.[55] The vast majority of ptosis cases fall in the category of involutional ptosis with good levator function and regardless of phenylephrine response, MMCR can be an appropriate first choice for these cases (**Fig. 3**).

Although MMCR has its advantages, there are situations in which ELR may be a better primary option. Severe ocular surface disease, including cicatricial conjunctival disease and other conditions leading to forniceal shortening, may be considered contraindications to MMCR for a number of reasons. The surgery itself may incite further scarring, leading to worsening of cicatrizing disease. It may also shorten the fornix critically, leading to scarring between the eyelid and the globe and resultant lagophthalmos and/or diplopia. In this scenario, an anterior approach ptosis surgery preserves the integrity of the conjunctiva and is thus preferred.

Patients with levator function less than 12 mm may not be the best candidates for MMCR. In this scenario, ELR is a more widely accepted approach (**Fig. 4**), although some may argue that neither surgery is perfectly effective in this group. Patients with particularly poor levator function may be better candidates for frontalis suspension, although maximal/supramaximal levator resection is an increasingly popular alternative.[87,88]

The severity of ptosis has been proposed as a criterion for surgical selection. It is widely accepted that cases of severe ptosis in which the MRD1 is <0 mm may be less amenable to MMCR, as classically the surgery is thought to achieve an eyelid elevation of only up to 3 mm.[19] In such cases, ELR is described as a better choice for primary surgery. However, recent studies suggest MMCR can be effective in such patients with severe ptosis,[89] and in our experience, these patients can have an excellent response to surgery

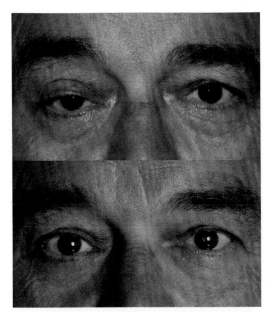

Fig. 3. MMCR for moderate involutional ptosis with good levator function. Top: Preoperative photograph demonstrating 2 mm of right upper eyelid ptosis. Bottom: Postoperative photograph after right MMCR demonstrating improvement in ptosis with good eyelid contour and symmetry.

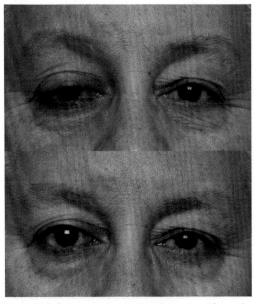

Fig. 4. ELR for severe involutional ptosis with moderate levator function. Top: Preoperative photograph demonstrating right upper eyelid ptosis. Bottom: Postoperative photograph after right ELR demonstrating improvement in ptosis and eyelid contour.

(**Fig. 5**). Thus, given relatively good levator function, we do use MMCR in these cases.

There are additional situations in which we prefer to perform MMCR despite falling outside of classic indications. Congenital cases with mild ptosis and good levator function can be managed with MMCR.[90] These are typically performed in young adulthood, as they were considered too mild for management as infants. Levator excursion of 12 mm or greater is likely ideal.

The mechanism of contact lens–associated ptosis has been proposed to be levator dehiscence due to repetitive mechanical eyelid stretching and rubbing between the eyelid and lens. Thus, these patients were historically thought to require ELR. However, MMCR has shown to be particularly effective in this patient population and would be a reasonable first-line choice[91] (**Fig. 6**).

Although classically contraindicated, we have had success performing MMCR in patients with glaucoma and superior filtering blebs (**Fig. 7**).[92] Many surgeons would prefer ELR because of risk of conjunctival surgery interfering with bleb function; however, in our studies we did not find a greater incidence of bleb failure or glaucoma progression in these cases, and MMCR was effective for management of ptosis.[92] Some would argue MMCR may be a more appropriate first-line

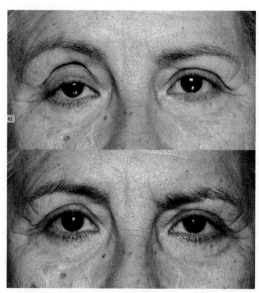

Fig. 6. MMCR for contact lens–associated ptosis with good levator function. Top: Preoperative photograph demonstrating right upper eyelid ptosis and increased tarsal platform show. Bottom: Postoperative photograph after right MMCR demonstrating improvement in ptosis.

surgery in patients with glaucoma with filtering blebs due to the decreased risk of overcorrection, to avoid the potentially more devastating complications associated with bleb exposure.

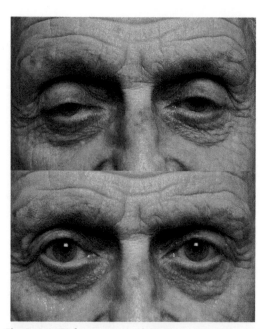

Fig. 5. MMCR for severe involutional ptosis with good levator function. Top: Preoperative photograph demonstrating bilateral upper eyelid ptosis with MRD1 of 0 mm. Bottom: Postoperative photograph after bilateral MMCR demonstrating marked improvement in ptosis.

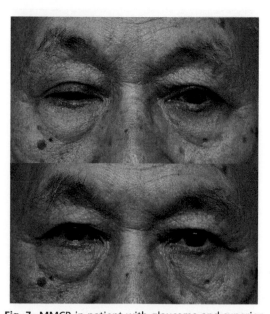

Fig. 7. MMCR in patient with glaucoma and superior filtering bleb with good levator function. Top: Preoperative photograph demonstrating right upper eyelid ptosis with flattening of the eyelid contour. Bottom: Postoperative photograph after right MMCR demonstrating improvement in ptosis and eyelid contour.

Horner syndrome is another circumstance in which MMCR surgery can be an effective first-line therapy. Although the denervated Muller muscle may be expected to have a reduced response to a plication procedure, empirically the opposite is true. Studies have long demonstrated MMCR surgery to be effective in achieving excellent elevation and symmetry in patients with Horner syndrome.[93]

Although patients with myasthenia gravis are ideally managed medically, surgery may be performed in some cases to correct residual ptosis when there is medication failure/intolerance. In addition, there are cases in which it is appropriate to treat ptosis partially with medical therapy and partially with surgery. We prefer MMCR as a first-choice surgery in these patients, as ptosis is prone to change, and patients may require a second surgery. In our experience, it is technically less complicated to perform a second operation on patients who have had previous MMCR as opposed to ELR, reserving the ELR option for progression of disease. In addition, anterior ptosis surgery involves transecting the orbicularis oculi muscle, which may worsen pre-existing orbicularis weakness and result in lagophthalmos in myasthenic patients.

Overall, based on the literature and our experience, MMCR is a good first option for most patients with ptosis who typically present with mild to moderate ptosis and good levator function.[56,86] There are certain situations in which ELR is preferred and these include severe ocular surface/cicatricial conjunctival disease, shortened fornices, and patients with poor levator function. Outside of these populations, we believe MMCR can be used safely and effectively in a wide range of special situations including patients with severe ptosis, mild congenital ptosis, contact lens–associated ptosis, glaucoma with superior filtering blebs, and myasthenia gravis.

SUMMARY

Ptosis surgery requires detailed knowledge of the eyelid anatomy, understanding of the pathophysiology, and careful preoperative planning. The decision of whether to perform surgery via an anterior/external or posterior/internal approach depends mainly on the surgeon's preference, although there are situations in which one may be preferable to the other. MMCR is a good first choice in most cases of mild to moderate ptosis with good levator function, regardless of phenylephrine response. A few specific circumstances may be more appropriately managed with ELR surgery, mostly related to other ophthalmic diseases. A thorough preoperative evaluation can guide the surgeon's decision, and surgery should be approached in an individualized manner tailored to the patient.

CLINICS CARE POINTS

- Posterior approach Muller muscle conjunctival resection (MMCR) surgery is an excellent first choice for most cases of mild to moderate ptosis with good levator function because it is predictable, provides a reliable cosmetic outcome, requires no patient cooperation during surgery, is associated with a lower rate of reoperation, and rarely leads to lagophthalmos and/or eyelid retraction.

- There are cases in which an anterior approach external levator resection (ELR) is preferred, including severe ocular surface/cicatricial conjunctival disease, shortened fornices, and in patients with poor levator function.

- There are circumstances in which the authors prefer MMCR and others may traditionally favor ELR. These include patients with mild congenital ptosis and good levator function, contact lens–associated ptosis, glaucoma with superior filtering blebs, and myasthenia gravis.

DISCLOSURE

Supported by an unrestricted grant from Research to Prevent Blindness, Inc.

REFERENCES

1. Sinha KR, Al Shaker S, Yeganeh A, et al. The relationship between eyebrow and eyelid position in patients with ptosis, dermatochalasis and controls. Ophthalmic Plast Reconstr Surg 2019;35(1):85–90.
2. Whitnall SE. Anatomy of the human orbit and accessory organs of vision. New York: Robert E. Krieger; 1979. p. 115–9, 259–288.
3. Lemke BN, Stasior OG, Rosenberg PN. The surgical relations of the levator palpebrae superioris muscle. Ophthalmic Plast Reconstr Surg 1988;4:25–30.
4. Kakizaki H, Takahashi Y, Nakano T, et al. Whitnall ligament anatomy revisited. Clin Exp Ophthalmol 2011; 39:152–5.
5. Anderson RL, Beard C. The levator aponeurosis. Attachments and their clinical significance. Arch Ophthalmol 1977;95:1437–41.
6. Kuwabara T, Cogan DG, Johnson CC. Structure of the muscles of the upper eyelid. Arch Ophthalmol 1975;93:1189–97.

7. Kakizaki H, Zako M, Nakano T, et al. The levator aponeurosis consists of two layers that include smooth muscle. Ophthalmic Plast Reconstr Surg 2005;21:379–82.

8. Kakizaki H, Madge SN, Malhotra R, et al. The levator aponeurosis contains smooth muscle fibers: new findings in Caucasians. Ophthalmic Plast Reconstr Surg 2009;25:267–9.

9. Ng SK, Chan W, Marcet MM, et al. Levator palpebrae superioris: an anatomical update. Orbit 2013; 32(1):76–84.

10. Sayoc BT. Plastic construction of the superior palpebral fold. Am J Ophthalmol 1954;38:556–9.

11. Berke RN, Wadsworth JA. Histology of levator muscle in congenital and acquired ptosis. AMA Arch Ophthalmol 1955;53(3):413–28.

12. Isaksson I. Studies on congenital genuine blepharoptosis. Morphological and functional investigations of the upper eyelid. Acta Ophthalmol Suppl 1962;72: 1–121.

13. Jones LT, Quickert MH, Wobig JL. The cure of ptosis by aponeurotic repair. Arch Ophthalmol 1975;93(8): 629–34.

14. Kakizaki H, Madge SN, Selva D. Insertion of the levator aponeurosis and Müller's muscle on the tarsus: a cadaveric study in Caucasians. Clin Exp Ophthalmol 2010;38(6):635–7.

15. Ahn HB, Oh HC, Roh MS, et al. The study of anatomic relationship between the Müller muscle and the tarsus in Asian upper eyelid. Ophthalmic Plast Reconstr Surg 2010;26(5):334–8.

16. Bang YH, Park SH, Kim JH, et al. The role of Müller's muscle reconsidered. Plast Reconstr Surg 1998; 101(5):1200–4.

17. Stasior GO, Lemke BN, Wallow IH, et al. Levator aponeurosis elastic fiber network. Ophthalmic Plast Reconstr Surg 1993;9(1):1–10.

18. Skibell BC, Harvey JH, Oestreicher JH, et al. Adrenergic receptors in the ptotic human eyelid: correlation with phenylephrine testing and surgical success in ptosis repair. Ophthalmic Plast Reconstr Surg 2007;23:367–71.

19. Felt DP, Frueh BR. A pharmacologic study of the sympathetic eyelid tarsal muscles. Ophthalmic Plast Reconstr Surg 1988;4(1):15–24.

20. Manson PN, Lazarus RB, Morgan R, et al. Pathways of sympathetic innervation to the superior and inferior (Muller's) tarsal muscles. Plast Reconstr Surg 1986;78(1):33–40.

21. Matsuo K. Stretching of the Mueller muscle results in involuntary contraction of the levator muscle. Ophthalmic Plast Reconstr Surg 2002;18:5–10.

22. Dutton JJ, Frueh BR. Eyelid anatomy and physiology with reference to blepharoptosis. In: Cohen AJ, Weinberg DA, editors. Evaluation and management of blepharoptosis. New York: Springer; 2011. p. 13–26.

23. Rootman DB. Pathophysiology of ptosis and mechanisms of repair: lessons from Muller's muscle conjunctival resection surgery. Adv Ophthalmol Optom 2017;2(1):421–34.

24. Cahill KV, Burns JA, Weber PA. The effect of blepharoptosis on the field of vision. Ophthalmic Plast Reconstr Surg 1987;3(3):121–5.

25. Meyer DR, Linberg JV, Powell SR, et al. Quantitating the superior visual field loss associated with ptosis. Arch Ophthalmol 1989;107(6):840–3.

26. Riemann CD, Hanson S, Foster JA. A comparison of manual kinetic and automated static perimetry in obtaining ptosis fields. Arch Ophthalmol 2000;118(1): 65–9.

27. Karesh JW, Putterman AM, Fett DR. Conjunctiva-Muller's muscle excision to correct anophthalmic ptosis. Ophthalmology 1986;93(8):1068–71.

28. Ban R, Matsuo K, Osada Y, et al. Reflexive contraction of the levator palpebrae superioris muscle to involuntarily sustain the effective eyelid retraction through the transverse trigeminal proprioceptive nerve on the proximal Mueller's muscle: verification with evoked electromyography. J Plast Reconstr Aesthet Surg 2010;63(1):59–64.

29. Matsuo K, Ban R. Surgical desensitisation of the mechanoreceptors in Muller's muscle relieves chronic tension-type headache caused by tonic reflexive contraction of the occipitofrontalis muscle in patients with aponeurotic blepharoptosis. J Plast Surg Hand Surg 2013;47(1):21–9.

30. Segal KL, Lelli GJ Jr, Djougarian A, et al. Proprioceptive phenomenon with involutional ptosis: evidential findings in anophthalmic ptosis. Ophthalmic Plast Reconstr Surg 2016;32(2):113–5.

31. Beaulieu R, Andre K, Mancini R. Frontalis muscle contraction and the role of visual deprivation and eyelid proprioception. Ophthalmic Plast Reconstr Surg 2018;34(6):552–6.

32. Vrcek I, Blumer R, Blandford A, et al. Histologic evaluation of nonvisual afferent sensory upper eyelid proprioception. Ophthalmic Plast Reconstr Surg 2020;36(1):7–12.

33. Donaldson IM. The functions of the proprioceptors of the eye muscles. Philos Trans R Soc Lond B Biol Sci 2000;355(1404):1685–754.

34. Gentle A, Ruskell G. Pathway of the primary afferent nerve fibres serving proprioception in monkey extraocular muscles. Ophthalmic Physiol Opt 1997;17(3): 225–31.

35. Kausar H, Antonios N. Combined thalamic ptosis and astasia. J Clin Neurosci 2013;20(11):1471–4.

36. Erdogmus S, Govsa F, Celik S. Innervation features of the extraocular muscles. J Craniofac Surg 2007; 18(6):1439–46.

37. Hwang K, Lee DK, Chung IH, et al. Patterns of oculomotor nerve distribution to the levator palpebrae superioris muscle, and correlation to temporary

ptosis after blepharoplasty. Ann Plast Surg 2001; 47(4):381–4.

38. Matsuo K, Osada Y, Ban R. Electrical stimulation to the trigeminal proprioceptive fibres that innervate the mechanoreceptors in Muller's muscle induces involuntary reflex contraction of the frontalis muscles. J Plast Surg Hand Surg 2013; 47(1):14–20.

39. Rootman DB, Shaker SA, Moreno TA, et al. The effect of loading on normal eyelid position. Presented at: American Society of Ophthalmic Plastic and Reconstructive Surgery (ASOPRS) 46th Annual Fall Scientific Symposium. Las Vegas, NV; November 12-13,2015.

40. Sinha KR, Rootman DB, Azizzadeh B, et al. Association of eyelid position and facial nerve palsy with unresolved weakness. JAMA Facial Plast Surg 2016;18(5):379–84.

41. Manta A, Dan J, Tran A, et al. Effect of external eyelid weighting on eyelid and eyebrow position in normal and ptosis patients. Presented at: American Society of Ophthalmic Plastic and Reconstructive Surgery (ASOPRS) 50th Annual Fall Scientific Symposium. San Francisco, CA; October 10-11,2019.

42. Dortzbach RK, Sutula FC. Involutional blepharoptosis. A histopathological study. Arch Ophthalmol 1980;98:2045–9.

43. Martin JJ, Tenzel RR. Acquired ptosis: dehiscences and disinsertions. Are they real or iatrogenic? Ophthalmic Plast Reconstr Surg 1992;8:129–33.

44. Wilkes TDE, Adams DF. Involutional (senile) ptosis. Geriatr Ophthalmol 1986;2:14–22.

45. Carroll RP. Cautery dissection in levator surgery. Ophthalmic Plast Reconstr Surg 1988;4:243–7.

46. Pereira LS, Hwang TN, Kersten RC, et al. Levator superioris muscle function in involutional blepharoptosis. Am J Ophthalmol 2008;145:1095–8.

47. Allen RC, Saylor MA, Nerad JA. The current state of ptosis repair: a comparison of internal and external approaches. Curr Opin Ophthalmol 2011;22(5): 394–9.

48. Putterman AM, Urist MJ. Muller muscle-conjunctiva resection - technique for treatment of blepharoptosis. Arch Ophthalmol 1975;93(8):619–23.

49. Buckman G, Jakobiec FA, Hyde K, et al. Success of the Fasanella-Servat operation independent of muller's smooth-muscle excision. Ophthalmology 1989;96(4):413–8.

50. Morris WR, Fleming JC. A histological analysis of the mullerectomy: redefining its mechanism in ptosis repair. Plast Reconstr Surg 2011;127:2333–41.

51. Zauberman NA, Koval T, Kinori M, et al. Müller's muscle-conjunctival resection for upper eyelid ptosis: correlation between amount of resected tissue and outcome. Br J Ophthalmol 2013;97:408–11.

52. Marcet MM, Setabutr P, Lemke BN, et al. Surgical microanatomy of the Muller muscle-conjunctival resection ptosis procedure. Ophthalmic Plast Reconstr Surg 2010;26:360–4.

53. Moore GH, Rootman DB, Karlin J, et al. Mueller's muscle conjunctival resection with skin-only blepharoplasty: effects on eyelid and eyebrow position. Ophthalmic Plast Reconstr Surg 2015; 31(4):290–2.

54. Rootman DB, Sinha KR, Goldberg RA. Change in eyelid position following Muller's muscle conjunctival resection with a standard versus variable resection length. Ophthalmic Plast Reconstr Surg 2018; 34(4):355–60.

55. Rootman DB, Karlin J, Moore G, et al. The role of tissue resection length in the determination of postoperative eyelid position for Muller's muscle-conjunctival resection surgery. Orbit 2015;34(2):92–8.

56. Ben Simon GJ, Lee S, Schwarcz RM, et al. External levator advancement vs Müller's muscle-conjunctival resection for correction of upper eyelid involutional ptosis. Am J Ophthalmol 2005;140:426–32.

57. Danesh J, Ugradar S, Goldberg RA, et al. Significance of early postoperative eyelid position on late postoperative result in Mueller's muscle conjunctival resection and external levator advancement surgery. Ophthalmic Plast Reconstr Surg 2018;34(5): 432–5.

58. Cohen LM, Katsev B, Esfandiari M, et al. The effect of early postoperative swelling on change in upper eyelid position after external levator resection and blepharoplasty. Ophthalmic Plast Reconstr Surg 2020;1–4. https://doi.org/10.1097/IOP.00000000000 01740.

59. Everbusch O. Zur operation der kongenitalen blepharoptosis. Klin Monatsbl Augenheilkd 1883;21: 100–7.

60. Lucarelli MJ, Lemke BN. Small incision external levator repair: technique and early results. Am J Ophthalmol 1999;127:637–44.

61. Frueh BR, Musch DC, McDonald HM. Efficacy and efficiency of a small incision, minimal dissection procedure versus a traditional approach for correcting aponeurotic ptosis. Ophthalmology 2004;111: 2158–63.

62. Ahuero AE, Winn BJ, Sires BS. Standardized suture placement for mini-invasive ptosis surgery. Arch Facial Plast Surg 2012;14(6):408–12.

63. Takahashi Y, Kakizaki H, Mito H, et al. Assessment of the predictive value of intraoperative eyelid height measurements in the sitting and supine positions during blepharoptosis repair. Ophthalmic Plast Reconstr Surg 2007;23:119–21.

64. Collin JR, O'Donnell BA. Adjustable sutures in eyelid surgery for ptosis and lid retraction. Br J Ophthalmol 1994;78:167–74.

65. Berris CE. Adjustable sutures for the correction of adult-acquired ptosis. Ophthalmic Plast Reconstr Surg 1988;4:171–3.

66. Meltzer MA, Elahi E, Taupeka P, et al. A simplified technique of ptosis repair using a single adjustable suture. Ophthalmology 2001;108:1889–92.

67. Nerad JA. Evaluation and treatment of the patient with ptosis. In: Techniques in ophthalmic plastic surgery: a personal tutorial. Philadelphia: Elsevier Inc.; 2010. p. 220.

68. Martin JJ Jr. Upper eyelid blepharoplasty with ptosis repair by levator aponeurectomy. JAMA Facial Plast Surg 2015;17(3):224–5.

69. Repp DJ, Rubinstein TJ, Sires BS. Role of algorithm-based levator aponeurectomy in small-incision external ptosis surgery for involutional ptosis. JAMA Facial Plast Surg 2017;19(6):490–5.

70. Radke PM, Rubinstein TJ, Repp DJ, et al. External levator resection for involutional ptosis: is intraoperative suture adjustment necessary for good outcomes? Orbit 2020;40(1):24–9.

71. Aakalu VK, Setabutr P. Current ptosis management: a national survey of ASOPRS members. Ophthalmic Plast Reconstr Surg 2011;27(4):270–6.

72. Scoppettuolo E, Chadha V, Bunce C, et al. British Oculoplastic Surgery Society (BOPSS) national ptosis survey. Br J Ophthalmol 2008;92(8):1134–8.

73. Young SM, Lim LH, Seah LL, et al. Prospective audit of ptosis surgery at the Singapore National Eye Centre: two-year results. Ophthalmic Plast Reconstr Surg 2013;29(6):446–53.

74. Ayala E, Galvez C, Gonzalez-Candial M, et al. Predictability of conjunctival-Muellerectomy for blepharoptosis repair. Orbit 2007;26(4):217–21.

75. Dresner SC. Fruther modifications of the Muller muscle conjunctival resection procedure for blepharoptosis. Ophthalmic Plast Reconstr Surg 1991;7(2):114–22.

76. Guyuron B, Davies B. Experience with the modified Putterman procedure. Plast Reconstr Surg 1988;82:775–80.

77. Mercandetti M, Putterman AM, Cohen ME, et al. Internal levator advancement by Muller's muscle–conjunctival resection. Arch Facial Plast Surg 2001;3:104–10.

78. Perry JD, Kadakia A, Foster JA. A new algorithm for ptosis repair using conjunctival Müllerectomy with or without tarsectomy. Ophthalmic Plast Reconstr Surg 2002;18:426–9.

79. Weinstein GS, Buerger GF. Modifications of the Muller's muscle-conjunctival resection operation for blepharoptosis. Am J Ophthalmol 1982;93(5):647–51.

80. Baldwin HC, Bhagey J, Khooshabeh R. Open sky Muller muscle-conjunctival resection in phenylephrine test-negative blepharoptosis patients. Ophthalmic Plast Reconstr Surg 2005;21:276–80.

81. Ediriwickrema LS, Geng J, Nair AA, et al. Single suture Müeller muscle conjunctival resection (ssMMCR): A modified technique for ptosis repair. Ophthalmic Plast Reconstr Surg 2019;35(4):403–6.

82. Gildener-Leapman JR, Sheps I, Stein R, et al. The sutureless mullerectomy. Ophthalmic Plast Reconstr Surg 2019;35(3):290–3.

83. Foster JA, Holck DE, Perry JD, et al. Fibrin sealant for Muller muscle-conjunctiva resection ptosis repair. Ophthalmic Plast Reconstr Surg 2006;22(3):184–7.

84. Ben Simon GJ, Lee S, Schwarcz RM, et al. Muller's muscle-conjunctival resection for correction of upper eyelid ptosis: relationship between phenylephrine testing and the amount of tissue resected with final eyelid position. Arch Facial Plast Surg 2007;9(6):413–7.

85. Carruth BP, Meyer DR. Simplified Muller's muscle-conjunctival resection internal ptosis repair. Ophthalmic Plast Reconstr Surg 2013;29(1):11–4.

86. Saonanon P, Sithanon S. External levator advancement versus Müller muscle-conjunctival resection for aponeurotic blepharoptosis: a randomized clinical trial. Plast Reconstr Surg 2018;141(2):213e–9e.

87. Cruz AA, Akaishi PM, Mendonça AK, et al. Supramaximal levator resection for unilateral congenital ptosis: cosmetic and functional results. Ophthalmic Plast Reconstr Surg 2014;30(5):366–71.

88. Mete A, Cagatay HH, Pamukcu C, et al. Maximal levator muscle resection for primary congenital blepharoptosis with poor levator function. Semin Ophthalmol 2017;32(3):270–5.

89. Patel RM, Aakalu VK, Setabutr P, et al. Efficacy of Muller's muscle and conjunctiva resection with or without tarsectomy for the treatment of severe involutional blepharoptosis. Ophthalmic Plast Reconstr Surg 2017;33(4):273–8.

90. Mazow ML, Shulkin ZA. Mueller's muscle-conjunctival resection in the treatment of congenital ptosis. Ophthalmic Plast Reconstr Surg 2011;27(5):311–2.

91. Teo L, Lagler CP, Mannor G, et al. Mullers muscle conjunctival resection for treatment of contact lens-associated ptosis. Ophthalmic Plast Reconstr Surg 2016;32(4):257–60.

92. Putthirangsiwong B, Yang M, Rootman DB. Surgical outcomes following Muller muscle-conjunctival resection in patients with glaucoma filtering surgery. Orbit 2019;39(5):331–5.

93. Glatt HJ, Putterman AM, Fett DR. Muller's muscle-conjunctival resection procedure in the treatment of ptosis in Horner's syndrome. Ophthalmic Surg 1990;21(2):93–6.

Transcutaneous Blepharoplasty with Volume Preservation
Indications, Advantages, Technique, Contraindications, and Alternatives

Andrew A. Jacono, MD[a,b,*]

KEYWORDS

- Blepharoplasty • Lower eyelid • Volume preservation • Aging lower eyelid anatomy

KEY POINTS

- Lower blepharoplasty requires precise diagnosis and appropriately directed surgical approach.
- Optimal rejuvenative results are achieved with transcutaneous lower blepharoplasty when orbicularis muscle is preserved and appropriate suspensory maneuvers are performed in conjunction with fat transposition or autologous fat grafting.
- Contraindications to the transcutaneous technique include a negative vector orbit, orbicularis muscle weakness and excess lower eyelid laxity, in which case a transconjunctival approach is preferred.

INTRODUCTION

Even though a patient presenting for eyelid rejuvenation may be displeased with the changes in the periorbital tissues creating a tired or baggy eyelid look, they are unwilling to trade improvement in this look for a change in the natural contour of their eyes. Patients and surgeons fear any distortion of the natural shape and aperture of the eye. This is especially true for patients, as they see too many postoperative friends, family members, or people on the street who look like they have had plastic surgery on their eyelids. Results often show "round" small eyes, distortion of the lateral canthus with a "cat eye" appearance, or ectropion. It is anxiety provoking for the surgeon, as these undesired changes seem to be difficult to control, with the same technique giving a very different outcome in different patients.

I have performed more than 3000 blepharoplasties and I have learned the hard way. There are techniques that I was taught that I now avoid. I have added techniques described more recently and have advanced the field of peri-orbital rejuvenation with modified techniques. Although these changes in technique are important to creating better outcomes and happier patients, I believe that there are 2 other considerations crucial to better blepharoplasty outcomes. First, it is of the utmost importance to choose the right surgical approach based on the patient's anatomy. An example of not matching the technique to the anatomy is performing a lower eyelid orbital fat reduction in a patient with a proptotic negative vector eye that creates deep set hollowed eyes that are not rejuvenated but actually more tired in appearance. The second is respecting the patient's eyelid appearance as it existed in youth.

[a] Department of Otolaryngology–Head & Neck Surgery, Division of Facial Plastic Surgery, Albert Einstein College of Medicine, New York, NY, USA; [b] Department of Facial Plastic and Reconstructive Surgery, Northwell Health (North Shore LIJ), Manhasset, NY, USA
* New York Center for Facial Plastic Surgery, 630 Park Avenue, New York, NY 10065.
E-mail address: drjacono@gmail.com

Facial Plast Surg Clin N Am 29 (2021) 209–228
https://doi.org/10.1016/j.fsc.2021.01.008

Because there are so many variables, and today so many techniques, it is important to have a clear understanding of the patient's anatomy now and in youth, what their desires are, and what pitfalls might exist with a chosen approach. Of all the procedures we perform as aging face surgeons, there is more art and judgment required when treating the eyelids than any other area in the face.

AGING LOWER EYELID ANATOMY

The lower eyelid is formed by 3 lamellae: the anterior, middle, and posterior lamellae. The anterior lamella is the skin and orbicularis oculi muscle, the middle lamella is the tarsal plate and orbital septum, and the posterior lamella is the conjunctiva and the lower lid retractors. The orbicularis oculi muscle is composed of 2 parts: the outer orbital and inner palpebral portion. The palpebral portion contains a pretarsal component and a preseptal component. The upper and lower pretarsal components of the orbicularis oculi muscle join medially and insert onto the lacrimal crest as the medial canthal tendon. The 2 lateral components of the pretarsal orbicularis join together to form the lateral canthal tendon, which inserts onto the Whitnall tubercle. Immediately deep to the preseptal orbicularis oculi muscle is the orbital septum, a continuation of the orbital periosteum. The lower eyelid retractors fuse with the orbital septum approximately 5 mm inferior to the inferior-most aspect of the tarsal plate.

Orbital fat is contained within the orbital septum. The lower eyelid has 3 fat pads: medial, central, and lateral. The inferior oblique muscle divides the medial and central fat compartments and is an important anatomic marker to identify and preserve. The medial fat pad is distinct in that it contains denser whiter-colored fat. Both genetics and aging play a role in the size of these fat pads, and these fat pads do not fluctuate in size with changes in body habitus.

Age-related changes in the periorbital area are multifactorial and are best understood by the contributing parts. The aged periorbital appearance is the result of cumulative changes in skin texture, volume depletion, loss of elasticity, formation of rhytids, drooping of the skin, and ptosis. This milieu of changes result in the characteristic findings of the aged lower eyelid, one that is marred by dermatochalasis, pseudoherniation of the orbital fat, malar festooning, and atonia of the lower eyelid that affects lid and canthal position.

Just like in upper eyelid aging, there are patients who accumulate more soft tissue and those who lose soft tissue. This is manifested as pseudoherniated fat compartments creating lower eyelid bag. Many patients develop devolumization of the lower eyelid with age and have no need for correction or reduction of the fat compartments. In fact, those with devolumization will need augmentation with autologous fat grafting to complete their eyelid rejuvenation.

The tear trough is an area of particular concern in the aging eyes. The tear trough is the concave area caudal to the inferior orbital fat. First described as the nasojugal fold by Duke-Elder and Wybar in 1961,[1] the modern day name "tear trough deformity" was coined in 1969 by Flowers[2] when it was observed that tears would track down this dependent area. The etiology of the tear trough deformity appears to be multifactorial.[3] Recent evidence suggests that the tear trough occurs as a result of skin tethering by an osteocutaneous ligament, situated between the origins of the palpebral and orbital parts of the orbicularis muscle. This ligament extends from the level of the insertion of the medial canthal tendon to the line of the medial pupil, where it continues laterally as the orbitomalar retaining ligament.[4] This tethering effect is exacerbated with aging due to increasing bulge of orbital fat from above, and atrophy with descent of the malar fat below[5–20] (Fig. 1). This ligament also tethers redundant orbicularis muscle that develops with age, creating malar festoons and mounding.

The midface is an important yet often overlooked contributing factor to periorbital aged appearance. Gravitational descent and volume depletion of the midface indirectly affects the periorbita and plays a significant role in the aged appearance of the lower lids. The midface descends with synchronous deflation of the suborbicularis oculi fat creating a deepening of the tear trough. The ptotic mid face creates another bulge inferior to the tear trough.

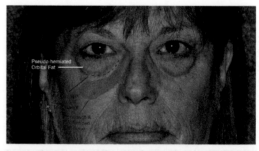

Fig. 1. The tear trough represents the area where the orbito-malar retaining ligaments tether the skin to the inferior orbital rim. As volume is lost in this region, and the pseudoherniated fat accumulates above the ligament and the midface hypertrophies and descends below it, the depth of the tear trough deepens in perspective.

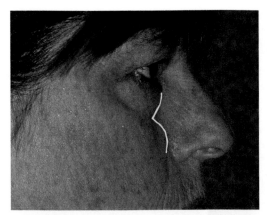

Fig. 2. A double convexity or "double bubble" is seen on profile view at the tear trough when orbital fat excess exists.

Pseudoherniation and apparent orbital fat excess accentuates the tear trough, volume loss and hollowing in the infraorbital and lateral orbital areas, and a midface bulge, creating a double convexity of profile view (**Fig. 2**).

Addressing the tear trough is important for successful rejuvenation of the lower periorbital area, which is why we recommend release of the orbitomalar retaining ligaments to allow for both redraping excess orbicularis muscle as well as volumizing the depth of the tear trough with transposed orbital fat. This ligament also tethers redundant orbicularis muscle that develops with age, creating malar festoons and mounding.

SURGICAL TECHNIQUES FOR REJUVENATION OF THE LOWER EYELID

There are 2 approaches to the lower eyelid I use, both involve volumizing the tear trough. I do not perform simple reductive blepharoplasty with fat pad removal anymore, as the patients will often need volume supplementation as early as 5 years after surgery, with continued volume loss with age, which magnifies the soft tissue deficit in the lower eyelid (**Fig. 3**). Even in younger patients who have less volume loss, I will transpose fat to give them more volume reserve for the future (**Fig. 4**).

One approach uses a transposition of excessive pseudoherniated lower eyelid orbital fat pads into the area of the tear trough, and the other approach adds supplemented autologous fat to the tear trough area in those patients who have a deflated orbit with modest fat pad volume. A deflated orbit also occurs in patients who had a reductive lower blepharoplasty performed prior. Many surgeons will combine removal of orbital fat pads with autologous fat injections to the tear trough. It is my preference to use the orbital fat because it is a vascularized fat flap and it always maintains its volume when transposed. Autologous fat is a free graft and has a failure rate of 20% to 25% with either incomplete or no graft take, so it is less predictable. With that being said, when there is no fat to transpose, autologous fat is the solution.

I use both a transcutaneous and transconjunctival approach to fat transposition and have specific indications for both. A transcutaneous approach to the fat in the lower eyelid in the wrong patient with contraindicated anatomy will increase the patient' risk for lower eyelid malposition and ectropion. It is our experience that even small changes in eyelid shape are extremely distressing to the patient and change their perception of their facial identity. In my practice, I have gone from performing transcutaneous blepharoplasty in 90% of my patients to 50% today to decrease the risk. It has become more of an issue in the past 5 to 7 years, with patients' use of selfie cameras on their cell phones that magnify even slight changes in eyelid shape. We are not talking about severe lateral canthal rounding or ectropion, but small changes. A recent study showed that selfie cameras increase nasal distortion by 30%.[1] When performing a transconjunctival approach I will still address skin excess with a skin pinch and tighten the orbicularis by tightening it with plication of the muscle to the orbital periosteum as described in the following.

PREOPERATIVE EVALUATION: INDICATIONS AND CONTRAINDICATIONS

Preoperative planning is lauded by some as the most important aspect of blepharoplasty, and is vital to achieving successful outcomes.[2,3] The eyes are a focal point of the face and serve as the natural transition between the upper and middle face.

Thorough preoperative evaluation will identify the best surgical candidates for blepharoplasty, as well as steer the surgeon and patient away from unwanted potential postoperative pitfalls. This evaluation is inclusive of patients' medical comorbidities, as well as their psychological well-being and emotional disposition. It is important to have a frank discussion with patients and record consultations with photographic documentation. This process is aimed toward setting realistic expectations, as well as pointing out any preexisting asymmetries for both patients and physicians to acknowledge. Smoking is discontinued for at least 2 weeks before surgery. All anticoagulants or

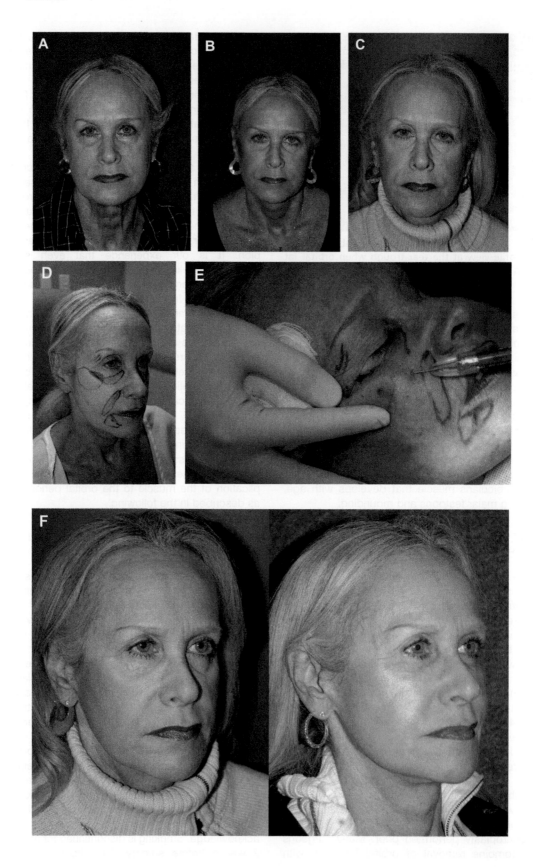

herbal medications that interfere with blood clotting are discontinued 2 weeks before surgery. Thyroid disorders are investigated and noted, as hypothyroid and hyperthyroid states cause disparate influences on the periorbital area that cannot be addressed with routine blepharoplasty. Any history of dry eye is investigated with comprehensive ophthalmologic assessment, including the Schirmer test, visual acuity, extraocular movements, intraocular pressure, and cornea and ocular adnexa evaluation. Even with normal Schirmer testing, ophthalmologic and systemic evaluation is indicated to rule-out collagen vascular or other autoimmune disease and provide treatment and an assessment of safety preoperatively.

Physical examination warrants special observation of all dermatologic and structural changes in the periorbital area. Volume changes in the orbit are evaluated, specifically the amount of orbital fat available to transpose. Insufficient volume in the orbital fat requires the use of autologous fat as an adjunct (**Fig. 5**). Volume excess in the pseudoherniation of the orbital fat accentuates the relative volume deficiency in the nasojugal groove and infraorbital hollows immediately inferior to the orbital fat pseudoherniation. In cases in which the lower eyelids have less dermatochalasis and orbicularis muscle redundancy, the transconjunctival approach is a more appropriate choice, leaving the orbicularis muscle untouched. Mild skin redundancy can then be treated with a skin pinch procedure or resurfacing with a peel or laser.

Excessive lower eyelid laxity should be assessed, defined as a snap test >1 second and distraction test (being able to distract the lower eyelid from the globe) >10 mm. On close inspection of those patients with excessive skin laxity, preoperative scleral show is often seen (**Fig. 6**).

Indications for transcutaneous lower blepharoplasty include excess skin and orbicularis muscle that requires redraping for adequate lid recontouring and lower eyelid rejuvenation. This approach also allows for broad exposure, for wide release of the orbitomalar retaining ligaments, and orbital fat transposition.

Today I have 3 absolute contraindications for using the transcutaneous approach. In the past, excessive laxity of the eyelid was a relative contraindication to transcutaneous lower blepharoplasty, but in my practice today it is an absolute contraindication. The transcutaneous approach in cases with increased laxity can lead to postoperative eyelid malposition on a spectrum from lateral canthal rounding to frank ectropion even when additional adjunctive procedures were included to prevent problems. In these cases, I would include a concomitant canthopexy, or horizontal lower eyelid tightening procedure (such as a lateral tarsal strip procedure), depending on the degree of laxity, and I would still wind up with malposition in 10% to 20% of cases. In cases of more extreme laxity with a lower eyelid tightening procedure, the eyes would appear smaller, distressing the patient. This problem was not reversible (**Fig. 7**). To avoid all this, I now use a transconjunctival approach and treat the skin and muscle less aggressively in cases with more significant eyelid laxity.

The other 2 absolute contraindications for transcutaneous blepharoplasty include patients with a negative vector and preoperative orbicularis weakness. A negative vector eyelid is noted when the patient's profile is examined (sagittal view) the cornea projects more anteriorly than the midface (**Fig. 8**). In these cases, I use a transconjunctival approach. These 2 preoperative physical findings have been noted in a study by Griffin and colleagues[4] on postblepharoplasty lower eyelid retraction patients to be present in 65% and 85%, respectively. When tightening the eyelid skin and orbicularis muscle, the tendency is for the redraped tissue to fall under the globe in a negative vector eyelid, similar to the way pants fall underneath a "beer gut." Patients with preoperative orbicularis weakness are also predisposed to lower eyelid retraction, and skin muscle flap surgery further weakens the muscle with denervation, loss of strength, and lower eyelid margin eversion. Orbicularis strength is assessed by trying to pry the patient's eyelids open during forceful closure by the patient. In a normal situation, the examiner cannot open the patient's eyelids. With more degenerative changes and age, the eyes are easily pried apart. In both of these situations, we elect to approach the orbitomalar ligament and orbital fat transconjunctivally and address the skin externally by pinch technique and suspending the orbicularis muscle redundancy with suture fixation to the orbital rim and/or plicating the lateral orbicularis muscle.

Fig. 3. Patient after reductive transcutaneous lower blepharoplasty. (*A*) Before. (*B*) 1 year postsurgery demonstrating removal of fat pockets but untreated tear trough, and (*C*) 7 years after blepharoplasty showing accentuation of tear trough with further soft tissue loss with aging requiring augmentation with autologous fat grafting. (*D*) Preoperative marking for areas of tear trough augmentation. (*E*) Autologous fat grafting with micro-canula injections. (*F*) Pre-autologous and post-autologous fat grafting at 1 year. The need for the autologous fat grafting could have been avoided by using an orbital fat repositioning at the time of the initial blepharoplasty.

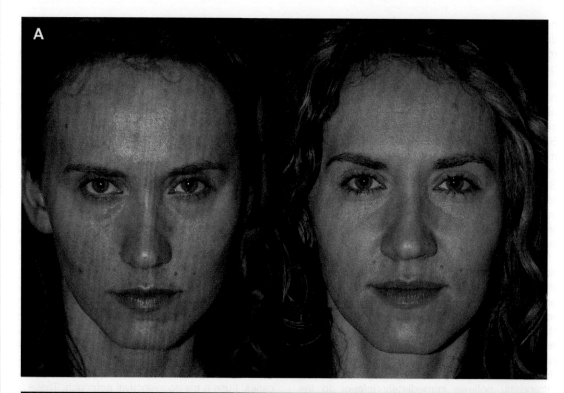

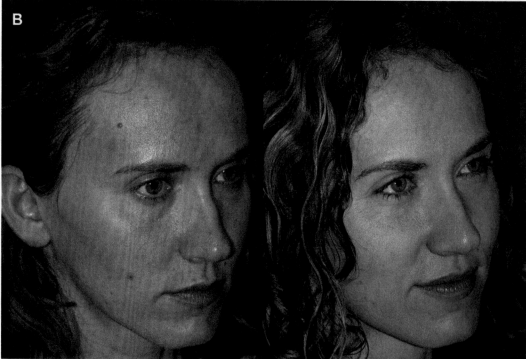

Fig. 4. Preoperative and postoperative (*A*) frontal and (*B*) three-quarter views of a 41-year-old patient with excess orbital fat pockets creating eyelid bags. Instead of removing the fat, a transconjunctival repositioning of orbital fat was performed to minimize the tear trough but more importantly to prevent the need for volume augmentation over the next 5 to 10 years.

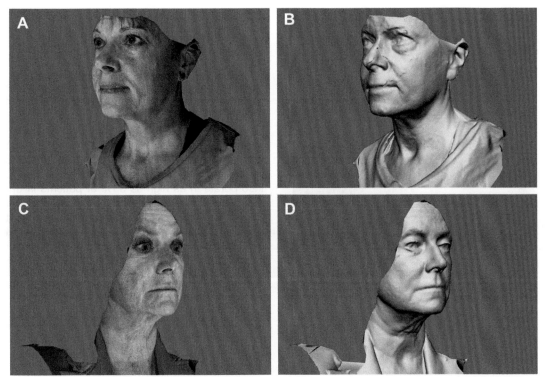

Fig. 5. (*A, B*) Preoperative evaluation of 59-year-old woman with 3-dimensional camera and surface contour image showing excess orbital fat available for fat transposition. (*C, D*) Preoperative evaluation of 62-year-old woman with 3-D camera and surface contour image showing insufficient orbital fat available for fat transposition. This case will require autologous fat supplementation.

TRANSCUTANEOUS BLEPHAROPLASTY SURGICAL PROCEDURE

Our transcutaneous lower blepharoplasty technique is an extended transcutaneous submuscular blepharoplasty with orbital-malar ligament release

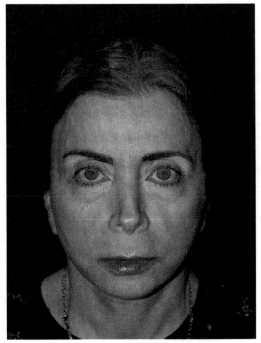

Fig. 6. Preoperative evaluation should look for patients with scleral show so it can be treated during the surgery.

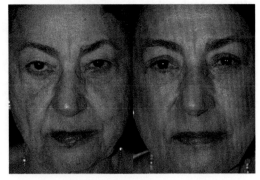

Fig. 7. Preoperative and postoperative view of a 72-year-old patient who underwent a transcutaneous lower blepharoplasty with fat transposition but required a lateral tarsal strip procedure due to excessive horizontal lower eyelid laxity and scleral show. The eyes appear smaller afterward due to the horizontal eyelid shortening.

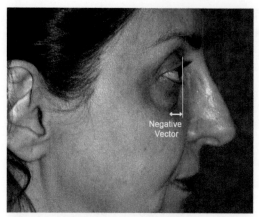

Fig. 8. A negative vector eyelid is noted when the patient's profile is examined (sagittal view). The cornea projects more anteriorly than the midface, and is associated with postoperative lower eyelid retraction.

and orbital fat repositioning (**Fig. 9**). Depending on the patient's preoperative degree of infraorbital volume loss, this approach is used including the infraorbital ligament release with fat removal, partial removal and transposition, or complete transposition. Using this method of periorbital volume replenishment is predicated on the presence of sufficient orbital fat volume for transposition. I prefer orbital fat transposition when orbital fat is available because it is a vascularized pedicled fat flap that has an essentially 100% take, whereas injected autologous fat is a free graft and fails to incorporate in as high as 35% of patients in our experience. To minimize the risk of lower eyelid malposition, our approach preserving a robust orbicularis oculi sling, and incorporates periosteal fixation of the lateral canthus and skin muscle flap. What follows is my description of the techniques in 6 steps.

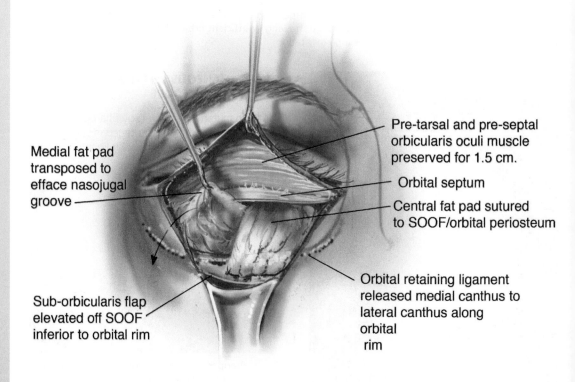

Medial fat pad transposed to efface nasojugal groove

Pre-tarsal and pre-septal orbicularis oculi muscle preserved for 1.5 cm.

Orbital septum

Central fat pad sutured to SOOF/orbital periosteum

Sub-orbicularis flap elevated off SOOF inferior to orbital rim

Orbital retaining ligament released medial canthus to lateral canthus along orbital rim

Fig. 9. The essential elements of the transcutaneous lower blepharoplasty technique is an extended submuscular dissection with orbital-malar ligament release and orbital fat repositioning.

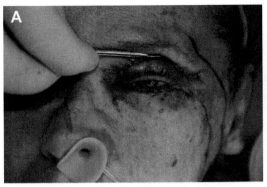 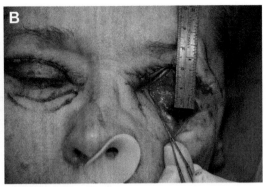

Fig. 10. (*A*) After the sub-ciliary incision is made, (*B*) a skin flap is elevated inferiorly with a sharp iris scissors for approximately 1.5 cm, preserving an intact sling of functional orbicularis muscle.

STEP 1. SKIN FLAP ELEVATION AND PRESERVATION OF ORBICULARIS MUSCLE

The patient is marked in the upright position, making note of the pseudoherniated orbital fat and the hollowed tear trough. The lower lid is injected with 1% lidocaine with epinephrine 1:100,000. The skin incision is incised with a #15 blade 1 mm below the lash line from 2 mm lateral to the punctum past the lateral canthus for approximately 10 mm in a crow's foot rhytid.

A retraction suture is placed through the midline lower eyelid and retracted superiorly. A skin flap is elevated inferiorly with a sharp iris scissors for approximately 1.5 cm preserving an intact sling of functional orbicularis muscle. In traditional skin muscle flap blepharoplasty only 2 to 3 mm of pretarsal orbicularis is preserved. We believe that maintaining this wider functional sling of orbicularis oculi and minimizing trauma to it muscle minimizes risk of lower lid retraction (**Fig. 10**).

STEP 2. SUBMUSCULAR DISSECTION AND RELEASE OF ORBITAL RETAINING LIGAMENTS

The orbicularis muscle is pierced just below the elevated skin flap at the level just superior to the orbital rim. The muscle is incised for the width of the orbit from medial to lateral. From this point inferiorly a composite skin muscle flap is elevated off the orbital septum to the orbital rim. At the orbital rim, the orbital retaining ligaments are released, using monopolar cautery in a plane just superficial to the sub-orbicularis oculi fat (SOOF),[2,3] with dissection extending further than the inferior-most aspect of the marked tear trough. Care is taken to preserve the infraorbital nerve. This space created inferior to the orbital rim is the recipient site for transposed orbital fat. Releasing the tear trough ligaments allows for repositioning of redundant orbicularis inferior to their insertion point and allows for better skin redraping than is accomplished in a transconjunctival approach (**Fig. 11**).

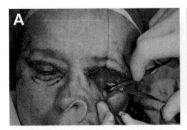 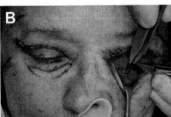 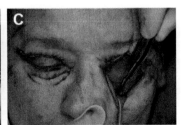

Fig. 11. (*A*) The orbicularis muscle is pierced just below the elevated skin flap at the level just superior to the orbital rim. The muscle is incised for the length of the orbit from medial to lateral. (*B, C*) At the orbital rim, the orbital retaining ligaments are released using bipolar cautery in a plane just superficial to the SOOF, leaving the periosteum down.

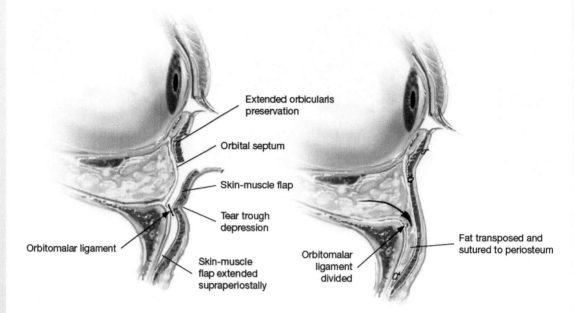

Fig. 12. Cross-sectional illustration showing the release or the orbitomalar ligament and transposition of the orbital fat into the tear trough depression.

STEP 3. VOLUMIZATION WITH FAT TRANSPOSITION

The skin muscle flap is retracted inferiorly with a Desmarre retractor, and gentle manual retropulsion of the globe helps to identify the orbital fat compartments. The medial, central, and lateral fat compartments are identified by blunt dissecting with a cotton tip applicator, identifying the inferior oblique muscle between the medial and central compartments. The orbital septum of the central and medial fat compartments is opened with a sharp scissors at its inferior-most point, teasing out the herniated fat pads. These fat pads are rotated inferiorly over the orbital rim into the tear trough and sutured to the supraperiosteal plane with interrupted 5 to 0 chromic

sutures (**Fig. 12**). More sutures are placed to sculpt the transposed fat to smoothly efface the tear trough and to blend the lower eyelid into the upper midface. This camouflages the boney inferior orbital rim that is a hallmark of aging.[4] The transposed fat also fills the medial tear trough defect[5] and smooths the lower eyelid-cheek contour[2,11] It is critical to make sure the fat flap fans out and is not lumpy or bumpy, as these irregularities will show through the rewrapped skin muscle flap. We usually melt away any irregularities by contouring with a bipolar cautery forceps(**Fig. 13**).

Excessive fat of the lateral fat pad is resected rather than transposed. In the authors experience the lateral fat pad is more fibrous and creates contour irregularities when transposed, so it is conservatively excised to the level of the superficial

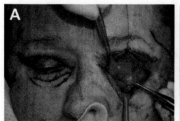
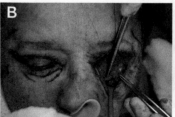
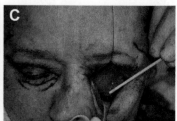

Fig. 13. (*A*) The medial and central orbital fat pads are dissected, and the inferior oblique muscle is identified. (*B*, *C*) They are rotated inferiorly over the orbital rim into the tear trough, and sutured to the supraperiosteal plane with interrupted 5 to 0 chromic sutures.

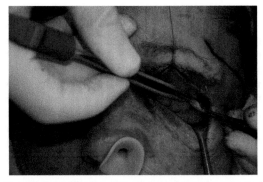

Fig. 14. Excessive fat of the lateral fat pad is resected rather than transposed, because the lateral fat pad is more fibrous and creates contour irregularities when transposed.

aspect of the orbital rim. Special care is taken in patients with prominent globes or hypoplastic malar eminences since they are at risk of having a deep sulcus postoperatively (**Fig. 14**). In these cases we will use the resected lateral fat pad and suture it to the orbital rim as an autograft or fill the lateral orbit with injected autologous fat.

STEP 4. SUPPORT OF LATERAL RETINACULUM WITH TARSAL FIXATION

Small sharp scissors are used to dissect down to the periosteum of the lateral orbital rim and then superiorly under the lateral aspect of the incision superior to the attachment of the lateral canthal tendon. Here, two 6 to 0 nylon sutures are passed through the periosteum of the internal superior aspect of the lateral orbital rim. A closed canthopexy is performed by passing one of these sutures through the lateral tarsal plate.[12] Overtightening of this suture is avoided to prevent lateral canthal distortion and buckling. Over tightening can also pull the lid margin below the globe creating scleral show (**Figs. 15** and **16**).

STEP 5. SUPERIOR MIDFACE ELEVATION WITH ORBICULARIS FLAP REDRAPING AND PERIOSTEAL FIXATION

The superior midface was released due to the dissection of the orbital retaining ligaments freeing the orbicularis oculi muscle. The second 6 to 0 nylon suture placed in the lateral orbital periosteum is sutured to the superior cuff of the skin muscle edge of the lower eyelid flap, elevating the superior midface (**Fig. 17**).

STEP 6. CONSERVATIVE SUPEROLATERAL SKIN RESECTION

The skin is redraped supero-laterally into the part of the skin incision lateral to the lateral canthus. Skin excess laterally ranges from 6 to 10 mm. As the skin flap is left to naturally approximate the cut skin edge beneath the lash line medially, only 1 to 2 mm of skin usually needs to be removed medially. Resecting most of the skin lateral to the canthus, and minimally subciliary further reduces the risk of lower eyelid margin retraction. The skin is closed with a 6 to 0 interrupted nylon suture lateral to the lateral canthus and with a 7 to 0 running locking silk suture medially (**Figs. 18** and **19**).

COMPLICATIONS AND MANAGEMENT

After experience with more than 2000 patients receiving transcutaneous blepharoplasty, we believe that this procedure can be performed safely and with an acceptable rate of complications. The key to performing the procedure safely is vigilant preoperative screening, incorporating intraoperative lateral canthal tightening procedures, and vigilant postoperative care and treatment. As stated previously in the indications/contraindications section, it is important to identify patients at high risk and use an alternative approach, that is, patients with a negative vector

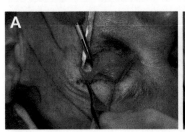
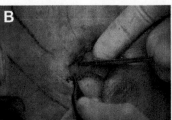
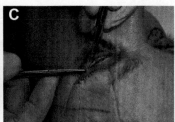

Fig. 15. (*A*) Small sharp scissors are used to dissect down to the periosteum of the lateral orbital rim and then superiorly under the lateral aspect of the incision superior to the attachment of the lateral canthal tendon. (*B*) A 6 to 0 nylon suture is passed through the periosteum of the internal superior aspect of the lateral orbital rim. (*C*) A closed canthopexy is performed by passing one of these sutures through the lateral tarsal plate.

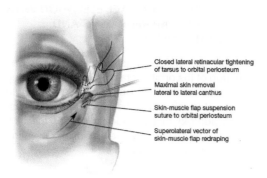

Closed lateral retinacular tightening of tarsus to orbital periosteum

Maximal skin removal lateral to lateral canthus

Skin-muscle flap suspension suture to orbital periosteum

Superolateral vector of skin-muscle flap redraping

Fig. 16. Illustration demonstrating the closed cantho-pexy suture creating lateral retinacular tightening of the tarsus to the orbital periosteum. The skin muscle flap suspension to the orbital periosteum in a superior-lateral vector is demonstrated as well.

complex and orbicularis weakness, where we will use a transconjunctival approach.

Ectropion from overaggressive skin excision may occur even in the absence of preoperative lower lid laxity,[21] and is another complication to be avoided. As noted previously, we remove a small margin of skin in the subciliary margin in the mid-pupillary line, and almost all skin gets removed lateral to the lateral canthus using a superolateral flap redraping vector.

Vigilant postoperative monitoring and early intervention prevents lower eyelid retraction. We see that postblepharoplasty lower eyelid retraction is the result of contraction and scar that develops within the orbicularis muscle and orbital septum postoperatively. We believe that the number 1 nidus for this process is excessive bruising and blood underneath the skin muscle flap after surgery. Because of this, we always see patients the day after surgery, and if excessive swelling and

bruising are noted, will evacuate a small amount of blood underneath the flap using a 14-gauge intravenous catheter and snaking it through the incision. We believe that even 1 mL of blood left behind can cause this problem, as the blood organizes and scar contracture ensues. In addition, we see patients every week for the first month after surgery to monitor whether any contracture is beginning to occur. This is evaluated using a force duction test, pushing the eyelids up superiorly and noting if any resistance is felt (**Fig. 20**). The earliest time some resistance is felt is 2 weeks after surgery, and we note this in 5% of patients. At this time, there is no eyelid malposition noted and intervention can prevent any problems. With a positive forced duction test we begin 5-Fluorouracil 50 mg/mL injections, usually 0.1 to 0.2 mL to modulate wound healing and minimize scar. The technique used is to inject into any fibrosis felt with a 30-gauge needle. We also begin the patient massaging the eyelids, forcing them upward as in a forced duction test for a minute 4 to 5 times daily. Depending on the progress, we will repeat the injections every 2 weeks.

With the preceding preoperative, intraoperative, and postoperative screening and measures, we have had no cases of ectropion and retraction. We see approximately a 1% to 2% rate of lateral central rounding that persists that often is not noted by the patient. In cases in which this is distressing to the patient, we will perform a second closed lateral canthal tightening procedure, as noted previously.

TRANSCONJUNCTIVAL BLEPHAROPLASTY SURGICAL PROCEDURE

In cases with excessive lower eyelid laxity, a negative vector orbit, or those with orbicularis oculi

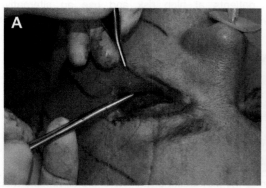
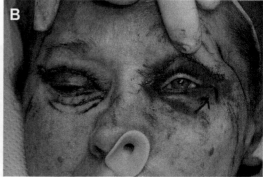

Fig. 17. (A) The second 6 to 0 nylon suture placed in the lateral orbital periosteum is sutured to the superior cuff of the skin muscle edge of the lower eyelid flap, elevating the superior midface. (B) The vector of the skin muscle flap repositioning is in a superolateral vector.

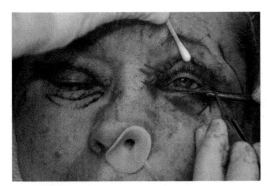

Fig. 18. Most of the skin excess is removed laterally, whereas medially only 1 to 2 mm of skin usually needs to be removed.

weakness, our preference is to perform a transconjunctival lower blepharoplasty with fat repositioning. Unlike in a skin muscle flap approach, which both dissects and partially denervates the orbicularis, this minimizes trauma to the muscle and decreases the risk of postoperative scarring and fibrosis that can lead to lower eyelid retraction. The skin is treated with this approach with a skin pinch and does not disturb the orbicularis muscle. In cases in which the orbicularis needs to be tightened, an "orbicularis hitch" procedure is performed, placing a plication suture on the surface of the muscle to the orbital periosteum without elevating a muscle flap.[5] As is described later in this article, it uses a single-suture suspension of preseptal muscle to lateral orbital rim.

I prefer a pre-septal approach to the orbital fat, but a retro-septal approach is perfectly acceptable. Preoperatively, the patient is marked in the upright position and the areas of fat excess are marked with small dots, and the depth of the infraorbital hollowing and nasojugal crease is marked with an oval (**Fig. 21**). Once the patient is prepped and draped, the eyelid is infiltrated transconjunctivally with 1% lidocaine with 1:100,000 epinephrine, and transcutaneous down to the nasojugal groove and premarked areas of infraorbital hollowing down to the periosteum. A Desmarres retractor is used to displace the eyelid inferiorly, and an incision is made with a Colorado tipped monopolar cautery on cutting approximately 5 mm below the tarsal border. Dissection proceeds in a plane between the orbicularis anteriorly and the septum posteriorly, continuing inferiorly to the arcus marginalis at the orbital rim. The

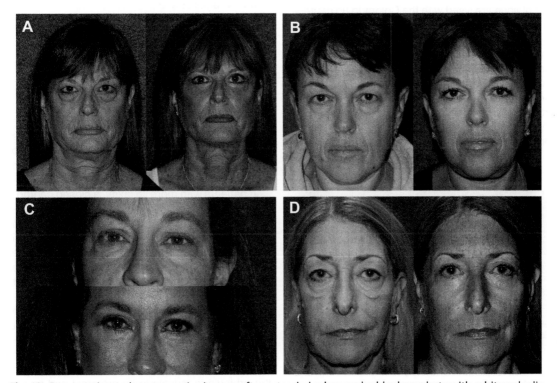

Fig. 19. Preoperative and postoperative images after extended submuscular blepharoplasty with orbitomalar ligament release and fat transposition: (*A*) a 63-year-old, (*B*) 56-year-old, (*C*) 59-year-old, and (*D*) 70-year-old. Notice the improvement in the orbicularis festooning in the 31D due to the extended submuscular flap redraping.

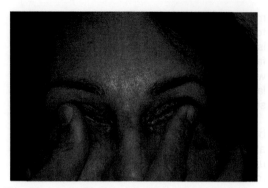

Fig. 20. Postoperative evaluation should include a force duction test, pushing the eyelids up superiorly and noting if any resistance is noted is a sign of early eyelid retraction that can be treated.

conjunctiva and retractors are then secured to the head drape with a traction (I use a 6–0 nylon suture), and a Desmarres retractor is used to displace the tarsus, muscle/skin inferiorly. The fat flaps are now created. They are contained behind the septum, and the orbital septum is entered with a small blunt scissors and the medial and central fat compartments are teased out with a Q-tip bluntly and the inferior oblique is identified between them. All connective tissue attachments of the fat pockets to the inferior orbital rim and inferior oblique are lysed with the Colorado tip cautery (**Fig. 22**). The fat flaps are grasped with a brown forceps and traction is applied inferiorly to ensure they have been released sufficiently. The temporal or lateral fat pad is dissected free next, and conservatively sculpted to reduce any degree of prominence; as stated previously, we have found attempting to transpose the more fibrous lateral fat pad often results in irregularities in the lateral orbit (**Fig. 23**).

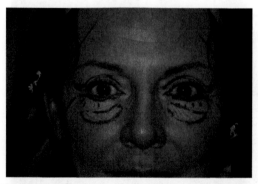

Fig. 21. Preoperatively, the patient is marked in the upright position and the areas of fat excess are marked as well as the depth of the infraorbital hollowing and nasojugal crease.

I prefer to transpose the fat sub-periosteally. A subperiosteal pocket is then created by entering at the orbital rim with the Colorado tipped monopolar cautery, and then elevating the periosteum with a Woodson elevator under direct visualization to prevent injury to the superior orbital, neurovascular bundle. The area is undermined inferiorly to the area of the preoperatively marked infraorbital hollows (**Fig. 24**). The medial and central fat compartments that have been released are then sutured to each other using a simple 5 to 0 chromic suture (**Fig. 25**). The confluent fat flap is then transposed and sutured with 2 sutures, 1 medially and 1 laterally to the undersurface of the elevated subperiosteal flap with a 5 to 0 chromic suture (**Fig. 26**). In the past, I used a transcutaneous bolster suture to fixate the fat, then remove the transcutaneous suture at postoperative day 7; I found that the fat would gravitate back superiorly and I would occasionally get recurrence of visible fat pockets. This does not happen with the internally fixated chromic suture described previously, because it will hold the fat flaps in place for 4 weeks and adequate scarification occurs to prevent the fat from translocating. The transposed fat is then inspected for smoothness and can be sculpted with a bipolar forceps to prevent any lumpiness. We close the conjunctival incision with one simple 5 to 0 chromic suture.

If the skin requires treatment, we perform a skin pinch procedure to minimize any trauma to the orbicularis muscle. We use a brown Adson forceps to pinch the skin immediately below the subciliary line and grasp the excess skin conservatively, and make sure the amount of skin grasped does not evert the lower lid margin. This proceeds from medial to lateral and is repeated until the skin stands up and can be excised. Excision is performed with small sharp iris scissors from lateral to medial at the base of the crushed skin (**Fig. 27**).

In patients with more lid laxity, a closed canthopexy is added, and if orbicularis muscle tightening is desired, an "orbicularis hitch" is performed. With the skin removed with the skin pinch, a buttonhole incision is made through the orbicularis in the lateral canthal region and the orbicularis is elevated superiorly from this point so the periosteum of the inner aspect of the superior orbital rim can be sutured. We use a 6 to 0 nylon suture to suture fixate the lateral aspect of the tarsus for the canthopexy as described previously. The orbicularis hitch is performed with a bite of the orbital periosteum but taking a bite of the orbicularis muscle in its pretarsal and upper preseptal portion. This requires elevation of a short skin flap laterally for approximately 6 or

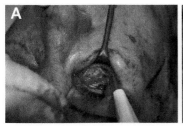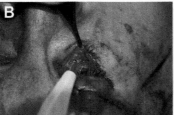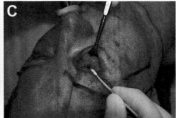

Fig. 22. (*A*) A Desmarres retractor is used to displace the eyelid inferiorly, and an incision is made with a Colorado tipped monopolar cautery on cutting approximately 5 mm below the tarsal border. (*B*) Dissection proceeds in a plane between the orbicularis anteriorly and the septum posteriorly. (*C*) The medial and central fat compartments are teased out with a Q-tip bluntly and the inferior oblique is identified between them.

7 mm to expose the orbicularis for the suture to be placed accurately. When the suture is tightened, extra skin will be elevated past the pinched excision so some additional often needs to be removed. This maneuver helps smooth orbicularis redundancy in a less aggressive way than elevating a skin muscle flap and reduces the risk of lower eyelid malposition as it supports the lower eyelid (**Figs. 28** and **29**).

COMPLICATIONS

Undercorrection or overcorrection of the transposed fat can create unsatisfactory outcomes, but with more experience, the surgeon will get better with contouring and have few if any problems. Undercorrection is treated with adjunctive filler or autologous fat grafting. Contouring the transposed fat with bipolar cautery will prevent overcorrection.

The most difficult problem to treat is symblepharon, where there is a partial or complete adhesion of the palpebral conjunctiva of the eyelid to the bulbar conjunctiva of the eyeball. This is prevented if the lower fornix is examined in the early postoperative period within the first 5 days. If

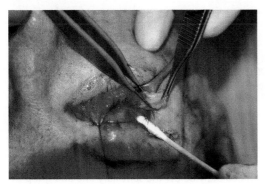

Fig. 23. The temporal or lateral fat pad is conservatively sculpted to reduce any degree of prominence.

adhesions are noted they can be easily broken up with a Q-tip. If detected within the first 2 weeks, these adhesions can be snipped after instilling tetracaine into the eye. I prescribe TobraDex drops and instruct the patients to look around the room 5 or 6 times a day to prevent the adhesions from reforming, If this opportunity is missed and the adhesions are thick, then a surgical procedure with release of these adhesions and placement of a hard palate mucosa graft may be required.

AUTOLOGOUS FAT GRAFTING TO THE LOWER EYELID

Many patients will age with loss of soft tissues of the lower eyelid and have deep nasojugal creases and infraorbital hollows but lack fat to transpose. Others have had a prior fat reductive blepharoplasty performed years ago, often a transconjunctival blepharoplasty, that now requires volume augmentation and treatment of skin redundancy that has developed. In these cases I combine autologous fat grafting with maneuvers to remove extra skin and tighten the orbicularis, as was described in the preceding section with transconjunctival blepharoplasty. I do not elevate a skin muscle flap in these cases because it would affect the ability of the injected fat to stay where it is placed. I inject fat deeply over the periosteum just under the orbicularis muscle, which is where skin muscle flaps are elevated.

There are a few important tenets to injecting fat in the lower eyelid complex. First, fat is injected supra-periosteally and deep to prevent palpation of nodules as the skin and muscle in the lower eyelids is often thin. I have seen many patients present with nodules and irregularities from fat grafting performed elsewhere because of superficial technique. Fat is not injected above the orbital rim, as fat becomes lumpy and visible because there is less soft tissue to camouflage it. Most importantly,

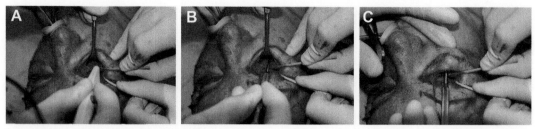

Fig. 24. (*A*) A subperiosteal pocket is created by entering at the orbital rim with the Colorado tipped monopolar cautery. (*B*) The periosteum is elevated with a Woodson elevator under direct visualization to prevent injury to the superior orbital neurovascular bundle. (*C*) The area is undermined inferiorly to the area of the preoperatively marked infraorbital hollows.

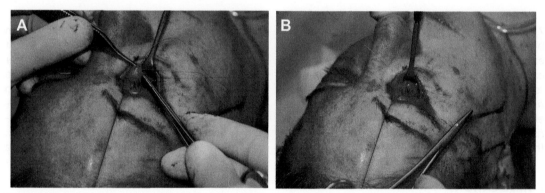

Fig. 25. (*A,B*) The medial and central fat compartments that have been released are sutured to each other using a simple 5 to 0 chromic suture.

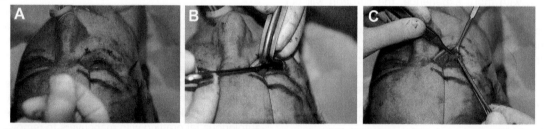

Fig. 26. (*A,B*) The confluent fat flap is then transposed and sutured with 2 sutures, 1 medially and 1 laterally to the undersurface of the elevated subperiosteal flap with a 5 to 0 chromic suture.

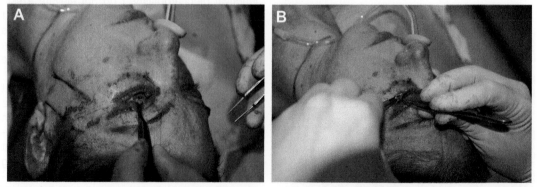

Fig. 27. (*A*) Brown Adson forceps is used to pinch the skin immediately below the subciliary line and grasp the excess skin conservatively, making sure the amount of skin grasped does not evert the lower lid margin. (*B*) Excision is performed with small sharp iris scissors from lateral to medial at the base of the crushed skin.

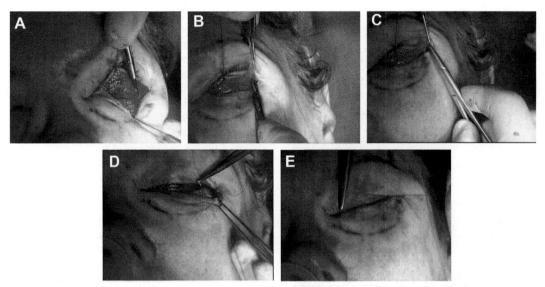

Fig. 28. Orbicularis hitch. (*A*) A short skin flap laterally for about 6 or 7 mm to expose the orbicularis for the suture to be placed accurately. (*B*) A button hole incision is made through the orbicularis in the lateral canthal region and the orbicularis is elevated superiorly from this point. (*C*) A 6 to 0 nylon suture I placed in the periosteum of the inner aspect of the superior orbital rim. (*D*) A bite of the orbicularis muscle in its pretarsal and upper preseptal portion is taken. (*E*) When the suture is tightened, extra skin will be elevated past the pinched excision, so some additional often needs to be removed.

I never overcorrect with fat grafting, assuming some will resorb, because in some cases it does not. I also will not correct more than 3 mL in each orbit. High-volume fat grafting has a tendency to form oil cysts and necrose because there is not enough intervening viable tissue to support the graft when larger volumes are used. This results in irregularities and depressions where the fat did not take (**Fig. 30**).

Unfortunately in the best of hands fat transfer take can be unpredictable, because it is a free graft that is, not vascularized and will need to have incorporation and ingrowth. In a recent review of 52 patients undergoing periorbital fat grafting in my practice, 14 patients, or 26%, had unsatisfactory outcomes because of undercorrection due to incomplete graft take. These cases require a secondary fat graft. Because of this high percentage, I discuss with all my patients

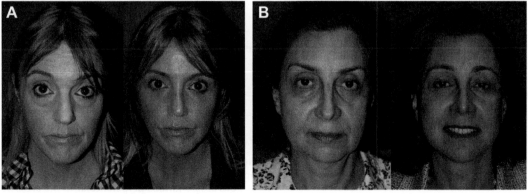

Fig. 29. (*A*, *B*) Preoperative and Postoperative images after transconjunctival fat repositioning with canthopexy and orbicularis hitch to support lower eyelid. Both patients have a negative vector and preoperative lateral canthal rounding.

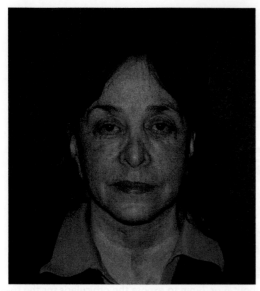

Fig. 30. Patient after fat grafting performed elsewhere with nodules and irregularities due to superficial injections and injecting superiorly above the orbital rim.

getting fat grafting preoperatively that a second local fat graft procedure may be required. This is why I prefer a predictable fat transposition.

I use the Tulip system (Tulip Medical, San Diego, CA) for fat transfer. I mark the patients preoperatively upright. I mark the central areas of hollowing to be corrected separately from the lateral orbital hollow. I do this because the fibrous attachments along the lateral orbital hollow are thicker and it makes it harder to inject fat. I want to keep myself mindful of injecting slower and with smaller amounts because this in this area even the slightest overcorrection is extremely visible (**Fig. 31**).

I always inject the fat before removing any skin, as the additional volume added reduces the amount of skin removal required. I inject the fat with the patient upright so that gravity is acting on the soft tissues. It is important to inject fat perpendicular to the areas being filled. Injecting parallel will create sausagelike or wormy fat pockets. I use an 18-gauge needle to pierce the skin in the cheek below the eyelid and inject small parcels of fat perpendicularly in 0.1 mL aliquots,

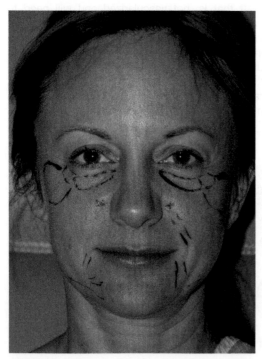

Fig. 31. The patient is marked preoperatively upright with the central areas of hollowing to be corrected marked separately from lateral orbital hollowing.

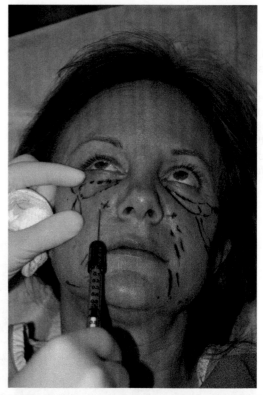

Fig. 32. Fat injections are performed with the patient upright so that gravity is acting on the soft tissues. Injections are performed perpendicular to the areas being filled to prevent sausage-shaped fat-filled irregularities that are created when injections are parallel to the depressed areas.

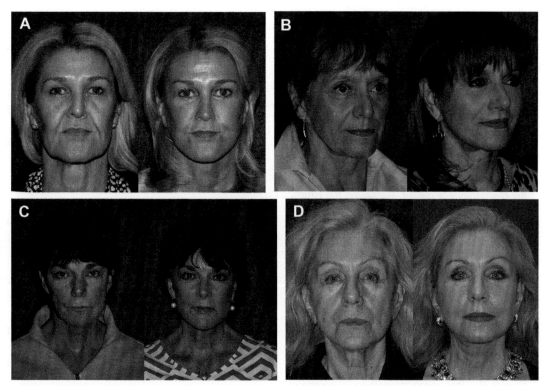

Fig. 33. Preoperative and postoperative examples of patients with a deflated orbit having primary lower blepharoplasty with autologous fat grafting, skin pinch, and orbicularis hitch (*A, B*), and examples of patients who had prior orbital fat reduction blepharoplasty years before now requiring fat augmentation and skin and orbicularis muscle tightening (*C, D*).

focusing on the medial nasojugal crease and central orbital hollow first. Small passes vertically disrupt the orbitomalar ligaments and the fat is injecting separating its attachments allowing the skin to be untethered from the bone. Most typically I will inject 1 to 1.5 mL in this region. Next I focus on the lateral orbital hollow, Injecting a total of 0.4 to 0.7 mL as required (**Figs. 32** and **33**).

COMPLICATIONS

The most common complication I see after autologous fat grafting is lack of fat graft take. This is treated with a subsequent fat transfer, More concerning are irregularities and overcorrection, which are difficult to treat. In my review of 52 patients, 6 patients had irregularities or overcorrection, comprising 11% of the cohort. These are usually treated with injections of an equal mixture of Kenalog 10 mg/mL and 5-fluorouracil 50 mg/mL. If this fails, then micro-liposuction is performed using an infiltration cannula; my preference is the Byron Coleman infiltration canula. A last resort is an open procedure, with an incision over the area to access the fat irregularity. I will melt the fat away with a bipolar forceps. The skin of the lower eyelid heals extremely well so the incisions and scar are well tolerated by the patient.

SUMMARY

Lower blepharoplasty is arguably the most complex procedure in aging face surgery, requiring precise diagnosis of anatomy and choosing the correct surgical approach to prevent complications. Transcutaneous blepharoplasty is a powerful rejuvenative technique when orbicularis oculi muscle is preserved and the lower eyelid is supported with suspensory maneuvers, including canthopexy and muscle flap suspension sutures. Volumization with orbital fat transposition and/or autologous fat grafting leads to more complete results. Most important is considering contraindications to the transcutaneous approach, which include the negative vector orbit, orbicularis weakness, and excessive lower eyelid laxity. In these cases, a transconjunctival approach is preferred with a less invasive approach to orbicularis tightening and skin removal, which include an orbicularis hitch and skin pinch excision.

DISCLOSURE

The authors have nothing to disclose.

REFERENCES

1. Ward B, Ward M, Fried O, et al. Nasal distortion in short-distance photographs: the selfie effect. JAMA Facial Plast Surg 2018;20(4):333–5.
2. Flowers RS, Flowers SS. Precision planning in blepharoplasty. The importance of preoperative mapping. Clin Plast Surg 1993;20(2):303–10.
3. Jelks GW, Jelks EB. Preoperative evaluation of the blepharoplasty patient. Bypassing the pitfalls. Clin Plast Surg 1993;20(2):213–23 [discussion: 224].
4. Griffin G, Azizzadeh B, Massry GG. New insights into physical findings associated with postblepharoplasty lower eyelid retraction. Aesthet Surg J 2014; 34(7):995–1004.
5. Little JW, Hartstein ME. Simplified muscle-suspension lower blepharoplasty by orbicularis hitch. Aesthet Surg J 2016;36(6):641–7.
6. Duke-Elder, S.W.K., The Eyelids. System of Ophthalmology: The Anatomy of the Visual System. Vol. 2. 1961, Mosby, Saint Louis, MO.
7. Flowers RS. Tear trough implants for correction of tear trough deformity. Clin Plast Surg 1993;20(2): 403–15.
8. Stutman RL, Codner MA. Tear trough deformity: review of anatomy and treatment options. Aesthet Surg J 2012;32(4):426–40.
9. Wong CH, Hsieh MK, Mendelson B. The tear trough ligament: anatomical basis for the tear trough deformity. Plast Reconstr Surg 2012;129(6):1392–402.
10. Lambros V. Observations on periorbital and midface aging. Plast Reconstr Surg 2007;120(5):1367–76 [discussion: 1377].
11. Haddock NT, Saadeh PB, Boutros S, et al. The tear trough and lid/cheek junction: anatomy and implications for surgical correction. Plast Reconstr Surg 2009;123(4):1332–40 [discussion: 1341–2].
12. Paul MD, Calvert JW, Evans GR. The evolution of the midface lift in aesthetic plastic surgery. Plast Reconstr Surg 2006;117(6):1809–27.
13. Hirmand H. Anatomy and nonsurgical correction of the tear trough deformity. Plast Reconstr Surg 2010;125(2):699–708.
14. Kpodzo DS, Nahai F, McCord CD. Malar mounds and festoons: review of current management. Aesthet Surg J 2014;34(2):235–48.
15. Baker SR. Orbital fat preservation in lower-lid blepharoplasty. Arch Facial Plast Surg 1999;1(1):33–7.
16. Quatela VC, Jacono AA. The extended centrolateral endoscopic midface lift. Facial Plast Surg 2003; 19(2):199–208.
17. Goldberg RA. Transconjunctival orbital fat repositioning: transposition of orbital fat pedicles into a subperiosteal pocket. Plast Reconstr Surg 2000; 105(2):743–8 [discussion: 749–51].
18. Ramirez OM, Maillard GF, Musolas A. The extended subperiosteal face lift: a definitive soft-tissue remodeling for facial rejuvenation. Plast Reconstr Surg 1991;88(2):227–36 [discussion: 237–8].
19. Hamra ST. The deep-plane rhytidectomy. Plast Reconstr Surg 1990;86(1):53–61 [discussion: 62–3].
20. Yoo DB, Peng GL, Massry GG. Transconjunctival lower blepharoplasty with fat repositioning: a retrospective comparison of transposing fat to the subperiosteal vs supraperiosteal planes. JAMA Facial Plast Surg 2013;15(3):176–81.
21. Hester TR Jr, Codner MA, McCord CD, et al. Evolution of technique of the direct transblepharoplasty approach for the correction of lower lid and midfacial aging: maximizing results and minimizing complications in a 5-year experience. Plast Reconstr Surg 2000;105(1):393–406 [discussion: 407–8].

Transconjunctival Lower Lid Blepharoplasty with and Without Fat Preservation and Skin Resurfacing

Deniz Sarhaddi, MD[a], Farzad R. Nahai, MD[b],*, Foad Nahai, MD[b]

KEYWORDS

- Transconjunctival lower lid blepharoplasty • Fat preservation • Croton oil peel • Skin pinch

KEY POINTS

- Transconjunctival lower lid blepharoplasty is a safe and effective procedure with a low complication rate.
- Success with this procedure depends on proper patient analysis and selection.
- The lower lid periorbital fat can be resected or preserved and draped or grafted over the orbital rim, depending on the clinical presentation.
- The lower lid skin can be resurfaced with a peel, with a laser, or by skin pinch depending on surgeon preference.

HISTORY AND DEVELOPMENT OF THE TRANSCONJUNCTIVAL APPROACH

The transconjunctival blepharoplasty, first introduced in the 1920s, gained widespread popularity in the 1990s with the work of Zarem and Resnick.[1] The transconjunctival approach was popularized as a technique to address periorbital aging while minimizing complications related to the traditional transcutaneous lower blepharoplasty.[2] The traditional lower blepharoplasty, performed through an external approach using a skin-muscle flap technique, was criticized heavily for its association with lower lid malposition and ectropion. In hindsight, this association was largely due to surgical technique and a failure to perform concomitant canthal support procedures.[3]

Continued advances in blepharoplasty techniques and an improved understanding of aging have increased the safety and efficacy of lower blepharoplasty overall. Contemporary blepharoplasty emphasizes lateral canthal support and re-creation of a youthful transition of the lower lid-cheek junction. Generally, the paradigm has shifted toward tissue preservation and augmentation.[4] Even so, when compared with a transcutaneous approach to lower blepharoplasty, the transconjunctival approach offers advantages, including less visible scarring and less downtime. When combined with ancillary techniques, such as skin resurfacing, skin pinch excision, and proper fat management, the transconjunctival approach addresses many of the signs of periorbital aging once thought to only be addressed with a transcutaneous approach.[2,3]

ANATOMY OF THE LOWER LID

An understanding and ability to visualize lower lid anatomy, inside out and outside in, are paramount to safely performing blepharoplasty and effectively smoothing the lid-cheek junction (**Fig. 1**).[5]

The lower lid can be divided into 3 lamellae, or layers, each of which has its own functional importance and surgical correlate: the anterior, middle, and posterior.

[a] Saint Louis Cosmetic Surgery, Inc, 17300 North Outer 40 Road, Suite 300, Chesterfield, MO 63005, USA; [b] The Center for Plastic Surgery at Metroderm, 875 Johnson Ferry Road Suite 300, Atlanta, GA 30342, USA
* Corresponding author.
E-mail address: drnahai@gmail.com

Facial Plast Surg Clin N Am 29 (2021) 229–241
https://doi.org/10.1016/j.fsc.2021.01.004
1064-7406/21/

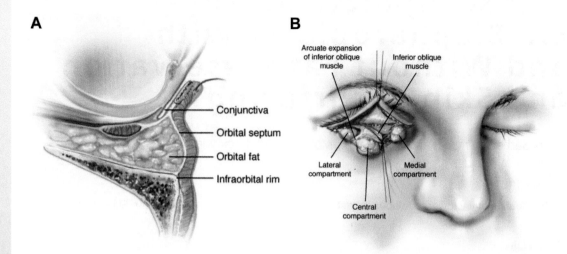

A

Conjunctiva

Orbital septum

Orbital fat

Infraorbital rim

B

Arcuate expansion of inferior oblique muscle

Inferior oblique muscle

Lateral compartment

Medial compartment

Central compartment

Fig. 1. (*A*) Sagittal section of the lower eyelid demonstrates the 3 layers: outer (skin and muscle), middle (orbital septum), and inner (lower lid retractors and conjunctiva). Note the confluence of the lower lid retractors and the orbital septum making the capsulopalpebral fascia immediately inferior to the lid margin. The preseptal approach pierces through the capsulopalpebral fascia and follows a relatively bloodless plane between the muscle and septum. Performing the procedure in the preseptal plane keeps the orbital fat out of the way for an easier dissection down to the orbital rim. At the point where the fat is removed, the septum is incised to expose the fat (see **Fig. 8**). (*B*) A transconjunctival view of the 3 fatty pads of the lower lid. The medial (or nasal) fatty pad is a lighter yellow, almost white color, and rests medial to the inferior oblique muscle. It is typically more sensitive during resection and may require a bit of extra lidocaine for the awake patient. The central fatty pad is typically the larger of the 3 and is lateral to the inferior oblique muscle. The lateral fatty pad rests below the lateral canthal ligament and can be a bit more challenging to resect via the transconjunctival approach. However, it is completely doable with a little effort and with the added assistance of marking the skin surface at maximum projection of the fatty pad to help locate it. (*From* Nahai F, et al. The Art of Aesthetic Surgery. 3rd Ed. New York: Thieme. 2020.; with permission.)

The anterior lamella, or outermost layer, consists of the thin lower eyelid skin and the concentric orbicularis oculi muscle.

The eyelid skin is the thinnest in the body, at about 0.7 mm thick. There is a delicate surgical plane between the lower eyelid skin and orbicularis oculi muscle.

The orbicularis oculi can be divided into 3 functional portions: pretarsal (overlying the tarsus), preseptal (overlying the septum), and preorbital (overlying the orbital bone). The pretarsal portion of the muscle helps in maintaining lower lid tone and involuntary blink. As such, it is preserved regardless of the type of procedure performed in order to minimize the risks of lid malposition and ectropion. The transition of the preseptal to preorbital portion of the orbicularis oculi is the transition from lid to cheek, defined by the orbicularis retaining ligament (ORL). A further division is made between the medial orbicularis and centrolateral portion of the muscle. This division is defined by innervation and thus function. The inner aspect is driven principally by the buccal branch of the facial nerve and is responsible for involuntary blinking and the function of the

lacrimal sac. The outer aspect of the muscle is mainly run by the zygomatic branch and is recruited during voluntary forceful lid closure.

The ORL, also known as the orbitomalar ligament, is a circumferential osteocutaneous ligament arising from the periosteum of the orbital rim, and, in the lower lid, it traverses the orbicularis oculi between the preseptal and preorbital portions to insert into the dermis of the lid-cheek junction. Medially, it is tightly bound to the periosteum and creates the inferior aspect of the nasojugal groove, or tear trough. This ligament can be released in the preperiosteal plane to smooth the lid-cheek junction and facilitate the mobility of the midface. Furthermore, this area often exhibits one of the earliest signs of facial aging and can be effectively treated with fillers to blend the transition from the lid to the cheek.[5]

The middle lamella consists of the orbital septum and is the landmark anatomic structure separating the inner and outer layers.

The orbital septum is a delicate, but distinct, fascial structure of the eyelid, which inserts directly onto the caudal edge of the tarsal plate. It is continuous with the periorbital periosteum and can be surgically followed as a plane to the midface periosteum. The septum serves as the anterior boundary containing the fat pads of the eye.

The lower lid has 3 intraorbital fat pads, lateral, central, and medial. They are managed in different ways to improve lid-cheek aesthetics. The lateral and central fat pads are separated by the arcuate expansion of Lockwood ligament, which inserts into the orbital rim anterolaterally. The central and medial fat pads are separated by the inferior oblique muscle, the injury of which will cause diplopia.[2]

The posterior lamella (the innermost layer of the eyelid closest to the globe) of the lower eyelid consists of the tarsal plate, lower lid retractors, and the conjunctiva.

The tarsal plate is a dense fibrous structure almost 1 mm thick at the superior aspect of the lower eyelid giving structure to the lid margin. In the lower lid, it is approximately 4 to 5 mm tall. It contains meibomian glands, which secrete the lipid layer of tear film.[2,5]

The lower lid retractors are a combination of muscle and fascial tissue that displaces the lower lid downward. The inferior tarsal muscle is a layer of smooth muscle that joins with the orbital septum and becomes a common ligament referred to as the capsulopalpebral fascia that inserts into the inferior tarsal border. When looking down, the inferior rectus muscle contracts, as do the lower lid retractors, retracting the lower lid to open the lower visual field. Cutting the lower lid retractors allows the lower lid margin to rise upward.[5,6]

The palpebral conjunctiva on the inner surface of the eyelid reflects onto the globe at the fornix to become the bulbar conjunctiva. Everting the lower lid, one will notice 2 vascular arcades: one overlying the tarsus, and one just above the fornix. These 2 arcades serve as useful markers during surgery when deciding where to place a transconjunctival incision.[2]

PREOPERATIVE EVALUATION

A history and examination focusing on the eye and eyelid function are an important part of the preoperative work up before lower eyelid surgery.[2,5,7,8]

One should note a history of hypertension and any anticoagulant medications, as these factors can increase the risk of postoperative hematoma. Preoperative visual acuity is recorded. A history of dry eye symptoms, or refractive/LASIK surgery within the last 6 months, predisposes patients to dry eye, exposure, and corneal complications. If dry eye is a consideration, these patients should undergo a Schirmer test to evaluate adequate

tear production, and/or tear film breakup time to evaluate for evaporative dry eye disease.

A thorough functional lower lid evaluation is very important and involves an evaluation of laxity with a lower lid distraction test (>0-mm distraction from the globe being the sign of significant laxity) and of orbicularis tone with a snap-back test. The snap test is positive if after the lid is distracted it does not reassume contact with the globe until a blink has occurred. If either finding is present, the need for a canthal tightening procedure is considered. Objectively, lower lid tone and scleral show should be evaluated by the margin reflex distance-2 (MRD2), the distance from pupillary light reflex to the lower lid margin. This distance should be less than 5 mm. The presence of the protective Bell phenomenon (globe rotates cephalad when the eyelids close) is noted, as an absence increases the risk of postoperative exposure keratitis.

Evaluation of the midface and globe position will help identify a preoperative predisposition to postoperative lower lid malposition. Patients with a negative vector (malar eminence lies posterior to the anterior-most point of the cornea on lateral view) are prone to lower lid malposition because of a relative deficiency of midface support. Patients with a prominent globe, measured with a Hertel exophthalmometer, are more likely to develop lower lid malposition if surgery is not carefully planned to account for this.

In addition to these functional considerations, patients are evaluated for the extent of lower lid fat pseudoherniation, lower lid skin excess, presence of a tear trough deformity, and degree of midface aging. To evaluate the degree of herniated fat, the patient looks upwards while the surgeon palpates the lid-cheek junction. Alternatively, the surgeon can gently press on the globe when the patient's eyes are closed, accentuating the pseudoherniated fat. The degree of midface aging is assessed by evaluating the lid-cheek junction, looking for skeletonization of the inferior orbital rim and making note of any malar bags or lateral edema.

INDICATIONS FOR TRANSCONJUNCTIVAL BLEPHAROPLASTY

The key to successfully treating the signs of aging of the lower eyelid and lid-cheek junction using the transconjunctival blepharoplasty lies in proper patient selection.[2,5] In patients with pseudoherniated fat, mild to moderate skin excess, and mild to moderate lid-cheek junction skeletonization, a variety of techniques can be combined with the transconjunctival approach. The typical candidate who is best for a transconjunctival approach is the one with prominent fat pads as the dominant feature of the lower lids. Patients with skin and muscle laxity may be good candidates for this approach; however, the degree of aesthetic improvement begins to diminish with more signs of aging. Therefore ancillary procedures, such as skin pinch, skin resurfacing, and/or fat repositioning, will maximize aesthetic outcomes. Of course, the other option is to select more invasive lower lid procedures; however, these will extend recovery times and increase morbidity.

PREOPERATIVE PLANNING
Skin Management

Skin pinch
A skin pinch technique, when performed concomitantly with transconjunctival blepharoplasty, can be used to manage mild lower eyelid skin excess with the use of a subciliary skin-only incision. This skin pinch technique preserves the orbicularis muscle and avoids middle lamellar scarring, with the nominal downside of adding a virtually imperceptible subciliary scar. Properly performed, this technique yields a stable postoperative lower eyelid position (no change in MRD2) when compared with a transconjunctival blepharoplasty without skin pinch.[9] If performing a skin pinch and an upper lid blepharoplasty, ensure that there are at least 6 mm of skin between the lateral limbs of the 2 incisions (see clinical case example; **Fig. 2**).

Skin undermining
A skin-only flap of the lower lid with conservative skin resection at the level of a subciliary incision can also be used to manage excess skin of the lower lid with transconjunctival blepharoplasty.

This "inside-outside" approach, which releases the attachments between orbicularis muscle and lower eyelid skin, was touted by Hidalgo[10] as superior in skin-smoothing potential when compared with the skin pinch technique. Using this approach, Hidalgo demonstrated lower lid malposition in only 3 of 248 consecutive patients. Similarly, Rosenberg and colleagues[11] showed no postoperative difference in MRD2 or lateral canthal rounding using this approach in 78 consecutive patients.

Skin resurfacing
To improve lower eyelid skin quality or dyschromia, skin resurfacing with peels or lasers can be used in conjunction with a transconjunctival blepharoplasty. Resurfacing is typically performed on the face as a whole to prevent demarcation, but the lower lid is an exception and can be treated alone with little risk of demarcation.[12] (See clinical case example; **Fig. 2**). A survey study of current practice trends among active American Society of Ophthalmic Plastic and Reconstructive Surgery members reported the use of laser skin resurfacing by 36% of the members and chemical peels by 29% of responding members.[4]

For laser or chemical skin resurfacing, it is important to realize that patients with Fitzpatrick skin types IV, V, and VI are at increased risk of developing dyspigmentation or hypertrophic scarring after treatment. For these patients, treatment should be limited to superficial peels if indicated. Typically, the darker the skin, the less severe the photoaging, and therefore, less need for resurfacing.

Skin preparation for a chemical peel includes 4 weeks of topical tretinoin, hydroquinone, and sun protection, all of which should be resumed once reepithelialization has occurred. For patients with a history of cold sores, herpes prophylaxis should begin 1 day preprocedure and continue for 4 days postprocedure.[13]

Medium-depth peels, such as a 20% to 30% TCA, are especially effective in improving advanced photoaging in the periorbital area. Deeper chemical peels, such as a 0.1% croton oil peel, can better address deeper rhytides. The senior authors most commonly use croton oil for skin resurfacing of the lower eyelid in their practice. However, deeper peels are also associated with more potential complications, including risk of scarring, textural changes, prolonged erythema, hyperpigmentation or hypopigmentation, and risk of ectropion. If an ectropion does develop and is not due to the surgical technique or midlamellar scarring, it tends to be self-limiting and corrects with conservative care.[12]

Laser resurfacing of the lower eyelid can improve texture and dyschromia and provides some skin tightening. Skin preparation is minimal, primarily requiring that the patient be diligent with sunblock and avoiding tanning. Antiherpes prophylaxis is recommended. Multiple options exist, including ablative devices, nonablative and radiofrequency devices, and fractional devices. It is important to note that ablative lasers, particularly the ablative CO_2, carry a higher risk of lower eyelid ectropion, particularly in patients undergoing secondary blepharoplasty. Clinical studies have shown that the ablative Er:YAG laser, although more superficial in penetration when compared with the CO_2 laser, is effective for both superficial and deep rhytides in the lower eyelid, probably owing to the thin skin in this area.[12] Segal and colleagues[6] combined transconjunctival blepharoplasty with erbium laser resurfacing without inducing lid retraction.

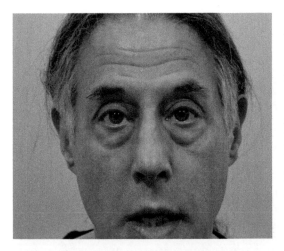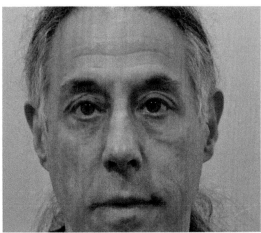

TC lower lid with skin pinch and 20% TCA peel (patient also had bilateral upper lid ptosis repair). Note the significant improvement in the disposition of his lower lids and the reduction in brow strain from the ptosis repair. The scar from the skin pinch is virtually imperceptible.

Fig. 2. Clinical example 3. A middle-aged man with severe fatty pad herniation and a flat mid face. He has lighter skin with sun damage and fine crepey lines. He underwent transconjunctival lower lid fat resection with a skin pinch and 20% TCA peel to the entire periorbital area. He also had concomitant bilateral upper lid ptosis repair. He is shown 1 year postoperatively. Note the significant improvement in the disposition of his lower lids and the reduction in brow strain from the ptosis repair. The scar from the skin pinch is virtually imperceptible, and the overlying skin is smoother. Transconjunctival lower lid with skin pinch and 20% TCA peel (patient also had bilateral upper lid ptosis repair). Note the significant improvement in the disposition of his lower lids and the reduction in brow strain from the ptosis repair. The scar from the skin pinch is virtually imperceptible. (*From* Nahai F, et al. The Art of Aesthetic Surgery. 3rd Ed. New York: Thieme. 2020.; with permission.)

Whichever resurfacing modality is chosen, the most important factor in avoiding complications and obtaining good results is operator comfort and proficiency with a given technique.

FAT MANAGEMENT

The transconjunctival approach allows the surgeon to address herniated orbital fat as well as midface volume loss. In manipulating the inferior orbital fat pads, a surgeon has options, including excision alone, augmentation with autologous fat grafts, or fad pad transposition.[7]

Fat Resection

For patients with isolated lower lid bags, little or no skin excess, and no inferior orbital rim volume loss, a transconjunctival approach to resecting the lower lid fat is potentially all that is needed. The transconjunctival approach is rarely associated with lower lid malposition and often has the added benefit of decreasing scleral show without a concomitant canthal procedure.[6] This is due to the incision through the lower lid retractors allowing elevation of the lower lid.[5] When fat is resected,

it should be done in all 3 compartments, and as a general rule, is trimmed back to the point where it is flush with the orbital rim (see clinical case examples; **Figs. 3–5**).

Fat Grafting

Fat grafting can be used to smooth the lid-cheek junction/tear trough deformity and to add volume to a skeletonized inferior orbital rim.

One technique is via micro–free fat grafts. These grafts are made from resected excess lower eyelid fat pads, which are cut down until they are 2 to 3 mm in size. After release of the ORL/tear trough ligament, these free fat grafts can be placed under direct vision using small forceps and can volumize the tear trough deformity. Miranda and Codner[14] demonstrated partial fat graft resorption in 9% of their patients, none of whom required revision or fillers.

Alternatively, autologous fat grafts from other parts of the body, most commonly harvested from the abdomen via manual syringe liposuction, are transplanted to the periorbital area with cannulas. These fat grafts can be used for deep malar augmentation and volumization of the tear trough

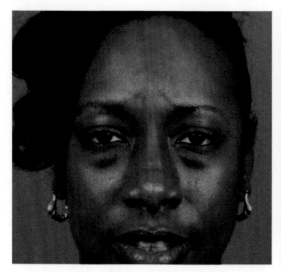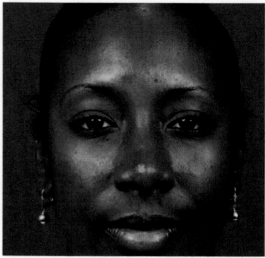

TC LL only. This is an optimal patient for trans-conjunctival fat removal. She is younger with good skin and muscle tone in the lower eyelid. Virtually no sun damage at all. The procedure alone has transformed the overall perception of her appearance.

Fig. 3. Clinical example 1. A younger dark-skinned woman, who is an ideal candidate for the transconjunctival approach to resect periorbital fat. Her skin and muscle are tight and do not need intervention. She is shown 1-year after the procedure with an ideal result. Transconjunctival lower lid only. This is an optimal patient for transconjunctival fat removal. She is younger with good skin and muscle tone in the lower eyelid. Virtually no sun damage at all. The procedure alone has transformed the overall perception of her appearance. (From Nahai F, et al. The Art of Aesthetic Surgery. 3rd Ed. New York: Thieme. 2020.; with permission.)

area. Although this can add an additional 5 to 7 days of recovery because of swelling and ecchymoses, in more than 300 cases, Rohrich and colleagues[15] did not have additional morbidity, nodularity, or irregularity. Furthermore, they reported improved skin texture and contour blending. Fat grafting is covered in more detail in Kenneth D. Steinsapir and Samantha Steinsapir article, "The treatment of post-blepharoplasty lower eyelid retraction," in this issue, and in the authors' opinion, is very operator and technique dependent.

Fat Pad Redraping

Rather than resecting herniating fat from the medial and central fat pockets, these fat pads can be pedicled and redraped to camouflage a skeletonized inferior orbital rim and volumize the tear trough deformity (**Fig. 6**). The lateral fat pad is typically conservatively excised. The downside of fat transposition is that it is limited by the reach of the pedicled fat pad and can be technically challenging because it is done through the transconjunctival incision, and the delicate tissues are difficult to suture to.[14]

Fat pad redraping is a common technique; the current practice trend among active American Society of Ophthalmic Plastic and Reconstructive Surgery members demonstrates that fat

repositioning is performed by 80% of respondents[4] and is the preferred technique of one of the authors (F.R.N.).

Fat pad repositioning, although not effective at decreasing the apparent length of the lower lid (which appears elongated with aging due to cheek volume deflation and inferior descent), does effectively efface the nasojugal fold (also known as the tear trough). Furthermore, this procedure does not affect the MRD2 when combined with transconjunctival blepharoplasty.[16]

OPERATIVE TECHNIQUE

Before surgery, with the patient awake and sitting up, mark the fat pads of the lower lid with a single dot on the center of each (you can have the patient close his/her eyes and gently press on the globe to help with this; **Fig. 7**) and mark the tear trough area with a few X's along the ligament. If you plan to perform fat grafting of the face, mark the areas that you are going to fat graft, mark the midface with an X at the point of maximal hollow and draw out the SOOF laterally as well. Hang preoperative photographs in the operating room (OR) in ready view of the surgeon for reference during the case. If resurfacing is going to be performed, the perimeter of the orbit is also marked with the

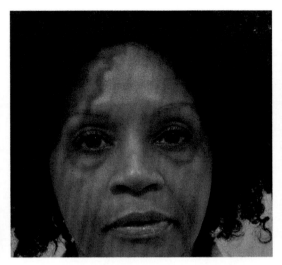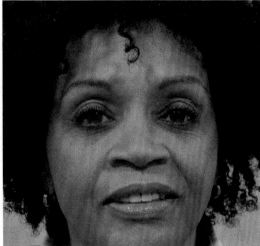

TC LL only. Similar to the previous case example but a bit older. Some laxity remains in the skin, but with her skin type the trans-conjunctival approach alone has yielded a very favorable result.

Fig. 4. Clinical example 2. Compare this to case 1. This woman is a bit older with a similar skin type. She has a bit more skin and muscle laxity, but less than would be expected in a person with lighter skin of the same age. She is still considered a very good candidate for the transconjunctival approach. She is shown 1-year after the procedure. Notice that compared with case 1, she does have some skin laxity after the procedure, but it is reasonable, and she was very pleased. Transconjunctival lower lid only. Similar to the previous case example but a bit older. Some laxity remains in the skin, but with her skin type, the transconjunctival approach alone has yielded a very favorable result. (*From* Nahai F, et al. The Art of Aesthetic Surgery. 3rd Ed. New York: Thieme. 2020.; with permission.).

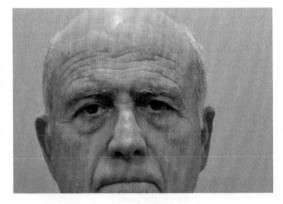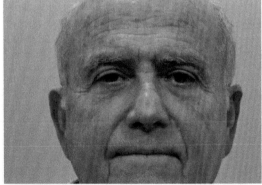

TC Lower lid (also had upper lids and direct brow lift).

Fig. 5. Clinical example 4. The final case is an older man in his early 70s that wanted improvement in the entire periorbital area. He has many of the signs of facial aging: brow ptosis, upper lid dermatochalasis, lower lid laxity with fatty pad herniation, and volume loss in the midface, to name a few. He had multiple procedures under local anesthesia in the office, including direct brow lift, upper lid blepharoplasty, and transconjunctival lower lid fat resection. Note the natural, less tired, and less heavy postoperative appearance. Transconjunctival lower lid (also had upper lids and direct brow lift). (From Nahai F, et al. The Art of Aesthetic Surgery. 3rd Ed. New York: Thieme. 2020.; with permission.)

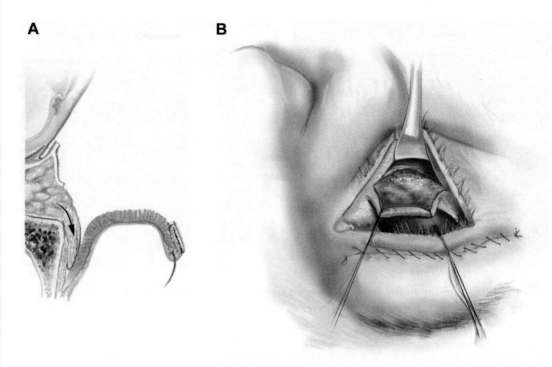

Fig. 6. Sagittal and transconjunctival views of lower eyelid fat transposition to blend the lid-cheek junction. The orbitomalar ligament must be released followed by a preperiosteal or postperiosteal dissection in order to create space for the transposed fat. The preperiosteal dissection leaves some tissue behind to which to secure the fat and to avoid percutaneous parachute sutures. It is a bit more of a technical dissection though. The subperiosteal dissection is a bit easier of a plane to dissect, but can lead to more postoperative swelling, making it harder to secure the transposed fat. Often temporary percutaneous sutures are needed to hold the fat down over the orbital rim. (*From* Nahai F, et al. The Art of Aesthetic Surgery. 3rd Ed. New York: Thieme. 2020.; with permission.)

patient sitting up, before intraoperative swelling effaces the anatomic landmarks.

Transconjunctival lower lid blepharoplasty may be performed under general anesthesia, conscious sedation, or local anesthesia with or without oral medications. In all situations, the cornea is protected with either corneal protectors or a stay suture on the proximal edge of the conjunctival incision that can be used to drape the conjunctiva over the globe for protection.

Once anesthesia is induced, infiltrate the fornices with 1 to 2 mL of 0.5% lidocaine with 1:200,000 epinephrine using a 30-guage needle on a 3-mL syringe. Use approximately 0.2 mL

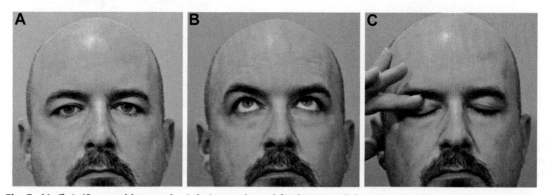

Fig. 7. (*A–C*) A 42-year-old man who is being evaluated for lower eyelid surgery. He does not like the bulging fatty pads and thinks they make him look tired (*A*). An effective method of assessing the fatty pad is to have the patient turn their gaze upwards (*B*) or gently pressing on the globe with the eye closed (*C*).

for the preseptal injection on each side and infiltrate a small amount of local anesthesia on the lateral orbital rim if performing a canthal procedure. Infiltrate the subciliary area with a small amount of local anesthesia if planning to excise skin. Allow the epinephrine to take effect as the patient is prepared and draped, and as you scrub and gown.

Regarding the local anesthetic, studies evaluating the use of tranexamic acid (topical, oral, or infiltrated) are shown in various aesthetic plastic surgery studies to decrease bleeding and postoperative edema and ecchymosis.[17–19] Although the authors have not yet adopted this practice, the literature thus far suggests promising outcomes.

Have your assistant gently retract the lower lid with Blair retractors and press the globe gently so the fornix becomes more prominent. Take a bite of the forniceal conjunctiva slightly medially with a 6-0 polypropylene suture and retract with a mosquito hemostat. Do the same with another suture slightly laterally, letting these hang gently over the forehead for retraction.

Next, identify the 2 vascular arcades of the lower lid, one superiorly by the tarsal plate, and one inferiorly near the fornix. Exposure can be obtained through either the preseptal or the postseptal approach (**Fig. 8**). For the preseptal approach, the incision is made just inferior to the superior arcade. For the postseptal approach, 2 incisions are made just above the lower arcade, a small incision to access the medial fat pad, separated by a bridge of intact conjunctiva, and a more lateral incision to access the central and lateral fat pads. The bridge of intact conjunctiva serves to protect the inferior oblique muscle from injury. The preseptal approach allows access to the midface for redraping the fat pads and preserves the fat pads during the dissection. With the septum intact during the initial part of the procedure, the view of the rim and local anatomy is easier. The postseptal approach allows direct access to the fat pads for excision.

The Bovie on cutting mode is used to incise the conjunctiva and retractors. A gentle spreading technique is used to open the preseptal plane down to the orbital rim.

Next, release the tear trough ligament medially. To do this, you can remain in the preperiosteal plane or deep to the periosteum. To divide the tear trough ligament in the preperiosteal plane, use the Bovie to dissect the orbicularis off of the periosteum. Do not cut through the orbicularis, because the buccal branch of the facial nerve, which controls blinking, travels through the muscle. Deep to the orbicularis, you will also note the origin of the lip elevators; -do not release these

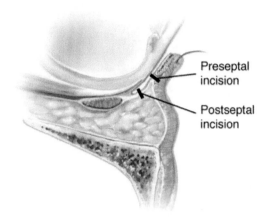

Preseptal incision

Postseptal incision

Fig. 8. Sagittal view of the lower eyelid with the 2 incision options to approach the periorbital fat. For the preseptal approach, the incision is 1 to 2 mm below the tarsus. This will then progress through the capsulopalpebral fascia and into the submuscular preseptal plane. This keeps the fat out of the way during the exposure and is the preferred approach of the lead author (F.R.N.). For a more direct approach, the postseptal technique can be used. The conjunctival incision is lower down the lid closer to the sulcus and goes directly into the fatty compartment. (*From* Nahai F, et al. The Art of Aesthetic Surgery. 3rd Ed. New York: Thieme. 2020.; with permission.).

off of the bone. Only release the medial orbicularis muscle off of the orbital rim.

Alternatively, to release the tear trough ligament in the subperiosteal plane, cut the arcus just outside the orbital rim and use a periosteal elevator to release the periosteum off the inferior orbital rim; -this will also release the tear trough ligament. Avoid injury to the inferior orbital neurovascular bundle.

Next, resect preseptal fat (**Fig. 9**). To access the fat pads, whether from the preseptal or postseptal approach, open the septum overlying each fat pad. Open the capsule of each fat pad and allow the fat to billow out, carefully teasing each fat pad out. A mild amount of pressure applied to the globe can help. If resecting, do so conservatively with the Bovie on coagulation. In both techniques, the lateral fat pad is the most difficult to access. Overresection creates a hollowed appearance. The endpoint of fat excision is assessed by applying gentle pressure on the globe and determining when the orbital fat is flush with the infraorbital rim. Redrape the skin and ensure that the contours are smooth and that fat is not overresected or underresected.

For redraping the medial fat pad, ensure that the fat pad reaches the tear trough deformity. The authors redrape and secure the fat with 6-0 Vicryl

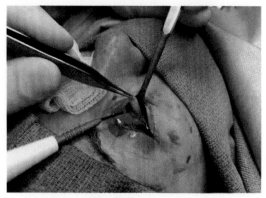

Pre-septal approach to the central fat pad of the lower eyelid. The orbital septum has been incised to express the fat pad before it is resected.

Fig. 9. View of the lower lid with expression of the central fatty pad through a transconjunctival incision and preseptal approach. The orbital septum is incised central to express the central fat pad. Take note of the blue skin marking on the lateral orbit indicating the location of the lateral fatty pad. This helps when looking for the fatty pad internally, which can be challenging from the transconjunctival approach. Preseptal approach to the central fat pad of the lower eyelid. The orbital septum has been incised to express the fat pad before it is resected.

transcutaneous mattress suture. If the fat pad does need to be trimmed, do so longitudinally rather than amputating at the tip, so the fat pad remains long and can reach.

In the authors' practice, they close the lower lid retractors with 2 simple buried 5-0 chromic sutures. Remove the stay stitches; you will use them again on the other side. If there is any chemosis during surgery, the authors place a temporary tarsorrhaphy stitch with a 5-0 chromic gut in line with the lateral corneal limbus.

TRANSCONJUNCTIVAL BLEPHAROPLASTY UNDER LOCAL ANESTHESIA

The authors have found that patient selection is key when considering blepharoplasty under local anesthesia in the office. If the patient expresses any hesitation or fear of pain during the procedure, such as with the local injection, then they recommend surgery in the OR under general anesthesia.

In the authors' practice, they use a combination of local anesthesia and oral sedation. The patient is given Phenergan (promethazine) intramuscularly 12.5 mg once they arrive in the office. Then, Percocet (oxycodone/acetaminophen) and Xanax (alprazolam) are given based on sex and body weight. The Pro-Nox nitrous oxide system is available for patients as well if needed. The lower eyelid and fat pads are anesthetized using 1% lidocaine with 1:100,000 epinephrine in a 3-mL syringe with

a 0.5-in 30-gauge needle. This can be typically done with approximately 3 mL of anesthetic on each side. The goal is mild sedation, whereby the patient is responsive to verbal and painful stimuli but is otherwise sleepy. It is important to note that the medial fat pad is particularly sensitive and needs additional local anesthetic before resection.

POSTOPERATIVE MANAGEMENT

Postoperatively, gel artificial tears are used nightly for 3 days. Preservative-free artificial tears are used during the day as needed. Prophylactic antibiotic eye drops are prescribed for 5 days postoperatively. Ophthalmic antibiotic ointment may also be used, but the patient's vision is impaired during use. Pain is controlled with acetaminophen and narcotics as needed. Edema and bruising are controlled with intermittent icing and head elevation and a Medrol dose pack when not contraindicated. Last, patients are instructed to limit screen time during recovery. Phones, computer, and TV screens strain the eyes, tend to make them dry, and extend the recovery. Limiting the screen time after surgery significantly shortens the recovery process. The first postoperative visit is in 5 to 7 days, at which time the temporary tarsorrhaphy suture, if it was placed during surgery, is removed.

In the authors' practice, skin resurfacing is most commonly performed with a croton oil peel. After the peel is complete, the area is occluded with zinc oxide tape (Hy-Tape) for 24 hours. After 24 hours, the tape is removed and replaced with a bismuth powder occlusive mask that remains in place for the next 7 to 8 days. The mask protects the skin during the peel and eliminates the need for caring for the peeled skin. During this time, the patient is instructed to keep this area dry (ie, no showering). The mask spontaneously separates around this time because of skin reepithelialization.

COMPLICATIONS AND MANAGEMENT
Complications Related to Management of Conjunctival Incision

The survey study conducted by Kossler and colleagues[4] evaluating current trends among active American Society of Ophthalmic Plastic and Reconstructive Surgery members demonstrated that the transconjunctival incisions are closed by only 45% of respondents. The most common suture used to close the transconjunctival incision was 6-0 plain gut (43%) followed by 6-0 fast absorbing gut (23%). Postoperative complications that argue in favor of leaving the conjunctiva unsutured are the possibility of suture abscess, pyogenic granuloma, additional edema and inflammation, and eyelid retraction. However, eyelid ointment granuloma formation without wound closure is a possibility as well; it is an unusual development resulting from introduction of topical ointment into the open conjunctival wound and presents as painless, firm, round lower eyelid masses. Management includes topical steroid ointment and drops, oral steroids and antibiotics, injection of intralesional steroids, or surgical excision.[20]

Overresection of Fat Pads

If periorbital fat is going to be removed, it should be sculpted until it is flush with the orbital rim. Fat pad overresection results in a hollowed appearance. If this is noted during surgery, make use of the resected fat as micro–free fat grafts to correct the contour. If this is noted postoperatively after all edema has resolved, consider autologous fat grafting (possible in-office) to correct the appearance or fillers to camouflage the skeletonized inferior orbital rim.

Lower Lid Malposition

Lower lid malposition is uncommon following the transconjunctival approach, but it can happen.[21–23] Malposition is one of the reasons the transconjunctival approach is popular. Common preoperative characteristics of patients with postoperative lower lid malposition are orbicularis weakness, a negative vector or prominent globe, and a volume-depleted inferior orbital rim. The first step to prevention is making note of these characteristics before undertaking lower blepharoplasty surgery and planning accordingly. Should malposition occur after a transconjunctival procedure, early identification and treatment are important and key to avoiding permanent deformity. Once identified, massage and squinting exercises are recommended immediately. If middle lamellar contraction is thought to be part of the cause, lid injections of kenalog-5 (5 mg/mL) and 5-Fluorouracil can help relieve the contractile force of the scar on the lid. Furthermore, administration of a hyaluronic acid gel filler (eg, Restylane) to the tear trough for lid support can also help correct lid retraction. Should these conservative maneuvers fail, corrective lid retraction surgery may be necessary. Details of lid retraction surgery are addressed in Hannah Landsberger and colleagues' article, "The prominent eye – what to watch-out for," in this issue.

Chemosis

Chemosis, subconjunctival edema, can be seen intraoperatively, early postoperatively (week 1), or later postoperatively (week 2–3).

The keys to prevention are protection of the sclera during surgery, minimizing thermal exposure, using a temporary tarsorrhaphy suture, pretreating the patient with steroid-containing ophthalmic ointment, and minimizing early postoperative lagophthalmos.

If intraoperative chemosis is noted, the authors routinely place a temporary tarsorrhaphy suture, which they have found limits its progression. If mild postoperative chemosis is noted, the authors treat with topical dexamethasone, phenylephrine, and lubricant drops or ointments. If chemosis is moderate, they patch the eye for 24 hours, and if persistent, they will consider temporary tarsorrhaphy suture placement in the office. If chemosis is severe but not inflamed, and prevents eyelid closing, the authors will incise the edematous conjunctiva and anterior tenons capsule under loupe magnification with a "one snip" to release the fluid, followed by steroid ophthalmic ointment and a 24-hour eye patch. If inflamed, they will treat with the above medications, patch until the inflammation is resolved, and then incise only if still necessary.

Hematoma

Retrobulbar hematoma is a possibility with any surgery of the eye, especially if the septum is violated. A hematoma in the retrobulbar space creates a compartment syndrome of the eye, where the blood is trapped within the orbit by the septum, with progressive pressure on the globe and intraorbital nerves and vessels.

The major risk factors are hypertension and use of anticoagulants. Prevention of this vision-threatening complication depends on proper patient selection and preparation, meticulous surgical hemostasis, particularly when resecting fat pads, blood pressure control intraoperatively and postoperatively, discontinuation of all antiplatelet medications, and patient instruction to avoid bending over and Valsalva (ie, straining when urinating or passing stool).

Symptoms of orbital hemorrhage include pain, pressure, diplopia, and possible vision loss. Signs include proptosis, chemosis, ophthalmoplegia, and loss of the pupillary light reflex. Treatment includes use of timolol or betaxolol ophthalmic drops to lower intraocular pressure, acetazolamide 500 mg orally to decrease aqueous production, mannitol 20% 2 g/kg intravenous (IV) to osmotically lower intraocular pressure, and prompt lateral canthotomy with inferior cantholysis until the lower lid is released and the hematoma is evacuated. In addition, methylprednisolone and dexamethasone IV can be used. Once the emergency is over and everything is under control, the lid is closed. Ophthalmology colleagues must be consulted.

Diplopia

Diplopia, or double vision, is often the way patients describe any visual disturbance. Binocular diplopia in the immediate postoperative period is likely due to diffusion of local anesthetic into the extraocular muscles. In days 1 to 7, monocular diplopia can be due to lubricating ointments or drops, in which case it improves when the patient wipes their eyes. Conversely, it can also be due to dry eye in the patient with postoperative lagophthalmos or poor compliance with lubricating drops/nighttime ointments. Furthermore, intraorbital edema (fat pad edema) can also cause self-limited visual disturbance during this time. However, in the patient with persistent binocular diplopia, injury to the inferior oblique muscle must be considered, and ophthalmology colleagues must be consulted. This injury is typically diagnosed by examination whereby there is lack of upward gaze during full adduction.

CLINICS CARE POINTS

- Even though transconjunctival blepharoplasty has an extremely low rate of lower eyelid malposition or retraction, in the authors' experience, almost zero, a full lower eyelid laxity examination is crucial, and with any sign of laxity, the authors recommend canthal anchoring.

- Canthal work may lead to chemosis. The authors recommend placing a temporary tarsorrhaphy suture at the level of the lateral limbus of the iris any time canthal work (canthopexy, canthoplasty) is undertaken, even if it is left in place for just 3 days, to help control chemosis and lower eyelid position during the height of postoperative edema.

- Lower eyelid surgery is not skin surgery. Proper evaluation of risk factors (negative vector, lax tarsoligamentous system, prominent globe, previous procedures, thyroid issues, and so forth), mitigation of these risk factors (by means of canthopexy or midface augmentation, for example), and minimal skin removal even in the scenario where a skin-flap is elevated and trimmed, can help avoid lower eyelid complications, such as malposition and ectropion.

DISCLOSURE

Dr D. Sarhaddi has nothing to disclose. Dr F.R. Nahai receives royalties from Thieme, is a consultant for MTF, and conducts clinical research with Galderma and Merz. Dr F. Nahai receives royalties from Thieme and Springer for books and QMP for videos.

REFERENCES

1. Zarem HA, Resnick JI. Expanded applications for transconjunctival lower lid blepharoplasty. Plast Reconstr Surg 1991;88(2):215–20.
2. Pacella SJ, Nahai FR, Nahai F. Transconjunctival blepharoplasty for upper and lower eyelids. Plast Reconstr Surg 2010;125(1):384–92.
3. Maffi TR, Chang S, Friedland JA. Traditional lower blepharoplasty: is additional support necessary? A 30-year review. Plast Reconstr Surg 2011;128(1):265–73.
4. Kossler AL, Peng GL, Yoo DB, et al. Current trends in upper and lower eyelid blepharoplasty among American Society of Ophthalmic Plastic and Reconstructive Surgery members. Ophthalmic Plast Reconstr Surg 2018;34(1):37–42.
5. Hashem AM, Couto RA, Waltzman JT, et al. Evidence-based medicine: a graded approach to lower lid blepharoplasty. Plast Reconstr Surg 2017;139(1):139e–50e.
6. Segal KL, Patel P, Levine B, et al. The effect of transconjunctival blepharoplasty on margin reflex distance 2. Aesthet Plast Surg 2016;40(1):13–8.
7. Murri M, Hamill EB, Hauck MJ, et al. Oculofacial plastic and reconstructive surgery: an update on lower lid blepharoplasty. In: Semin Plast Surg, Vol. 31, No. 1. Thieme Medical Publishers; 2017, February. p. 46.
8. Davison SP, Iorio M, Oh C. Transconjunctival lower lid blepharoplasty with and without fat repositioning. Clin Plast Surg 2015;42(1):51–6.
9. Taban M, Taban M, Perry JD. Lower eyelid position after transconjunctival lower blepharoplasty with versus without a skin pinch. Ophthalmic Plast Reconstr Surg 2008;24(1):7–9.
10. Hidalgo DA. An integrated approach to lower blepharoplasty. Plast Reconstr Surg 2011;127(1):386–95.
11. Rosenberg DB, Lattman J, Shah AR. Prevention of lower eyelid malposition after blepharoplasty: anatomic and technical considerations of the inside-out blepharoplasty. Arch Facial Plast Surg 2007;9(6):434–8.
12. Glaser DA, Kurta A. Periorbital rejuvenation. Facial Plast Surg Clin North Am 2016;24(2):145–52.
13. Bensimon RH. Croton oil peels. Aesthet Surg J 2008;28(1):33–45.

14. Miranda SG, Codner MA. Micro free orbital fat grafts to the tear trough deformity during lower blepharoplasty. Plast Reconstr Surg 2017;139(6):1335–43.

15. Rohrich RJ, Pezeshk RA, Sieber DA. The six-step lower blepharoplasty: using fractionated fat to enhance blending of the lid-cheek junction. Plast Reconstr Surg 2017;139(6):1381–3.

16. Ramesh S, Goldberg RA, Wulc AE, et al. Observations on the tear trough. Aesthet Surg J 2020; 40(9):938–47.

17. Rohrich RJ, Cho MJ. The role of tranexamic acid in plastic surgery: review and technical considerations. Plast Reconstr Surg 2018;141(2):507–15.

18. Couto RA, Charafeddine A, Sinclair NR, et al. Local infiltration of tranexamic acid with local anesthetic reduces intraoperative facelift bleeding: a preliminary report. Aesthet Surg J 2020;40(6):587–93.

19. McGuire C, Nurmsoo S, Samargandi OA, et al. Role of tranexamic acid in reducing intraoperative blood loss and postoperative edema and ecchymosis in primary elective rhinoplasty: a systematic review and meta-analysis. JAMA Facial Plast Surg 2019; 21(3):191–8.

20. Belinsky I, Patel P, Charles NC, et al. Ointment granulomas following sutureless transconjunctival blepharoplasty: diagnosis and management. Ophthalmic Plast Reconstr Surg 2015;31(4):282–6.

21. Patel A, Wang Y, Massry GG. Management of post-blepharoplasty lower eyelid retraction. Facial Plast Surg Clin 2019;27(4):425–34.

22. Nahai F, Wojno TH. Problems in periorbital surgery a repair manual. New York: Thieme; 2019.

23. Codner MA, McCord CD Jr. Eyelid and periorbital surgery. New York: Thieme; 2016. p. 262.

Periorbital Fat Grafting
A New Paradigm for Rejuvenation of the Eyelids

Timothy Marten, MD*, Dino Elyassnia, MD

KEYWORDS

- Fat grafting • Fat injections • Autologous fat grafting • Fat transfer • Microfat grafting • Lipofilling
- Secondary blepharoplasty • Stem cell blepharoplasty

KEY POINTS

- Traditional blepharoplasty procedures do not always address the changes that occur with age in the orbital area and can actually degrade the appearance of the eye.
- Fat grafting represents the most important new addition to surgical procedures to rejuvenate the orbit since the inception of the "blepharoplasty" technique.
- Fat grafting is an artistically powerful method to rejuvenate the periorbital orbital area that often provides a more healthy, fit, youthful, and sensual appearance than traditional blepharoplasty procedures.
- Periorbital fat grafting is easier and faster to perform than "septal reset" and eyelid fat transpositioning and provides the opportunity for comprehensive improvement of the entire orbital region, not just spot filling of the tear trough.
- Fat grafting is often more important to rejuvenating the periorbital areas of the secondary blepharoplasty patient than traditional eyelid surgery.

THE AGING ORBIT AND THE NEED FOR FAT GRAFTING

Why perform periorbital fat grafting? Why not just perform traditional blepharoplasty? The answer to these questions lies in the multifactorial origin of periorbital aging and the fact that fat is predictably lost from the periorbital area and the orbit and adjacent areas often become hollow as one ages. Acknowledging this, and recognizing the components of the aging change of the periorbital area and appreciating the underlying anatomic abnormalities, is essential to recommending appropriate treatment and the planning of proper surgical repair. Careful analysis will reveal that most patient problems seen in the aging periorbital area fall into the following categories (**Box 1**).

Our traditional surgical procedures allow treatment of the first 5 changes. Fat grafting allows us to treat atrophy—an important new element in

creating natural and attractive periocular appearance and something we could not do in the past.

Patients primarily concerned with *surface aging* of their periocular skin may not require blepharoplasty surgery and may achieve the improvement they desire through salon care and dermatologic surface treatments of their periorbital skin. These treatments include skin peels, intense pulsed light and broadband light treatments, laser skin resurfacing, and various cutaneous laser and other treatments designed to remove or reduce "age spots," skin wrinkles, and other age-associated skin surface imperfections.

Patients primarily concerned with palpebral skin excess, fatty accumulation and fat "herniation," relaxation and/or dehiscence of ligaments and musculoaponeurotic structures, and *loss of youthful periocular contour* achieve little, if any, improvement if surface treatments of the skin

Marten Clinic of Plastic Surgery, 450 Sutter St Suite 2222, San Francisco, CA 94108, USA
* Corresponding author.
E-mail address: tmarten@martenclinic.com

Facial Plast Surg Clin N Am 29 (2021) 243–273
https://doi.org/10.1016/j.fsc.2021.02.003
1064-7406/21/© 2021 Elsevier Inc. All rights reserved.

only are used. These patients require formal forehead lift and blepharoplasty procedures to reposition ptotic tissue, excise excess tissue, and surgically reinforce weakened ligamentous and musculoaponeurotic structures if these problems are to be properly treated and an attractive and natural appearing improvement is to be obtained. The misapplication of surface skin treatment to problems of forehead ptosis, eyelid skin excess, fatty accumulation, and weakening of ligamentous/musculoaponeurotic structures to eyes that have lost youthful shape and optimal function will produce smooth lid skin with no improvement in contour.

Patients with significant periorbital *atrophy* and age-associated hollowing and loss of periorbital volume will generally achieve suboptimal improvement from both surface treatments of periorbital skin and traditional blepharoplasty procedures. Smoothing skin will not hide an aged, gaunt, or ill appearance due to loss of periorbital fat, nor will removing tissue from already depleted orbital areas create natural and attractive periocular contours. Restoring lost periorbital volume by fat grafting is a powerful technique that is acknowledged by many surgeons engaged in treating the aging eyelid as the "missing link" in periorbital surgery and the most important advance in periorbital aesthetic surgery in several decades or more. Properly performed, the addition of fat to a periorbital region that has atrophied due to age or disease can produce a significant and sustained improvement in appearance unobtainable by traditional eyelid surgery (**Fig. 1**).

WHAT DOES THE YOUNG EYE REALLY LOOK LIKE, WHAT SHOULD OUR PRIORITIES BE IN REJUVENATION OF THE PERIORBITAL AREA, AND HOW CAN WE BEST MEET THOSE AESTHETIC GOALS?

Simply stated, the young eye is clear, smooth skinned, neatly creased, elongated with a slight canthal tilt, and aesthetically framed by a well-positioned and appropriately shaped eyebrow.

The hallmark of the young, attractive orbit is *fullness*, and we must ask ourselves "do our traditional blepharoplasty procedures produce results that look like these?" (**Fig. 2**).

Fig. 3 shows a group of patients who have previously undergone blepharoplasty procedures. Are these really good results? Do these eyes seem youthful? Healthy? Attractive? Rejuvenated? Surgeons seeking to rejuvenate the eyelids must ask themselves "should we be removing or adding fat to achieve the most aesthetic result?" Should a blepharoplasty be more than a traditional partial blepharectomy? Do we need to rethink our approach to our blepharoplasty procedures? Can fat grafting help us achieve better outcomes?

IF LID FULLNESS IS GOOD, WHY NOT JUST USE FILLER?

Fillers have certain advantages and are a viable alternative to periorbital fat grafting. Fillers have helped patients and surgeons understand volume loss as part of the aging process. They are nonsurgical, have a quick recovery, are long-lasting in orbital area, easily adjustable, and reversible (hyaluronic acid gel [HAG] products). These advantages must be weighed against disadvantages including that they require ongoing maintenance and that the treatments are time-consuming for busy patients, uncomfortable or painful, expensive, can be uneven or unnatural, and can precipitate a Tyndall effect. Over time patients often get "filler face"—an overfilled, heavy, unfeminine, "old," and unattractive appearance. Many patients will also develop "filler burn-out" and come in requesting something that produces a more long-lasting and natural appearance. Perhaps the biggest disadvantage and lost opportunity of filler is its lack of "stem cell" tissue effects.

WHY NOT JUST TRANSPOSE EYELID FAT?

Why not just transpose eyelid fat or perform a "septal reset"? These procedures are technically difficult, time-consuming open surgeries that entail a long recovery and carry a significant potential for irregularities and serious problems and complications. More importantly, only limited fat is typically available and these procedures largely treat the "tear trough" only. No improvement is obtained in lateral orbit, cheek, midface, temple, and upper orbit.

ADVANTAGES OF PERIORBITAL FAT GRAFTING

Fat grafting allows surgeons to treat atrophy and improve outcomes over traditional excisional procedures in which tissue is removed. It comprises a

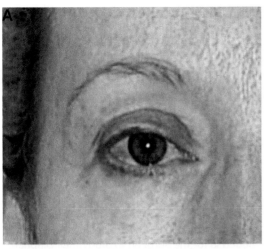 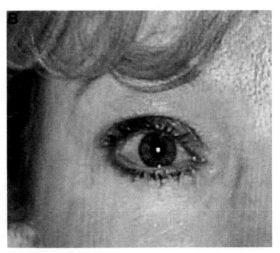

Fig. 1. Periorbital fat grafting. (*A*) Patient seen after facelift and upper and lower blepharoplasty. Despite technical excellence in the excision of skin and fat the eye has an aged and unhealthy appearance (previous procedure performed by an unknown surgeon). (*B*) Same patient seen 11 months after secondary facelift and periorbital fat grafting, but no blepharoplasty has been performed. The eye now has a more youthful, healthy, and alluring appearance. (Procedure performed by Timothy Marten, MD, FACS – courtesy of Marten Clinic of Plastic Surgery.)

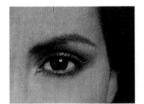 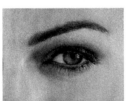 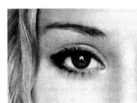 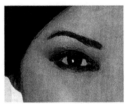

Fig. 2. *Characteristics of the young healthy eye.* The young eye is clear, smooth skinned, neatly creased, elongated with a slight canthal tilt, and aesthetically framed by a well-positioned and appropriately shaped eyebrow. But the hallmark of the young, attractive orbit is *fullness.* (Courtesy of Timothy Marten, MD - Marten Clinic of Plastic Surgery.)

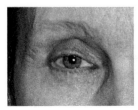 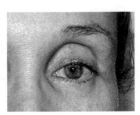 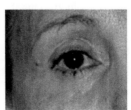 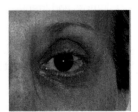

Fig. 3. *Postoperative blepharoplasty patients.* Are these really good results? Do these eyes appear youthful? Healthy? Attractive? Rejuvenated? (all procedures performed by unknown surgeons). (*Courtesy of* Timothy Marten, MD - Marten Clinic of Plastic Surgery.)

volumetric rejuvenation—a new dimension for surgeons seeking to rejuvenate the periorbital area. It is autologous and provides for comprehensive treatment of the entire orbital area—not just the eyelids. Unlike nonautologous fillers, fat produces long-lasting and sustained improvement with a stem cell regenerative effect.

VOLUMETRIC REJUVENATION, TISSUE INTEGRATION, AND STEM CELL EFFECT

Fat grafting provides previously unavailable advantages for the surgeon rejuvenating the periorbital area by providing a means to obtain volumetric rejuvenation—a new and different means to improve periocular and facial appearance and a new dimension for surgeons to work in. Before fat grafting, surgeons performing blepharoplasty procedures were largely engaged in exalted technical exercises focused on what they could remove. Fat grafting provides a means for us to look at surgical rejuvenation of the orbit more broadly and appropriately and at how we can best create a truly youthful, healthy, and attractive appearance.

Unlike injectable fillers, fat is autologous, integrates with facial tissues, and becomes a part of the face, promoting a more natural appearance during facial movement, avoiding a Tyndall effect, and producing a sustained and long-lasting improvement. In addition, mounting scientific evidence now supports the often-cited clinical observation that fat injections actually induce an improvement in facial tissue quality through a "stem cell" effect and when performed in the periorbital area may achieve rejuvenation in the true sense of the word.

DRAWBACKS OF FAT INJECTIONS

Performing periorbital fat grafting in conjunction with blepharoplasty has disadvantages including the learning curve associated with any new procedure, the time spent and needed to harvest fat, increased postoperative edema, a longer period of recovery, uncertain graft take, and the potential for problems and complications such as asymmetries, lumps, and irregularities. In addition, patient and surgeon misconceptions must be overcome, including the misguided belief of some that injected fat can migrate or fall, that fat injections will make the face "look fat," or that it does not last.

IDENTIFYING THE PATIENT WHO NEEDS PERIORBITAL FAT GRAFTING

Areas in need of treatment vary from patient to patient, and planning fat grafting procedures requires looking at the face more as a "sculptor" and less as a "tailor" as we have done in the past. Any area that is treatable with nonautologous injectable fillers is potentially treatable with fat grafting, including, but not limited to, the temples, forehead, brow, glabella, radix, upper orbit ("upper eyelid"), lower orbit ("lower eyelid"), cheeks, midface, and "tear trough", and experience with fillers is a useful point of reference for planning fat additions to the face. A key element in restoring a harmonious and youthful appearance is for the surgeon to look beyond spot rejuvenation of the eyelids and to consider the entire periorbital area (temples, forehead, cheeks. midface) as an aesthetically integrated whole.

Perhaps the best way to decide where fat is needed is for the surgeon to study their blepharoplasty outcomes and identify areas where the procedure has fallen short. Usually the biggest shortcoming for the experienced surgeon is the failure to replenish lost volume, and the areas in need of treatment will be obvious.

Examining nonsmiling photographs of patients when they were younger are very helpful and provide a way to gain an appreciation of volume loss in the periorbital area and its contribution to aging changes in the orbital area. Old photos are also very helpful in educating patients as to how their orbital area has changed with age and in explaining the need for fat grafting. In almost all cases old photos of prospective patients taken when they were younger show a full upper and lower orbit, full midface and cheek, and a palpebral skin fold that rests only a few millimeters from their lashes. After thoughtful review over time one gains a deeper appreciation of periorbital (and facial) atrophy and the desire to correct it (**Fig. 4**).

PERIORBITAL FAT GRAFTING APPLICATIONS

How can fat grafting help surgeons rejuvenate the periorbital area? What can the fat be used for and where should the fat be injected?

Some of the ways fat grafting is used to improve orbital appearance and blepharoplasty results are discussed in the following section.

Cheeks

Fat grafting the cheek enhances a patient's facial shape, proportion, and cheek projection; corrects age-associated loss of cheek volume; and thus improves periorbital appearance (**Fig. 5**). Often fat grafting can rival or even exceed the improvements obtained when Terino malar, Binder submalar, and combined malar–submalar shell style cheek implants are placed (see **Figs. 1**, **5-7**, **13-17** see also patient

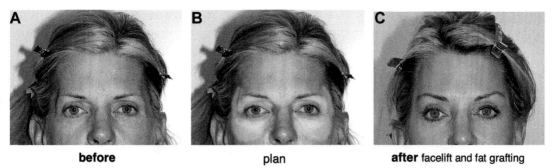

before   **plan**   **after** facelift and fat grafting

Fig. 4. (*A*, *B*, *C*) Patient before and after simultaneous facelift and periorbital fat injections. (*A*) Patient before procedure. No prior surgery. (*B*) Shaded areas showing where fat was placed: 3 mL were placed in each upper orbit, 5 mL was placed in each temple, 1 mL was placed in each tear trough, 3 mL was placed in each infraorbital area, 4 mL in each cheek, and 2 mL in the glabella. (*C*) Same patient 2 years and 4 months after high SMAS facelift, neck lift, lower blepharoplasty, and 34 mL of periorbital fat injections. (Procedure performed by Timothy Marten, MD, FACS – Courtesy of Marten Clinic of Plastic Surgery.)

examples 1–5). In many instances fat grafting results in a softer more natural appearing, integrated cheek than cheek implants provide and produces a softer and less harsh appearance.

How Atrophy of the Cheek and Midface Affects the Appearance of the Lower Eyelid and Its Relevance in Procedures to Rejuvenate the Periorbital Area

As the cheek atrophies, the lower eyelid orbital fat ("fat bags") becomes more exposed and prominent in a process known as *pseudohernia-tion*. Removing lower eyelid fat in such circumstances as is often done in traditional blepharoplasty procedures, can create a hollow, elderly, and even ill "nursing home eye" appearance and a low-lying lid–cheek junction. A better strategy for many patients is to reconstitute the cheek with fat grafts and integrate the pseudoherniated fat with the cheek, rather than removing it, raising the lid–cheek junction to create a smooth and more youthful transition from the lower eyelid to the cheek (**Figs. 6** and **7**).

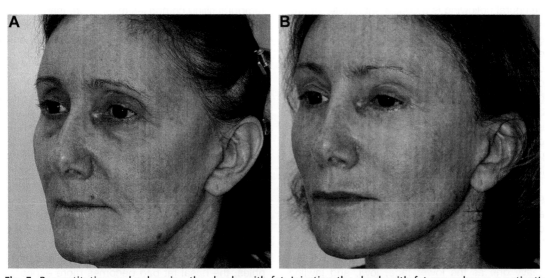

Fig. 5. Reconstituting and enhancing the cheeks with fat. Injecting the cheek with fat can enhance a patient's facial shape and proportion, increase cheek projection, and correct age-associated loss of cheek volume. (*A*) Patient with atrophic cheek and face before facelift and fat grafting. (*B*) Same patient seen 1 year and 8 months after high SMAS facelift, forehead lift, neck lift, and pan-facial fat grafting. Fat grafting often results in a softer more natural appearing, integrated cheek mass than cheek implants provide and can produce a softer and less harsh appearance. Note also fill in temple, upper orbit, tear trough, lower orbit and midface areas. (Procedure performed by Timothy Marten, MD, FACS – Courtesy of Marten Clinic of Plastic Surgery.)

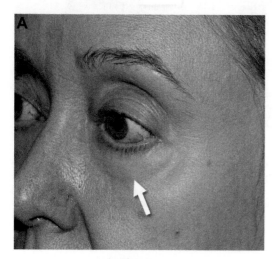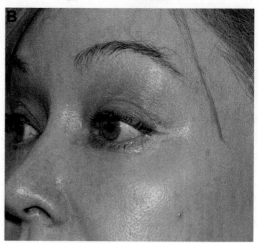

(1 y and 9 mo post-op)

before

after facelift and fat grafting

(<u>no</u> blepharoplasty was performed)

Fig. 6. Reconstituting the cheek and midface with fat grafting and treating pseudoherniation of lower eyelid fat. As the cheek atrophies, the lower eyelid "fat bags" become more exposed and prominent (pseudoherniation). Removing lower eyelid fat creates a hollow, elderly, and even ill appearance. A more appropriate and attractive rejuvenation is often obtained when the cheek is reconstituted by fat grafting it. (*A*) Patient with atrophic cheek. The lower lid fat is exposed (*white arrow*) and seems as a "bag" (pseudoherniation) that surgeons traditionally remove. (*B*) Same patient seen 1 year and 9 months after fat grafting to the nasojugal groove, midface, and cheeks with *no* blepharoplasty. Protruding lower eyelid fat is disguised by building and reconstituting the cheek and produces a more youthful, fit, and attractive appearance than removing lower lid fat would have. (Note: fat grafting was performed in the upper orbit, temple, glabella, radix, columella, piriform, and nasolabial crease). (Procedure performed by Timothy Marten, MD, FACS – Courtesy of Marten Clinic of Plastic Surgery.)

Temples

Temporal hollowing is a consistent marker of one entering their 40s that is readily improved with fat grafting (**Fig. 8**). Even skillfully performed eyelid surgery results in marginal improvement in overall orbital and upper facial appearance if the outcome of blepharoplasties is viewed against the background of a hollow, elderly and hard-appearing, bony, atrophic, empty temple. Restoring lost volume in the temples is arguably an important and essential part of contemporary "blepharoplasty" procedures performed by surgeons willing to look beyond the eyelids.

Fat grafting the temples is important to facial shaping and is typically sought by surgeons with a sharp aesthetic eye for detail in their facelift procedures. The ideal youthful, attractive female face has an inverted oval shape that with aging typically changes to be more rectangular and bottom-heavy one as the lower face, jowl, and jawline sags. Temporal atrophy and hollowing contributes to facial rectangularization, and when advanced a "peanut" facial shape results. Although a well-performed facelift corrects the lower facial square-ness, temporal filling by fat grafting provides a wider intertemporal distance producing an inverted oval shape. Seen from this perspective, temporal filling comprises much more than simple filling of the temporal hollow or even more than a comprehensive rejuvenation of the eyelids and orbital area, it provides a more youthful, feminine, and beautiful appearing facial shape.

Upper orbit/"upper eyelid" area

Whether the result of illness, aging, or an overzealous previous surgical procedure, filling the hollow upper orbit can produce a remarkable rejuvenation of the upper eyelid and eliminate an unnaturally hollow and elderly appearance sometimes referred to by patients as "nursing home" or "owl eyes" (**Figs. 9** and **10**).

Pseudoherniation of the upper eyelid nasal fat pad

As the temporal fat pad of the upper eyelid atrophies, the nasal fat pad becomes more exposed and prominent—a sequence of events known as *pseudoherniation*. Removing fat from the nasal compartment in such circumstances as is traditionally taught usually creates a hollow, elderly, and unhealthy appearance or exacerbates such an appearance if already present. A more

(1 y and 9 mo post-op)

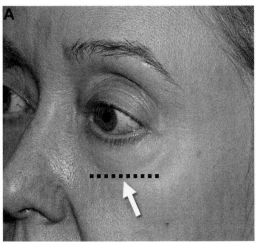 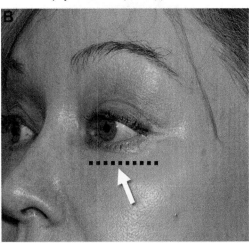

before   **after** facelift and fat grafting

(<u>no</u> blepharoplasty was performed)

Fig. 7. Effect on position of lid–cheek junction when lower blepharoplasty versus midface and cheek fat grafting is performed. (*A*) Patient with atrophic cheek and pseudoherniated orbital fat. If lower lid fat is removed as traditionally taught, a low lid–cheek junction will result (*white arrow* and *black line*). A low lid–cheek junction is a feature of the unaesthetic, aged, or ill-appearing orbit. (*B*) Same patient 1 year and 9 months after facelift and fat grafting to the nasojugal groove, midface, and cheeks but *no* blepharoplasty. Protruding pseudoherniated lower eyelid fat is integrated into the cheek resulting in a high lid–cheek junction (*white arrow* and *black line*). A high lid–cheek junction is a feature of youth and vitality. (Note: fat grafting was performed in the upper orbit, temple, glabella, radix, columella, piriform, and nasolabial crease). (Procedure performed by Timothy Marten, MD, FACS – Courtesy of Marten Clinic of Plastic Surgery.)

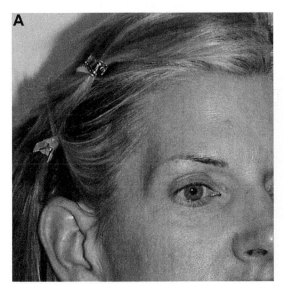 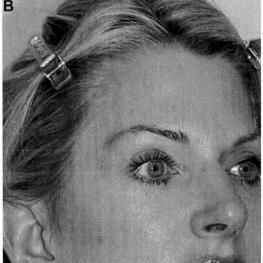

Fig. 8. (*A, B*) Filling of the temple hollow with fat. Temporal hollowing is a consistent marker of the fourth decade of life readily improved with fat injections. (*A*) Patient aged 45 years before surgery. (*B*) Same patient 2 years and 4 months after high SMAS facelift and grafting of 5 mL of fat into the temple region on each side (fat was injected in the upper and lower orbit, midface, and cheek). (Procedure performed by Timothy Marten, MD, FACS – Courtesy of Marten Clinic of Plastic Surgery.)

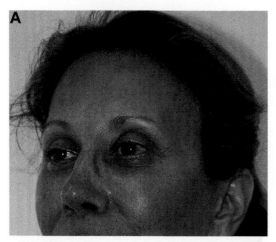 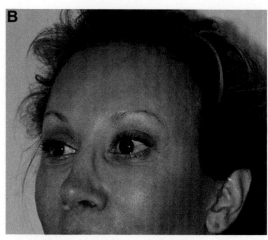

Fig. 9. (*A, B*) Correcting age-associated upper orbital hollowing. (*A*) Patient who underwent facelift and related procedures elsewhere has hollow upper eyelids from prior eyelid surgery. Note atrophy in temple, radix, infraorbital, midface, and cheek areas. (Procedure performed by an unknown surgeon). (*B*) Same patient seen 1 year after secondary facelift and related procedures including fat grafting to the upper orbit. No blepharoplasty was performed. The upper lid is filled and restored, and a healthier, more youthful appearance is seen. Note comprehensive improvement in periorbital appearance achieved by filling adjacent temple, infraorbital, midface, and cheek areas. These improvements cannot be obtained by traditional excisional blepharoplasty. (Procedure performed by Timothy Marten, MD, FACS – Courtesy of Marten Clinic of Plastic Surgery.)

appropriate and attractive rejuvenation of the upper orbit is obtained under these circumstances when the atrophic lateral fat compartment is refilled and restored by fat grafting (**Fig. 11**). In most cases *the problem is not that the nasal fat pad has grown. It is that the temporal fat pad has atrophied.*

Restoration of the upper eyelid palpebral skin fold

As the temporal fat pad of the upper eyelid atrophies, lid skin is retracted into the upper orbit

obliterating the normal palpebral skin fold. Removing fat from the nasal compartment as is traditionally taught accentuates a hollow, elderly, and unhealthy appearance and does nothing to restore the normal palpebral lid skin fold, essential to a youthful, healthy, and attractive appearance. A more appropriate and attractive rejuvenation of the upper orbit is obtained when the atrophic lateral fat compartment is reconstituted by fat grafting. When the upper orbital volume is restored, upper eyelid skin retracted up into the upper orbit preoperatively descends to form a

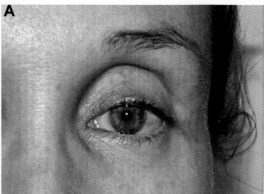 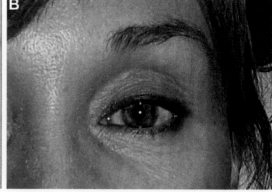

Fig. 10. (*A, B*) Correcting iatrogenic upper orbital hollowing and "owl eye." (*A*) Patient with hollow upper eyelid and unnaturally hollow and elderly ocular "owl eye" or "nursing home" appearance following blepharoplasty performed by an unknown surgeon. (*B*) Same patient seen after 3 mL of fat injections to the upper orbit. Although the upper lid is incompletely filled and restored, a healthier, more youthful appearance is seen. (Procedure performed by Timothy Marten, MD, FACS – Courtesy of Marten Clinic of Plastic Surgery.)

"large" nasal fat pad   atrophy of lateral fat pad   "large" nasal fat pad   lateral fat pad restored

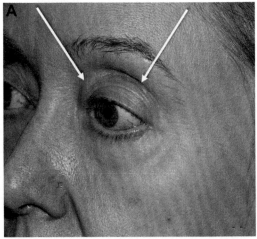
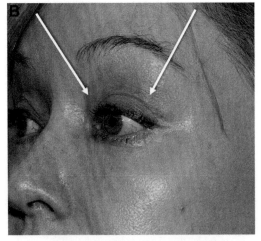

before   **after** facelift and fat grafting

(<u>no</u> blepharoplasty was performed)

Fig. 11. Pseudoherniation of the upper eyelid nasal fat pad. As the temporal fat pad of the upper eyelid atrophies, the nasal fat pad becomes more exposed and prominent in a process known as pseudoherniation. Removing fat from the nasal compartment in such circumstances as is traditionally taught creates a hollow, elderly, and unhealthy appearance. A more appropriate and attractive rejuvenation of the upper orbit is often obtained when the atrophic lateral fat compartment is reconstituted by fat grafting. (*A*) Patient with atrophy of the temporal fat pad in the upper orbit. The upper lid nasal fat pad is exposed and seems ostensibly as a "bag" (pseudoherniation) that surgeons were traditionally taught to remove. Removing nasal fat under such circumstance will actually degrade the appearance of the eye. (*B*) Same patient seen 1 year and 9 months after fat grafting of the upper orbit but *no* blepharoplasty or reduction of the nasal fat pad. Protruding eyelid fat in the nasal compartment has been disguised by building up and restoring the lateral compartment and filling in the lateral upper orbit (note that the nasal fat pad is unchanged in size and its outline still visible). This produces a more youthful, fit, and attractive appearance than removing upper eyelid nasal compartment fat would have (note: fat grafting has also been performed in the nasojugal groove, infraorbital area, midface, cheek, temple, glabella, radix, columella, piriform, and nasolabial crease). (Procedure performed by Timothy Marten, MD, FACS – Courtesy of Marten Clinic of Plastic Surgery.)

youthful and natural appearing palpebral lid skin fold (**Fig. 12**).

Lower orbit/"lower eyelid" area

Fat grafting the infraorbital ("lower eyelid") area is in some ways analogous to augmenting the upper orbit, and the artistic payoff is very high if the procedure is carried out correctly (**Fig. 13**).

Fat grafting the infraorbital area allows correction of age-associated atrophy and hollowness that lends the face an ill or haggard appearance; "shortens" the apparent length of the lower eyelid; and produces a youthful, attractive, and highly desirable smooth transition from the lower eyelid to the cheek that is generally unobtainable by traditional lower eyelid surgery, fat transpositions, "septal resets," midface lifts, free fat grafts, and other procedures.

"Tear trough"

Where the infraorbital area ends and the nasojugal "tear trough", midface, and cheek areas begin is

hard to define and in practice the treatment of the infraorbital, cheek, and nasojugal areas must be undertaken concurrently, and in most situations the treated areas will overlap each other to a certain extent. In addition, it must be remembered that the ultimate goal of the procedure is creating youthful and attractive *contour*, not simply filling a specific area, and doing so requires treating multiple areas.

Fat grafting the tear trough (**Fig. 14**) is simpler and faster to perform than fat transposition and septal reset, and we have largely abandoned these blepharoplasty procedures as have Little, Tonnard and Verpale, and others. And unlike when septal reset and fat transpositioning are performed, fat grafting allows one to fill not only the tear trough but also the infraorbital region, the cheek and midface, the upper orbit, the temple, forehead, and the radix and glabella and *comprehensively rejuvenate the entire periorbital region*. Fat grafting is

lid fold not   atrophy of
present   lateral fat

lid fold   lateral fat pad
restored   restored

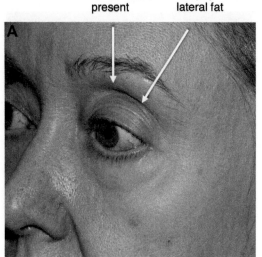

before

after facelift and fat grafting

(<u>no</u> blepharoplasty was performed)

Fig. 12. Restoring the upper eyelid palpebral skin fold. As the temporal fat pad of the upper eyelid atrophies, lid skin is retracted up into the upper orbit obliterating the palpebral lid skin fold that should be present. Removing fat from the nasal compartment in such circumstances as is traditionally taught creates a hollow, elderly, and unhealthy appearance and does not restore palpebral lid skin fold that is essential to a youthful, healthy, and attractive appearance. A more appropriate and attractive rejuvenation of the upper orbit is often obtained when the atrophic lateral fat compartment is reconstituted by fat grafting. When upper orbital volume is restored, skin retracted up into the upper orbit preoperatively forms a more youthful and natural appearing palpebral lid skin fold. (*A*) Patient with atrophy of the temporal fat pad in the upper orbit. The upper orbit is empty, upper eyelid skin is retracted up into the orbit, and no upper eyelid lid palpebral skin fold is present. This lends the eye an aged and "nursing home" appearance. (*B*) Same patient seen 1 year and 9 months after fat grafting of the upper orbit (and midface and cheek) but *no* blepharoplasty or reduction of the nasal fat pad. Skin retracted up into the upper orbit preoperatively now forms a more youthful and natural appearing palpebral lid skin fold. This produces a more youthful, fit, and attractive appearance than removing upper eyelid nasal compartment fat would have. (Procedure performed by Timothy Marten, MD, FACS – Courtesy of Marten Clinic of Plastic Surgery.)

aesthetically far more powerful and superior to a limited correction of the tear trough only.

Midface

The midface is a loosely defined triangular area bound by the infraorbital rim superiorly, the nasolabial fold medially, and the zygomaticus major muscle laterally. For several decades the aging change in this area has been mischaracterized as one of descent and mistakenly referred to as "midface ptosis" and as a result a variety of failed and/or largely abandoned procedures were conceived over the course of that time to "lift" what was mistakenly thought of as a "fallen" area. Often the early outcomes of these procedures looked satisfactory due to swelling but surgeons and patients were typically disappointed that once healing was complete and swelling had subsided a discernible improvement was not seen.

As experience with midface lifts accumulated, surgeons realized that *the aging change in the*

midface consisted largely of deflation, and not descent, and a rethinking of how the midface is best treated occurred. It is now more widely recognized that one cannot lift an empty space, but instead must fill it, and fat grafting has taken a preeminent role in treatment of this aesthetically important area. Indeed, Tonnard and Verpale, Little, and others who all once advocated "lifting" the midface have abandoned it and acknowledged that the midface is best rejuvenated by fat grafting alone (**Fig. 15**).

Practically speaking, the midface overlaps the infraorbital region, the tear trough, and the cheek (see **Fig. 22**), and when these adjacent areas are treated separate filling of the midface may not be needed. Fat grafting the midface when indicated corrects a hollow, ill, and unaesthetic orbital appearance that occurs with age by filling and strengthening it in ways that a midface lift cannot.

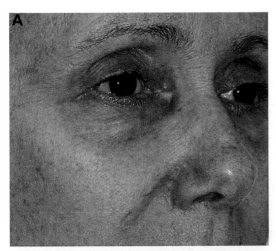
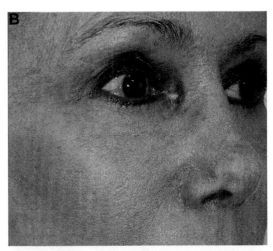

Fig. 13. (*A, B*) Filling the hollow lower orbit with fat. (*A*) Patient with hollow lower eyelid and unnaturally hollow and elderly infraorbital appearance. The lower eyelid seems long, and there is a distinct line of demarcation between the lower eyelid and the cheek. (*B*) Same patient seen after facelift and fat grafting of the infraorbital area. There is a smooth transition from the lower eyelid to the cheek, and the patient has a more healthy, youthful, and attractive appearance (note: the upper orbit, radix, cheek, and nasolabial crease have also been treated with fat injections, and the patient has undergone senile ptosis correction). (Procedure performed by Timothy Marten, MD, FACS – Courtesy of Marten Clinic of Plastic Surgery.)

Special Circumstances that Demand Periorbital Fat Grafting

Proptotic ocular globe

The proptotic ocular globe or "negative vector" eye has presented a challenge to surgeons performing blepharoplasty since the inception of the procedure. Traditional upper blepharoplasty in which skin and fat is removed from the upper eyelid often results in a hollow upper orbit, overly high palpebral skin fold, and a distinctive "bug eye" stare or "frog eye" appearance. Traditional lower blepharoplasty in which fat was removed from the lower eyelid often compounds these appearances and precipitates lower lid retraction

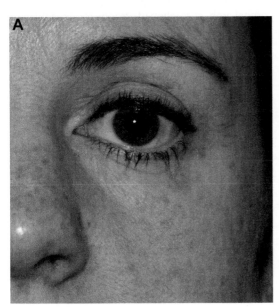
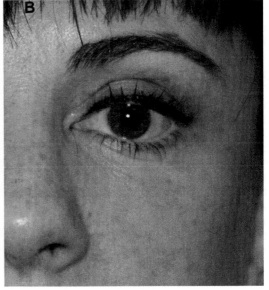

Fig. 14. (*A, B*) Filling the nasojugal ("tear trough") with fat. (*A*) Patient with hollow nasojugal groove ("tear trough") and unnaturally hollow and elderly infraorbital appearance. (*B*) Same patient seen after fat grafting. (Procedure performed by Timothy Marten, MD, FACS – Courtesy of Marten Clinic of Plastic Surgery.)

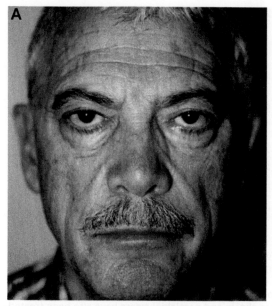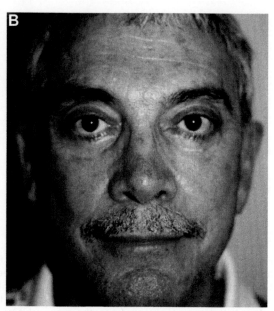

Fig. 15. (*A, B*) Filling the hollow midface with fat. (*A*) Patient with deflated and hollow midface and unnaturally hollow and elderly infraorbital appearance. The lower eyelid seems long, and there is a distinct line of demarcation between the lower eyelid and the cheek. (*B*) Same patient seen 1 year and 4 months after facelift, neck lift, foreheadplasty, upper and lower blepharoplasty, and fat grafting of the midface and infraorbital area. There is a smoother transition from the lower eyelid to the cheek, and the patient has a more healthy, fit, and youthful appearance. This change could not be obtained by a midface lift, as there is simply no midface to lift. (Procedure performed by Timothy Marten, MD, FACS – Courtesy of Marten Clinic of Plastic Surgery.)

and scleral show and a "polar bear" look. In addition, canthopexy is generally ineffective in these patients. Periorbital fat grafting is often a better way to improve these patients' ocular appearance and can disguise this problem and create a "neutral" vector oculomalar relationship (**Fig. 16**). Treating the proptotic globe calls on the surgeon's ability to recognize and treat multiple areas and not just spot treat one site.

Secondary blepharoplasty patient

The secondary blepharoplasty patient whose age-related fat loss was not replaced at their primary procedures, or whose periocular fat was inappropriately removed during previous procedures, are cases in which all sites previously discussed need fat grafting. For these patients fat grafting is often more important than the secondary blepharoplasty itself, which is performed largely to tighten canthal laxity or correct levator dehiscence (bilateral senile ptosis). In most secondary blepharoplasty cases, fat grafting provides the most consequential share of the improvement and is capable of truly transforming the patient in a way that traditional blepharoplasty procedures cannot (**Figs. 17, 29** and cases 3 and 4).

The secondary blepharoplasty patient stands as compelling evidence that correction of facial atrophy requires the addition of volume to the face, not a subtraction, lifting, or tightening, demanding a rethinking of the traditional approach to rejuvenation of the orbital area. Unlike problems corrected by a subtraction of tissue from the orbital area, correction of atrophy requires the surgeon to use techniques that "fill" and "sculpt" the orbit and surrounding areas. Fat grafting, when properly performed in these patients, produces soft and natural contours and afford the surgeon the opportunity to correct problems that a traditional eyelid surgery cannot. Treating the secondary blepharoplasty patient calls on the surgeon's ability to recognize and treat multiple areas and not just spot treat one site.

FAT INJECTION TECHNIQUE

The technique for preorbital fat grafting is well described,[1–8] and Coleman's principles are adhered to when fat injections are performed.

Needed Equipment

Special instruments are required to harvest and inject fat in addition to specialized equipment to process and organize it (**Figs. 18–20**). Poor outcomes are typically obtained if sharp hypodermic needles are used to harvest fat, if fat is not

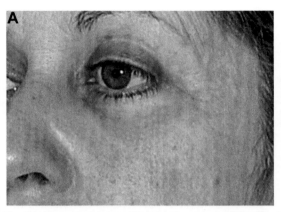
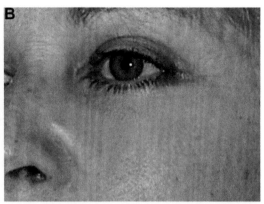

Fig. 16. Periorbital fat grafting for the proptotic ocular globe. (*A*) A patient seen preoperatively with a proptotic ocular globe and "negative vector" eye. The eye has an unaesthetic prominent "frog eye" or "bug eye" appearance. A traditional upper and/or lower blepharoplasty can be expected to make this problem worse and actually degrade the appearance of the eye. (*B*) Same patient seen 1 year and 5 months after facelift, neck lift, forehead lift, and periorbital fat grafting. The upper eyelid has a more youthful, healthy appearance, and the upper lid palpebral skin fold has been pushed closer to the ciliary margin to a more normal and aesthetic position. The lower orbit can be seen to be fuller due to filling of the midface, and the lower eyelid makes a smoother and more youthful and aesthetic transition to the cheek. The illusion is completed by filling of the temple and the cheek, essentially recessing the proptotic globe and creating a neutral vector eye by augmenting and strengthening the surrounding anatomy. (Procedure performed by Timothy Marten, MD, FACS – Courtesy of Marten Clinic of Plastic Surgery.)

processed, or if the fat is injected in a manner similar to that used to inject nonautologous facial fillers. If sharp hypodermic needles are used to *inject* fat, there is increased potential for intravascular injection, fat embolization, tissue infarction, visual impairment, and blindness, and therefore their routine use is not recommended.

Reusable cannulas (see **Fig. 18**A) have been the standard for many years and continue to be widely used by many surgeons. They suffer the drawback that they must be cleaned and sterilized and are not approved for use in some countries. The smaller and most useful cannulas are also very fragile and can break if not used and cared for carefully.

In many practices disposable, single-use cannulas are supplanting reusable cannulas (see **Fig. 18**B). These cannulas come in a variety of diameters and lengths and do not need to undergo cleaning, processing, and resterilization.

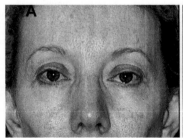
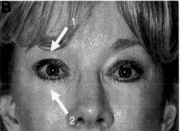
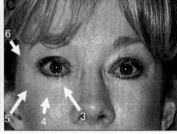

Fig. 17. Periorbital fat grafting in the patient requesting secondary blepharoplasty. (*A*) Preoperative views of a woman who has had previous facelift, neck lift, and overly aggressive blepharoplasties performed by an unknown surgeon. (*B*) Same patient, seen 11 months after secondary facelift; forehead lift; and fat grafting of the temples, glabella, radix, upper orbit, lower orbit, "tear trough", cheek, and midface. No excisional eyelid surgery (blepharoplasties) was performed. Note fullness in upper (*arrow 1*) and lower (*arrow 2*) orbital areas and restoration of youthful orbital-eyelid contours. (*C*) Note that correction has not only been made in the upper and lower orbit (*arrows 1 and 2* in *B*) but also in the "tear trough (3)," midface (4), cheek (5), and temple (6). Comprehensive filling of the entire periorbital area had been achieved, not just spot filling of the tear trough that would have been obtained had orbital fat transpositioning or septal reset been performed instead. (Procedure performed by Timothy J Marten, MD, FACS – courtesy of Marten Clinic of Plastic Surgery.)

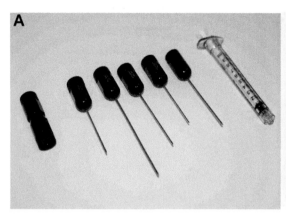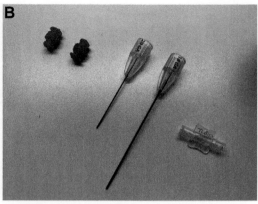

Fig. 18. (*A*, *B*) Fat injection cannulas. Special blunt-tipped cannulas are required to properly perform fat injections, and poor outcomes are typically obtained if sharp hypodermic needles are used. Sharp needle injection also poses a serious risk of fat embolization and related problems. Cannulas used to treat the orbital area range in size from 0.7 mm (20 ga) to 0.9 mm (19 ga) in diameter. (*A*) Reusable cannulas. Shown from left to right are Luer to Luer transfer coupling, injection cannulas ranging in diameter from 0.7 mm (20 ga) to 0.9 mm (19 ga) and 4 to 6 cm long, and Luer lock syringe. (*B*) Single-use disposable fat injection cannulas. High-quality single-use disposable cannulas and supplies make fat grafting convenient and preclude the need for time-consuming cleaning, reprocessing, and resterilization of reusable equipment. These are available in a variety of diameters and lengths (not shown are single-use harvesting cannulas). Shown from left to right are disposable syringe caps to cap the ends of syringes during centrifuging, 0.7-mm (20-gauge) 4-cm long single-use disposable injection cannula, 0.9-mm (19-gauge) 6-cm long single-use disposable injection cannula, single-use disposable Luer lock transfer coupling for transferring fat from 10-mL syringes to 1-mL syringes. (*Courtesy of* Timothy Marten, MD, FACS— Marten Clinic of Plastic Surgery.)

Choosing a Fat Donor Site

Currently there is no clinical or scientific unanimity as to where the "best" fat for grafting is obtained, and scientific literature variously claims several areas as the optimal donor site. Because of this donor sites are typically chosen and marked in accord with the patient to improve their figure. For women this typically includes the hips, waist, flank, outer thigh, and abdomen and for men the "love handle" and "spare tire" areas.

It is prudent to examine the patient at the time of their consultation to ensure they have

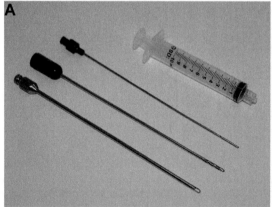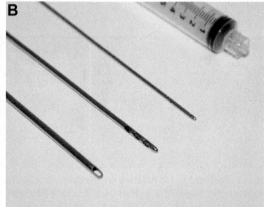

Fig. 19. (*A*, *B*) Fat harvesting cannulas. (*A*) Special harvesting cannulas are attached to 10 cc Luer Lock syringes and are used to atraumatically extract fat from donor sites using gentle hand applied suction. Fat harvested with these cannulas easily passes through injection cannulas as small as 0.7 mm (20 ga). Shown from top down: (1) 10 cc Leur lock syringe, (2) 1.6 mm by 20 cm local anesthetic infiltration cannula, (3) 2.4 mm Tulip "tri-port" harvesting cannula, and (4) 2.4 mm Coleman harvesting cannula. (*B*) Close-up of instrument tips. Shown from top down: (1) 10 cc Leur lock syringe, (2) infiltration cannula, (3) Tulip harvesting cannula, and (4) Coleman harvesting cannula. (*Courtesy of* Timothy Marten, MD, FACS – Marten Clinic of Plastic Surgery.)

A **B**

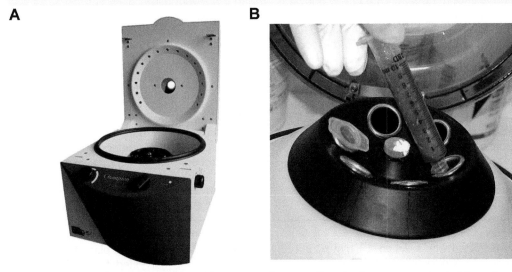

Fig. 20. (*A, B*) Centrifuging fat. Harvested fat is generally not uniform in character as extracted from donor sites, as each syringe will contain a variable amount of fat, blood, local anesthetic, and ruptured fat cells ("oil") and some type of processing is necessary to obtain uniform material for injection. Centrifugation allows separation of the "oil" and "water" fractions from the fat cells. (*A*) Small portable countertop centrifuge. (*B*) Close-up view of centrifuge rotor being loaded with unprocessed fat in 10 cc syringes. Note that the syringe tip has been sealed with a disposable plastic cap. The removable and sterilizable metal sleeves shown fit into rotor to keep syringe barrels containing fat sterile and allow them to be handled on the sterile field after spinning. Other centrifuges are designed to allow the entire rotor to be sterilized. (*Courtesy of* Timothy Marten, MD, FACS – Marten Clinic of Plastic Surgery.)

adequate fat for harvest, unless it is obvious that plentiful donor fat is present. Thin patients with limited fat stores or patients who have undergone prior body lifts, liposuction, cryolipolysis, or noninvasive fat reduction procedures may have compromised donor fat and often present significant challenges when harvesting fat. Extra time and effort is required to obtain fat from them. Anesthesia and operating room (OR) times, and the anesthesiologist, surgeon, and facility fee, are adjusted accordingly.

Preoperative Marking of the Face

Fat injections cannot be made arbitrarily, and a careful plan must be marked preoperatively with the patient seated in the upright position. It is not possible to optimally mark the patient supine after anesthesia has begun. Creating an initial plan on a life-sized laser print of a photograph of the patient's face in yellow "highlighter" marker is helpful in organizing one's thoughts and facilitates discussions with the patient as to which areas are to be treated. In most cases marks are made with the patient while they hold a hand mirror. The goal is to create a topographic map of the deficient and atrophic areas of the orbital and periorbital areas to guide the surgeon during the procedure (a reverse

plan as marked for liposuction). Marking prominences and facial landmarks that do not need fat is helpful.

Harvesting Fat

Fat should be harvested in a thoughtful and artistic manner that improves the patient's figure. It is generally removed bilaterally and in a symmetric fashion unless body contours dictate otherwise. Patients are advised that fat harvest is not a formal liposuction and that the small instruments used to harvest fat are not capable of making large improvements in body contour.

Fat is harvested after anesthesia is induced but before the facial prep. Rarely is a complete prep of the torso necessary. In most cases a limited prep of the marked area is made and a sterile field is established about the prepped area with adhesive-edged sterile blue paper drape towels. The surgeon and assistant need not wear a gown for this part of the procedure, as sterile gloves are adequate in maintaining sterile technique for this part of the procedure.

In the deeply sedated or general anesthetic patient, areas from which fat is to be harvested are conservatively infiltrated with 0.1% lidocaine with 1:1,000,000 epinephrine solution using a specially designed multiholed 1.6 mm × 20 cm-long local anesthetic infiltration cannula (see **Fig. 19**), and an adequate time is allowed for anesthetic and hemostatic effect. Approximately 1 mL of this local anesthetic solution is injected for every 3 mL of anticipated fat removal. It is not necessary or desirable to infiltrate in a tumescent fashion, as overwetting the donor site will result in an overdilute harvest and more time spent in the harvesting process. Local anesthetic is injected, even if a deep sedation or a general anesthetic is used, to limit the overall amount of anesthetic and narcotic given. In the awake or lightly sedated patient, the skin puncture site is anesthetized with a small amount of 0.5% lidocaine with epinephrine and the harvest area with 0.25% lidocaine with epinephrine.

Fat is harvested with a 2.1 to 2.4 mm "Carraway", "Tri-port", "Coleman", or others as harvesting cannula attached to a 10 mL syringe using gentle, gradually applied syringe suction to avoid vacuum barotrauma to the fat. In the awake or lightly sedated patient the smaller 2.1 mm harvesting cannula is used. Fat harvested with these cannulas will easily pass through 0.7 mm (20 ga) injection cannulas, and the use of a smaller harvesting cannula is not necessary and will needlessly slow the harvesting process. In general, a 30% to 50% "overharvest" is made to ensure an adequate supply of processed (centrifuged and separated) fat for use in the periorbital areas, as centrifuging (see later discussion) typically reduces the fat volume by 30% to 50%.

Once fat harvest is complete, the stab incisions made for fat harvest are closed with interrupted 6-0 nylon or other suture of choice. The harvest site is cleansed of prep solution and the sutured site dressed with a TegaDerm dressing. Attention is turned to the opposite side where a similar harvest is made.

Processing Harvested Fat

Harvested fat is not uniform in character and concentration as extracted from donor sites. Each syringe contains a variable amount of fat, blood, local anesthetic, and ruptured fat cells ("oil"). Processing is necessary to obtain homogeneous material (uniform number of fat cells per unit volume) for injection. Although fat can be separated from the oil and water fractions using a "tea strainer" type sieve or by rolling on Telfa gauze, most of the "growth factors" and "cellular messengers" are likely lost when this is done. It is also now known that not all fat cells are the same and that the "high-density adipocytes" are the most "stem cell" rich. Processing fat through a sieve or by

rolling it on Telfa gauze does not segregate and concentrate these high-density fat cells.

Centrifugation as advocated by Coleman however allows removal of the "oil" (fat cells ruptured during the harvest process) and "water" (blood and local anesthetic) fractions from the fat cells while concentrating these other potentially important components and has been our favored method of fat processing for 3 decades. Centrifugation also concentrates the high-density adipocytes, allowing the surgeon to use this fat, which is thought to be superior in quality and richer in "stem cells" for grafting into critical areas such as the orbits and lips or even the entire face if an adequate "overharvest" of fat is made.

Before centrifugation is begun a sterile disposable plastic Leur Lock cap is placed on each syringe tip to keep harvested fat inside, and the syringe plunger is removed from the syringe barrel. Capped syringe barrels containing unprocessed fat are loaded into the centrifuge rotor in a balanced fashion and spun for 1 to 3 minutes at 1000 to 3000 RPM. Most small, portable centrifuges available for this purpose are inexpensive and have rotors that can be sterilized so that the syringe barrels containing the fat remain sterile and can be brought back on the sterile surgical field after centrifugation is complete. Others centrifuges have sterilizable sleeves that are inserted into the rotor (see **Fig. 20**).

After centrifugation syringe barrels containing centrifuged fat are removed and contain an upper oil (ruptured fat cells), central fat (the material the surgeon seeks), and lower "water" (blood and local anesthetic) components (see **Fig. 21**).

The "water" component is separated by simply removing the syringe tip cap and allowing it to run out. The cap is then replaced. Alternatively, the "platelet plug" is sequestered and mixed back with the fat or injected separately into areas of the face, hands, and chest that have sustained solar and environmental damage over time. The oil fraction is poured off from the top of the syringe. Telfa sponges can also be placed inside the syringe barrel to wick up the residual oil present after the most of it is poured off. If fat overharvest is made, this wicking off of residual oil with Telfa sponges is not performed, and the top 1 or 2 mL of fat from each syringe is discarded, or in the very thin patient it is reinjected back into the body at an appropriate site and "banked." A rack to hold the syringes containing fat greatly facilitates fat processing activities. This rack also holds 1 mL syringes and other equipments used in the fat grafting procedure.

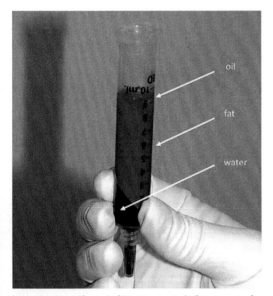

Fig. 21. Centrifuged fat. Harvested fat seen after centrifugation. Three layers can be seen in the centrifuged material: an upper "oil" layer (ruptured fat cells), a middle layer of intact fat cells, and a bottom layer of blood and local anesthetic. Unlike straining of fat through a "tea strainer" sieve or rolling it on Telfa gauze, centrifugation is believed to allow separation of the "oil" and "water" fractions from the fat cells with minimal loss of "stem cells," "PRP," "growth factors," and "cellular messengers." Centrifugation also allows high density fat (bottom 2 cc of fat in center of syringe) with increased "stem cell" activity to be separated and preferentially used if desired. (*Courtesy of* Timothy Marten, MD, FACS – Marten Clinic of Plastic Surgery.)

Patients with Previous Filler Use

Patients who have undergone previous filler injections present a challenge to the surgeon performing fat grafting procedures in the periorbital area and are arguably recognized as suboptimal candidates for surgery. Often more filler is present than patients are aware of or admit to, and the filler hides the extent of the actual deformity. The presence of residual filler also likely compromises graft survival, makes a uniform take less likely, and compromises the outcome of the procedure. Experience has shown that even fillers placed several years previously in the periorbital area make procedures more difficult and the outcomes less predictable.

Filler patients are a "moving target" and can be difficult to assess and treat. Hyaluronic acid get (HAG) fillers can be dissolved with hyaluronidase (Vitrase, Wydase, Hylenex), and it is recommended that HAG filler be dissolved several days or more before surgery. If filler is removed at the

time of the procedure, the patient does not have the opportunity to see what they really look like without it, and the extent of the problem is not evident to the surgeon. When HAG filler is dissolved with hyaluronidase, the patient has residual inflammation and is still arguably a suboptimal candidate for fat grafting. Unfortunately, in current times, this situation describes a large group of patients.

Patients with a history of using nonhyaluronic acid–based fillers such as calcium hydroxylapatite (CaHA, Radiesse) polymethylmethacrylate, and silicone typically present an even more perplexing problem. Poly-L-lactic acid (PLLA) filler use is particularly problematic because of the chronic inflammation, internal fibrosis, and related tissue compromise this material causes. Past and present filler patients should be informed that they are more likely to have impaired fat graft survival, uneven fat take, and need multiple staged fat graft treatments.

Injecting Fat

After centrifugation and removal of the oil and water fractions (and high-density fat segregated, if desired), the fat is transferred into 1 mL Luer lock syringes using a transfer coupling or other method, as proper injection in very small aliquots as required cannot be made with a 10 cc, 5 cc, or 3 cc syringe.

Anesthesia for the Face

Nerve blocks are performed on the periorbital face with 0.25% bupivicaine with epinephrine 1:200,000 local anesthetic solution, and an adequate time is allowed for anesthetic and hemostatic effect. It is typically not necessary to directly infiltrate areas to be grafted with local anesthetic if nerve blocks are performed correctly and sedation is administered, and fat is typically infiltrated into "dry" recipient areas. In the awake or lightly sedated patient areas to receive fat are conservatively infiltrated with 0.5% lidocaine with epinephrine to ensure patient comfort.

Once nerve blocks and local anesthetic are administered, 0.7 mm (20 ga) and 0.9 mm (19 ga) cannulas are used to infiltrate fat into the periorbital area transcutaneously through small stab incisions depending on the areas being treated (see **Figs. 24-28**).

Fat infiltration is preformed in multiple passes, in specific planes appropriate for the area being treated, injecting on the in- and out-strokes while moving the cannula rapidly back and forth and feathering into adjacent areas. Injecting from at least 2 separate injection sites allows "crisscrossing" of cannula passes during graft placement and smoother and more uniform fat infiltration and helps avert a "corn row" effect that might result if injection is from only one site.

Determining How Much Fat to Inject

Unless one is willing to submit to a long process of trial and error, determining how much fat needs to be injected at a given site requires empirical information provided by others who have experience with the procedure. One cannot simply rely on one's intuition or what one sees in the OR. There is a tendency to treat most areas too conservatively if fat volumes are decided by intuition and observation alone, and some "overcorrection" is needed, as not all of the graft will survive. A larger volume of fat is also needed than one would use to fill a similar defect with nonautologous filler.

A prudent strategy for determining the amount of fat that is injected at a given site is to rate the severity of the atrophy for each periorbital region based on the preoperative photos and then use empirical published data to choose the amount administered to each area. As a practical matter this amounts simply to rating or categorizing the severity of atrophy at each proposed site of treatment as "small", "medium," and "large," and then using published data as a guide for the volume

needed for treatment of each area. If the degree of atrophy is "small" one would choose an amount from the low end of the recommended range. If the degree of atrophy is "large" one would choose an amount from the high end and if "medium" somewhere in between. The authors' recommended ranges for amounts of fat needed in the periorbital area for the technique described herein are provided in **Fig. 22** and **Table 1**.

These parameters are guidelines and not absolutes. Considerations such as what equipment was used, how the fat was harvested, how it was processed, how it was injected, and the condition of the tissues receiving the fat all influence the amounts needed and eventual outcomes. Patients who are smokers or previous smokers and patients who have undergone previous noninvasive radiofrequency and ultrasonic "skin shrinking" procedures may have compromised subdermal microcirculation and are suboptimal candidates for fat grafting. They will likely need more fat than nonsmokers and patients who have not undergone these treatments. Similarly, patients who are longstanding filler users, especially inflammatory fillers such as PLLA, are likely to have internal facial fibrosis and inflammatory changes rendering them suboptimal candidates as well for fat grafting. These patients also will require larger fat volumes to obtain an equivalent result. It is also the

Marten Clinic of Plastic Surgery – Peri-orbital Fat Grafting Region and Volume Guidelines

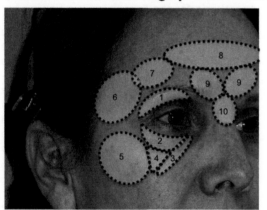

Anatomic Region	Volume of Fat[a]
1) supra-orbital	1-3 cc per side
2) infra-orbital	1-3 cc per side
3) naso-jugal groove ("tear trough")	0.5-1.5 cc per side
4) mid-face	1-3 cc per side
5) cheek	3-7 cc per side
6) temple	3-7 cc per side
7) supra-brow	1-3 cc per side
8) forehead	4-8 cc (total both sides)
9) glabella	1-3 cc (total both sides)
10) radix	1-3 cc (total both sides)

[a] amounts listed above are for fat harvested with a 2.1 to 2.4 mm harvesting cannula centrifuged for 1-3 min at 1,000 rpm administered to average sized female head in 0.5 cc or less aliquots using a 0.7 to 0.9 mm injection cannula. Larger amounts may be required for un-centrifuged or "tea strained" fat is used

Fig. 22. Anatomic regions and summary of range of volumes typically used to treat facial areas. Amounts listed are for fat harvested with a 2.1 to 2.4 mm harvesting cannula centrifuged for 1 to 3 min at 1000 rpm administered to average-sized female head in 0.5 cc or less aliquots using 1 cc syringe as part of a facelift procedure. Larger amounts may be required for uncentrifuged or "tea strained" fat, larger female faces, male patients, and patients not undergoing facelift procedures. The strategy for determining the amount of fat needed for a given site is to *rate the severity of atrophy based on what is seen in the preoperative photos* at each proposed site of treatment as "small," "medium," and "large" and then using data above to determine the amount typically needed for treatment of each area. If the defect is "small" one would choose an amount from the low end of the recommended range. If the defect is "large" one would choose an amount from the high end and if "medium" somewhere in between. (*Courtesy of* Timothy Marten, MD, FACS – Marten Clinic of Plastic Surgery.)

Table 1
Marten clinic of plastic surgery—periorbital fat grafting OR reference guidelines

Area (Region on Illustration)	Cannula Size/Length	Tissue Plane	Amount (per Side) (Except as Noted)	Special Considerations (Parenthetic Comment Is Degree of Difficulty)
Forehead (20)	0.7 mm (20 ga)/5 cm	preperiosteal preferred subcutaneous if forehead lift	2–4 cc	Most often treating depression in mid-central area and not entire forehead (intermediate)
Supra-brow (2)	0.7 mm (20 ga)/5 cm	preperiosteal preferred subcutaneous if forehead lift	1–3 cc	Goal is to blend prominent brow with forehead (intermediate)
Glabella (3)	0.7 mm (20 ga)/4 cm	Subcutaneous	1–3 cc* (total)	GF lines are not effectively treated wAFG unless neurotoxin also used (intermediate)
Radix (4)	0.7 mm (20 ga)/4 cm	Preperiosteal to skin	1–3 cc* (total)	Can be continued on bridge of nose if inverted V or rhinoplasty irregularities present (19) (intermediate)
Temples (1)	0.9 mm (19 ga)/5 cm	Subcutaneous	3–7 cc	Larger cannula less likely to perforate temporal veins. If vein perforated hold pressure on area for 3–5 min and may then resume injections (intermediate)
Brow-supraorbital ("upper eyelid") (5)	0.7 mm (20 ga)/4 cm	Preperiosteal/ suborbicularis oculi	1–3 cc	Conceptualize as *lowering the supraorbital rim* not filling the eyelid. Must protect ocular globe during fat infiltration (advanced)
Infraorbital ("lower eyelid") (6)	0.7 mm (20 ga)/4 cm	Preperiosteal/ suborbicularis oculi	1–3 cc	Important to inject perpendicularly from below rather than parallel to defect. Must protect ocular globe during fat infiltration (advanced)
Nasojugal groove ("tear trough") (7)	0.7 mm (20 ga)/4 cm	Preperiosteal/ suborbicularis oculi	0.5–1.5 cc	Important to inject perpendicularly from below rather than parallel to defect (advanced)

(*continued on next page*)

Table 1
(continued)

Area (Region on Illustration)	Cannula Size/Length	Tissue Plane	Amount (per Side) (Except as Noted)	Special Considerations (Parenthetic Comment Is Degree of Difficulty)
Cheeks (9)	0.7 mm (20 ga)/5 cm	Preperiosteal to skin	3–7 cc	Must consider shape of forehead, prominence of chin, and width of mandible. If temples are hollow and not treated filling cheeks will look unnatural. Some of this fat will typically be encountered during subsequent SMAS dissection (beginner)
Midface (8)	0.7 mm (20 ga)/4 cm	Preperiosteal to skin	1–3 cc	Overlaps infraorbital, tear trough, and cheek areas (beginner)

Important notes regarding recommended amounts:

(1) Amounts listed in table are amount administered *per side* except where noted with asterisk and "(total)."

(2) Amounts listed in table are for fat harvested with a 2.1–2.4 mm harvesting cannula centrifuged for 1–3 min at 1000 rpm administered to average-sized female head in 0.5 cc aliquots as part of a facelift procedure. Larger amounts may be required for uncentrifuged or "tea strained" fat, larger female faces, male patients, patients who have had radio-frequency and ultrasonic "skin shrinking" treatments, and patients not undergoing facelift procedures.

(3) A prudent strategy for determining the amount of fat needed for a given site is to *rate the severity of atrophy present based on what is seen in the preoperative photos and then to use empirical data (above) to chose the amount to be administered.* As a practical matter this amounts to simply rating the severity of the problem at each proposed site of treatment as "small," "medium," and "large" and then using data above to determine the amount typically needed for treatment of each area. If the amount of atrophy present is "small" one would choose an amount from the low end of the recommended range. If the amount present is "large" one would choose an amount from the high end and if "medium" somewhere in between.

Abbreviation: SMAS, superficial musculoaponeurotic system.

case that the thoughtful surgeon performing fat grafting compensates for a large and small face and adjusts the amounts administered accordingly.

The strategy outlined earlier, and the range of recommended volumes to administer, serves as a time-tested starting point that will shorten the learning curve for the surgeon learning fat grafting and serves as a point of reference from which one develops their own range of volumes with experience and over time.

Injection Technique

Approximately 0.05 mL or less is injected per back-and-forth cannula pass. This corresponds to 20 to 40 back and forth passes for each 1 mL syringe of centrifuged fat. The goal is to inject the fat in a way that scatters it in planes and place of administration that optimizes its chance of developing a blood supply and surviving. Fat injected in a bolus fashion leaves fat cells bunched together, and only those on the periphery will have

tissue contact and are likely to survive. The centrally situated fat particles will only have contact with each other and are less likely to survive and may lead to oil cysts and contour irregularities. The procedure should be thought of as analogous to "spray painting," not "caulking."

The beginning injector typically moves the cannula back and forth too slowly as fat is infiltrated, but as familiarity with the technique is acquired the movements can and should be made faster.

All other things being equal, faster back and forth movements and when the injection cannula is kept in constant motion, a significant intravascular injection is less likely, and an accidental bolus injection into one area is avoided. Rapid back and forth movements ensure the smoothest, safest, and most uniform infiltration and distribution of fat.

How the syringe is held is also important in controlling the volume expressed from the cannula with each pass and avoiding overinjection. If the syringe is held in the manner one would typically use to give a filler or other injection (with the thumb on the end of the syringe plunger) it is easy to un-intentionally inject too much fat if tissue resistance suddenly changes. More control is maintained, and overinjection more easily avoided, if the sy-ringe is held with the end of the plunger in the palm of the hand (**Fig. 23**). With practice, a slight closing of the hand when the syringe is held this way results in a small amount of fat being expressed from the cannula, and overinjection of any one area is more readily avoided. The flow of fat can be further controlled when the syringe is held in this way if thumb pressure is placed on the syringe plunger where it enters the syringe bar-rel (see **Fig. 23**B); this is particularly useful in the periorbital area where uniform and precise infiltra-tion of fat is of greater importance. Smaller can-nulas also help avoid bolus injection, as their small diameter physically limits how fast fat is extruded from the syringe.

Cannula obstruction is very uncommon if fat is harvested and processed as described. If a can-nula becomes blocked additional injection pres-sure should *not* be applied; this is the most common cause of a sudden and unintentional bolus injection. In such circumstances the blocked cannula should be withdrawn and passed to the surgical assistant to clear, and the surgeon should continue with a different one. Typically, the cause of the obstruction is a particle of fat or subcutane-ous debris inside of the cannula hub that is most readily cleared by removing the cannula and extracting the particle of fat or fragment of tissue debris from inside the cannula hub with a fine-tipped forceps.

In what plane is fat placed?

Fat injections are made in different planes depend-ing on the areas and problems being treated. In areas of the face where multiple tissue layers are present and the overlying skin is thick, injection is made "full thickness" at the treated site from periosteum to the subdermal layer. These areas include the geniomandibular groove (prejowl groove), piriform, midface, cheek, and the chin. In the periorbital area injections are necessarily placed more specifically due to the anatomic char-acteristics of the treated sites, if optimal results are to be obtained and if irregularities are to be avoided. These areas include the temples, which are typically injected subcutaneously, and the up-per orbit, lower orbit, and "tear trough" that are injected in a preperiosteal/suborbicularis oculi deep plane.

Sequencing Fat Injections in Blepharoplasty Procedures

When fat grafting is best performed during surgery the rejuvenate the periorbital area is scientifically unanswered but as a practical matter it is most expedient to inject fat at the *beginning* of the pro-cedure before the forehead lift and blepharoplasty. It is easier to harvest the fat at the beginning of the procedure before the face is prepped or draped and when the patient is in a deeper plane of anes-thesia. In the beginning of the procedure the tissue planes of the upper face and periorbital areas have not been opened, the face is not swollen, and pre-operatively made pen marks and facial landmarks are easier to see. Surgical principles suggest that it

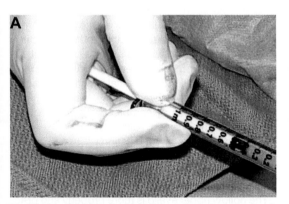 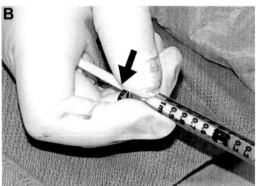

Fig. 23. (*A, B*) Method of holding syringe to control volume released during injection. (*A*) If the syringe is held in the way one would typically use to give an injection, it is easy to infiltrate too much fat if tissue resistance sud-denly changes. More control can be maintained, and overinjection better avoided, if the syringe is held with the end of the plunger in the palm of the hand. Held in this manner a slight closing of the hand results in a small amount of fat only being expressed. (*B*) The flow of fat can further be controlled when the syringe is held in this way if thumb pressure is placed on the syringe plunger (white plastic in this photo) at the point where it en-ters the syringe barrel (clear plastic) at the point designated by the black arrow. (*Courtesy of* Timothy Marten, MD, FACS – Marten Clinic of Plastic Surgery.)

is best to inject the fat before the incisional part of the procedure to limit the time the graft is out of the body. The most important reason to perform fat grafting first is that the surgeon is more technically and artistically energetic at the beginning of the procedure and will do a better job. If one waits until the end of the procedure (particularly a long facelift procedure), fat grafting will likely be performed with less patience and care.

Particulars of Sites of Treatment

Cheek
Treatment of the cheek is usually performed using access incisions on the cheek and the perioral areas (**Fig. 24**). A 5-cm long 0.7 (20 ga) cannula is used, and fat is placed in all tissue layers between the periosteum and skin. Typically 3 to 7 mL of centrifuged fat is placed in the cheek area, depending on the degree of atrophy present. Occasionally more or less is indicated. Often an asymmetrical placement of fat is required due to malar asymmetry. A guideline for the placement of fat in the cheek area is for the surgeon to imagine filling the area in which one would place a cheek implant. The cheek is a forgiving area and is a good area for the beginning injector to treat.

Midface
Fat grafting of the midface is typically performed with a 4-cm long 0.7 mm (20 ga) cannula from stab incisions on the midinferior medial cheek, and fat is placed in all tissue layers between the periosteum and skin.

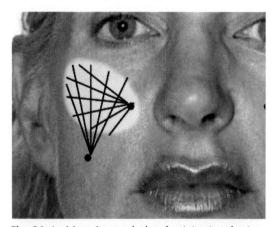

Fig. 24. Incision sites and plan for injecting fat into the cheek area. Fat grafting of the cheeks is typically performed with a 5-cm long 0.7 mm (20 ga) cannula, and fat is placed in all tissue layers between the periosteum and skin in most cases. Typically 3 to 7 cc of centrifuged fat is placed in each check. Level of difficulty: beginner. (Illustration courtesy of Marten Clinic of Plastic Surgery.)

Typically 1 to 3 mL of centrifuged fat is placed in each side, depending on degree of atrophy present. Occasionally more or less is indicated. Fat grafting the midface is intermediate in difficulty.

Temple
The temple areas are usually grafted in a subcutaneous plane from small stab incisions just within the temporal hairline (**Fig. 25**).

Typically 3 to 7 mL of centrifuged fat is placed in the temple area. Occasionally more or less is indicated. In most cases a slightly bigger and blunter 6-cm long 0.9 mm injection cannula is superior to sharper and smaller diameter cannulas preferred elsewhere. Using slightly larger cannulas helps minimize perforation of temporal veins present in the temporal area and allows fat to be placed around them to conceal them.

The injection cannula is not inserted specifically superficial or deep to the temporal veins but passes into the plane of least resistance in the temporal area. Should a temporal vein be inadvertently punctured during injection is a simple matter to hold pressure on the temporal area for a few moments with a surgical sponge. After applying uniform and continuous pressure for a few minutes bleeding stops and treatment of the area is completed. Treating the temple is intermediate in difficulty.

Upper orbit/"upper eyelid"
What layers fat should be placed in the upper orbit ("upper eyelid") is the subject of some debate. Subcutaneous, suborbicularis oculi, and even subseptal (intraorbital) locations have all been advocated and used safely and effectively by various surgeons. For the beginning injector it is safest to avoid the subseptal area due to the risk of intraorbital and retrobulbar bleeding and other problems. It is also wise to avoid a purely subcutaneous injection in this area due to the extremely thin skin present and limit initial injections to a preperiosteal/suborbicularis oculi location. After almost 4 decades of combined experience both authors still inject almost strictly in a preperiosteal–preseptal location.

A common misconception in treating the hollow upper orbit is that the fat is needed and should be injected in the preseptal portion of the eyelid itself. The hollow upper eyelid is more properly and practically restored by placing fat in a preorbital position along the anterior-inferior margin of the supraorbital rim. The process is best conceptualized as a *lowering of the inferior margin of the supraorbital rim* and filling the upper orbital area, lowering skin that has retracted up into the orbit down onto the preseptal eyelid. This process

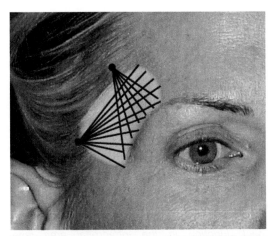

Fig. 25. Incision sites and plan for injecting fat into the temple areas. Injection of the temples is performed with a 5-cm long 0.9 mm (19 ga) cannula, and fat is placed in a subcutaneous plane. The medium-sized 0.9 mm cannula reduces the likelihood that temporal veins are inadvertently perforated. Typically 3 to 7 cc of centrifuged fat is placed on each side. Level of difficulty: intermediate. (Illustration courtesy of Marten Clinic of Plastic Surgery.)

creates a full and appropriately creased and youthful appearing upper eyelid. Once one accepts that improvement is obtained by injection of the orbit, and not the eyelid itself, it becomes apparent that larger volumes than might otherwise be expected are required. The smaller injection cannulas now available make injecting the upper orbit easier and more predictable, as they are advanced more smoothly and accurately through tissues and allow the deposition of very tiny aliquots of fat per pass. It is highly recommended that small cannulas be used to treat this area. A 4-cm long 0.7 mm (20 ga) cannula Is preferred, and 1 to 3 mL of centrifuged fat is placed in each upper orbit to achieve the improvement typically required. On occasion more or less is indicated.

When fat grafting the upper orbit, it should always be kept in mind that one is working in very close proximity to the eye. Although the injection cannulas are blunt tipped, they are small and capable of perforating the ocular globe. In light of this, injections puncture sites are placed in such a way that the injection cannula is passed parallel to the globe and the supraorbital rim and not perpendicular to it **(Fig. 26)**.

Directing the cannula toward the globe when injecting the upper orbit is potentially dangerous and is avoided. In addition, the surgeon should always have the index finger of the nondominant (noninjecting) hand held firmly on the inferior margin of the supraorbital rim as the cannula is passed into

tissues and injection is made, and this finger is always kept between the tip of the cannula and the globe.

The finger is positioned so that the cannula hits against it instead of penetrating the globe if inadvertently misdirected. Having one's finger in this position also gives important feedback to the injector as to where the tip of the cannula is and helps one place fat as accurately as possible. A shorter 4-cm long cannula is easier to control and keep in the correct plane on the inferior margin of the supraorbital rim and is used in preference to longer instruments.

Fat grafting the upper orbit and "eyelid" is intermediate to advanced in difficulty, and treatment of this area should be made after experience has been gained treating more forgiving areas. The key to avoiding problems is to stay deep in a suborbicularis oculi/preperiosteal plane and not to make any superficial injections. As surgeons come to appreciate the utility and gain familiarity with fat grafting the upper orbit, it will be recognized as one of the most artistically rewarding uses of autologous fat and one that is likely to become a routine part of rejuvenating the upper eyelid.

"Tear trough"

Fat grafting of the "tear trough" area is performed through peri-alar stab incisions on the medial midface using a 4-cm 0.7 mm (20 ga) injection cannula

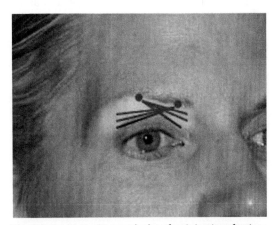

Fig. 26. Incision sites and plan for injecting fat into the upper orbital ("upper eyelid") area. Injection of the upper orbital area is performed with a 4-cm long 0.7 mm cannula, and fat is placed in a suborbicularis oculi/preperiosteal plane. Typically 1 to 3 cc of centrifuged fat is placed in each upper orbit but occasionally more is indicated. The process is best conceptualized as one of *lowering the inferior margin of the supraorbital rim,* not filling the eyelid itself. Level of difficulty: intermediate. (Illustration courtesy of Marten Clinic of Plastic Surgery.)

and fat placed deep in a preperiosteal/suborbicularis oculi plane as when the infraorbital area is treated (**Fig. 27**A). Typically 0.5 to 1.5 mL of centrifuged fat is placed on each side depending on how far inferiorly and laterally the "tear trough" extends onto the cheek. A smoother effect is obtained and an unaesthetic "sausage" roll or "banana" bulge less likely when fat is injected perpendicular rather than parallel to the defect (**Fig. 27**B).

Another guideline for the placement of fat in the tear trough area is for the surgeon to imagine filling the area in which one might place a tear trough implant, as the goal of treatment is essentially the same. Treating the tear trough area is advanced in difficulty and is best undertaken after the surgeon has gained experience in treating less demanding areas. It is best to practice on other less demanding areas before trying to treat this site. It is key to stay deep in a suborbicularis oculi/preperiosteal plane and not to make any superficial injections. Treating the tear trough is advanced in difficulty.

Lower orbit/"lower eyelid" area

Injecting the infraorbital (lower eyelid) area is analogous to injecting the upper orbit in that there are similar misconceptions as to where the fat should be placed, similar technical considerations as to which tissue layers fat should be injected into, and similar concerns regarding potential injury to the ocular globe. In addition, and as is the case in treating the upper orbit, fat need not and should not be injected in the pretarsal eyelid. Fat is injected deep in a suborbicularis oculi/

preperiosteal plane, and *the technical goal of the procedure is raising up and anteriorly projecting the infraorbital rim rather than filling the lid itself.* And like the upper orbit, volumes required to obtain corrections in the lower orbit are more than one might intuitively expect, with 1 to 3 mL usually necessary to produce the desired effect. Unlike the upper orbit, experience shows that fat is best and most easily injected, and a "banana" or "sausage roll" (unaesthetic bulge) is less likely to occur, if injection is made from injection sites on the midcheek *perpendicular* to the infraorbital rim (**Fig. 28**). When fat is injected in this manner lumps and irregularities are also less common.

Fat should not be injected parallel to the lid–cheek junction in the infraorbital area (see **Fig. 28**B). It is our observation that surgeons injecting fat parallel to the infraorbital rim have more trouble getting fat into the proper plane and location and have more problems with irregularities, "lumps" and "bumps," "sausage-" and "banana"-shaped bulges, and other untoward results.

As is the case in injecting the upper orbit, when injecting the lower orbit the surgeon should place their index fingertip of the noninjecting hand firmly on the infraorbital rim to protect the ocular globe while injections are made. This fingertip is always kept between the tip of the cannula and the globe.

The idea is to position the fingertip so that the cannula would hit against it instead of penetrating the globe if inadvertently overadvanced. Having one's fingertip in this position also gives important feedback to the injector as to where the tip of the cannula

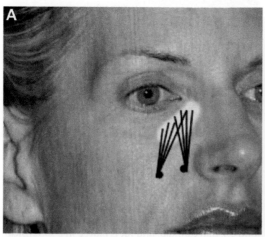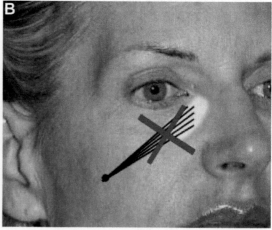

Fig. 27. (*A, B*) Correct (*A*) and incorrect (*B*) plan for injecting fat into the nasojugal ("tear trough") areas. (*A*) Fat grafting of the nasojugal "tear trough" area is typically performed with a 4-cm 0.7 mm (20 ga) injection cannula, and fat is placed deep in a preperiosteal/suborbicularis oculi plane. Typically 0.5 to 1.5 cc of centrifuged fat is placed on each side depending on how far inferiorly and laterally the "tear trough" extends onto the cheek. A smoother effect is obtained and a "sausage" roll (unaesthetic bulge) less likely when fat is injected perpendicular (*A*) rather than parallel (*B*) to the defect. Level of difficulty: advanced. (Illustration courtesy of Marten Clinic of Plastic Surgery.)

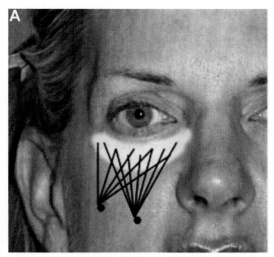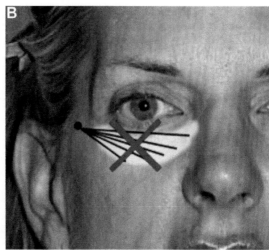

Fig. 28. (*A*, *B*) Correct (*A*) and incorrect (*B*) plan for injecting fat into infraorbital ("lower eyelid") area. Fat grafting of the infraorbital area is typically performed with a 4-cm long 0.7 mm (20 ga) cannula, and fat is placed deep in a suborbicularis oculi/preperiosteal plane. More superficial injections should be avoided. Typically 1 to 3 cc of centrifuged fat is placed on each side, but occasionally more or less is indicated. A smoother effect is obtained, and a "banana" or "sausage" (unaesthetic bulge) is less likely when fat is injected perpendicular (*A*) rather than parallel (*B*) to the infraorbital rim. Level of difficulty: advanced. (Illustration courtesy of Marten Clinic of Plastic Surgery.)

is and helps one place fat as accurately as possible. And as is the case when injecting the upper orbit, a shorter 4-cm long cannula is easier to control and keep in the correct plane on the infraorbital rim and is used in preference to longer instruments.

As the injection cannula is advanced perpendicular to the orbit and toward the fingertip in a suborbicularis/preperiosteal plane through infraorbital tissues, the origin of the zygomatico cutaneous and orbicularis retaining ligaments can be felt along the infraorbital rim and the cannula tip allowed to penetrate them. Typically after multiple back and forth cannula movements used in the placement of fat in this manner no resistance is felt along the course of the ligaments, and it is assumed that the multiple passes used to place the graft have effectively partially released them, improving the overall outcome. Another guideline for the placement of fat in the infraorbital area is for the surgeon to imagine filling the area in which one might place an infraorbital implant, as the goal of treatment is similar.

It is wise to avoid any subcutaneous injection in the infraorbital area due to the extremely thin skin present and the likelihood of creating visible lumps and irregularities and to limit injections to a preperiosteal/suborbicularis oculi plane until considerable experience is obtained. Treating the infraorbital area is advanced in difficulty and is best undertaken after the surgeon has gained experience in treating less demanding areas. The key to avoiding problems is to stay deep in a

suborbicularis occuli/preperiosteal plane and not to make any superficial injections.

Final touches

Periorbital fat injections are continued until the preoperatively determined volume of fat is added to each target area. A 1- to 3-fold "overcorrection" is made as compared with volumes one would use if HAG fillers are used, but typically the patient does not look overfilled on the OR table and before swelling sets in. In all, the process is technically and artistically demanding, and its difficulty must be acknowledged. That said, because of its aesthetic importance and the comprehensive treatment of the aging change of the periorbital area missed by traditional blepharoplasty procedures, fat transfer should become enjoyable for the surgeon and yield great benefits to patients so treated.

After fat is infiltrated, treated areas are palpated to ensure that the fat is distributed smoothly in the target tissue, and any lumps or irregularities are gently pressed out. The ocular globe is gently depressed and irregularities checked for in the infraorbital area.

Completion of Concurrently Planned Procedures

On completion of periorbital fat injections attention is turned to the forehead, and other planned procedures are subsequently performed, as indicated. Because properly performed periorbital fat injections are placed in a preseptal location, transconjunctival reduction of protruding ocular fat is performed after fat injections, as is lid skin excision, canthopexy, and even ptosis correction when indicated.

Dressings

No dressing is required or applied.

POSTOPERATIVE CARE

Patients are asked to rest quietly and apply cool compresses applied to their eyes and other treated areas for 15 to 20 minutes of every hour they are awake for the first 3 days after surgery or use a commercially available thermostatically regulated water-cooled mask (Aquecool [www.aqueductmedical.com/]). For most patients, edema peaks on the third or fourth day. Patients are advised *not* to place ice or ice cold compresses directly on their face, as this is likely to be injurious to grafted fat and to compromise outcomes. Patients are provided nonmedicated preservative-free ophthalmic ointment for use at bedtime for 3 weeks and nonmedicated preservative-free tear drops used during the day as required.

RECOVERY AND HEALING

When patients will return to work and their social lives depends on how aggressively their procedure are performed (how much fat injected and where), their tolerance for surgery, their capacity for healing, the type of work they do, the activities they enjoy, their need for secrecy, and how they feel overall about their appearance. Patients are asked to set aside 7 to 10 days, to recover from surgery, and additional time off is recommended before an important business presentation, family gathering, vacation, or like event.

If the patient is doing well and not experiencing problems, they are allowed to travel and return to light office work and casual social activity 7 to 10 days after surgery. If a patient's job entails more strenuous activity or physical labor, a longer period of convalescence is advisable. Patients are advised not to drive for the first 10 days after surgery and until they are feeling well, their vision is clear, and they are no longer taking pain medication. Patients are informed that in some cases it may take 2 to 3 months to have a natural appearance in a photograph or attend an important function.

RETREATMENT

The improvement in contour in the patient's periorbital area seen 4 to 6 months after surgery is due to living fat and comprises a persistent improvement. Patients are generally informed that "what they see is what they get" at that point, as swelling and induration must have largely resolved by that time. Four to six months after surgery is also the point where retreatment is considered, should it be indicated and the patient requests it. Because there is a limit to the amount of fat that is properly infiltrated into the thin atrophic face, the need for secondary fat grafting is not viewed as a failure of the primary procedure, it is simply an inherent limitation of the technique in some circumstances. If the patient achieved improvement with the primary treatment, a secondary procedure is typically equally or more beneficial and often need be far less comprehensive. We advise our patients that although "take" of fat varies, and some patients seem to hold on to more than others, we have never seen a patient receive no benefit from a fat grafting procedure and that even if most of the fat is somehow lost, tens of thousands of "stem cells" are transferred to treated areas, and these would trigger a regenerative effect arguably as important as the volume addition.

COMPLICATIONS

No major complications attributable to fat injections have been seen while performing the procedure over a combined experience of more than 30 years, with no infection, embolization, tissue infarction, visual impairment, or blindness. These devastating problems are reported and are known to occur however when fat injections are performed. Clinical experience has shown that embolization is extremely uncommon when fat is injected in accord with currently recommended technique in which the injection is made with a blunt cannula and the cannula is kept rapidly moving. Embolization and most of the related complications including blindness are reported with sharp needle injection, and these and other complications of fat injections are discussed by Coleman[8] and others.

Complications of fat injections in the periorbital area attributable to the procedure fall largely under the heading of "aesthetic problems" and include lumps, "oil cysts", asymmetries, undercorrection, overcorrection, and donor site irregularities. These are more accurately considered inherent risks of the procedure however in that even if the procedure is technically performed properly and with care, variations in "take" that occur with any graft are beyond the surgeon's control; this is particularly true in the case of a fat graft, as fat is a comparatively fragile tissue.

Certain patients seem to be at higher risk for problems and complications as a result of compromised fat donor and recipient sites. These patients include smokers and former smokers, patients who have undergone previous radiotherapy, and patients who have undergone radiofrequency and ultrasound "skin-shrinking" treatments. Unlike laser resurfacing procedures, where energy is dispersed on the skin surface, these latter procedures disperse energy subcutaneously, which can damage tissue microcirculation and microlymphatics and seem to compromise graft take and healing. Patients who have undergone multiple "skin shrinking" treatments are likely to experience more prolonged edema and swelling with fat grafting. Compromise of a similar sort seems to be present in patients who have had large volumes of inflammatory fillers placed (such as PLLA, CaHA microspheres) and in patients who have had HAG fillers chronically present. Simply dissolving HAG fillers enzymatically with hyaluronidase does not seem to eliminate this problem, as residual inflammation is still present, which can result in suboptimal graft take. All such patients are approached with caution, and it is prudent that they be informed that they are likely to be at an increased risk of problems and complications.

Most complications are small and easily managed if fat injections are performed properly and conservative additions are made. "Oil cysts" are usually simply aspirated or unroofed. Lumps have been exceedingly rare in our practices, but are now being increasingly seen in patients who have been treated by other physicians. These are treated by microliposuction, direct excision, or overgrafting with more fat. Asymmetries and undercorrections are generally treatable by additional fat injections and donor site irregularities with touch-up liposuction and/or fat grafting.

Overcorrection is very uncommon after single treatments and typically only occurs when patients undergo multiple fat grafting procedures. When a patient returns after a single session fat grafting procedure with an overfilled appearance, one should be suspicious that the patient received filler injections from another physician or injector, which is particularly the case if a Tyndall effect (fullness and bluish discoloration in the tear trough and infraorbital area) is present, ridges are seen in the nasolabial creases, or if excess fullness is present in untreated or lightly fat grafted areas. In such cases, it is prudent to consider hyaluronidase administration, as it has been our experience that this may resolve the problem, even if the patient denies having filler recently placed.

When overcorrection occurs following fat grafting, improvement can usually be obtained by judicious extraction of fat from overcorrected areas. In the orbital area, when overcorrection or irregularities are present, treatment depends on the nature of the problem and most importantly, the location of the excess or irregular fat. If fat has been incorrectly placed superficially or in multiple layers in the eyelid, open exploration of the lid will likely be necessary and excess fat removed or reduced as appropriate. When this is carried out in the lower lid it is prudent that a canthopexy and temporary intermarginal tarsorrhaphy be performed and/or a Frost suture be placed (**Fig. 29**).

If fat was appropriately placed deeply in a suborbicularis oculi/preperiosteal plane, excess is removed with judicious microliposuction (placing a 0.7 mm or 0.9 mm infiltration cannula on a 3 cc syringe). Alternatively, the lid is opened, and the surgeon directly contours the suborbicularis oculi/preperiosteal plane using open technique. Typically this is far less disruptive and risky than the necessary delamination of the eyelid when

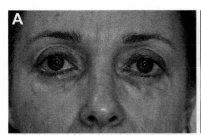 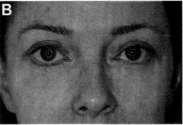 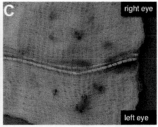

Fig. 29. (*A*) A 57-year-old patient who has undergone previous blepharoplasties and infraorbital fat grafting complicated by lumps and irregularities in the infraorbital area (procedure performed by an unknown surgeon). (*B*) Same patient 1 year and 4 months after lower eyelid exploration, direct excision of fat lumps, canthopexy, and overgrafting with additional fat. Smooth and more regular infraorbital contours are now present. Iatrogenic hollowing of the upper eyelids has also been corrected by fat grating. (The patient has also had facelift, forehead lift, and canthopexy.) (*C*) Fat lumps and particles removed during lid exploration. (Procedure performed by Timothy Marten, MD – courtesy of the Marten Clinic of Plastic Surgery.)

one is removing fat that was injected superficially or in multiple layers (see **Fig. 29**).

The best way to treat complications is to avoid them altogether, and the surgeons with the fewest complications are likely to be the ones who take the time to learn to perform the procedure properly, obtain the necessary equipment to do so, and who introduce fat grafting into their practice in a gradual, conservative manner.

COMMON MISCONCEPTIONS ABOUT THE PERIORBITAL FAT GRAFTING
Doesn't the Fat Go away?

Although many surgeons have come to recognize volume loss as part of the periorbital aging process, some cling to the excuse that "the fat does not last" as a way of not having to learn and perform the fat grafting procedure. This assertion is proved to be meritless and is no longer a valid justification for denying patients the important benefits fat grafting offers. Unlike temporary fillers, fat is living autologous tissue that vascularizes and establishes itself as part of the face. It is analogous to hair transplantation and other grafts performed by surgeons. Furthermore, if the grafts did not persist, there would not be overcorrected patients, and unwanted lumps and irregularities would simply vanish with time.

Isn't the Fat Lumpy?

Asserting that fat grafts are "lumpy" is a common excuse the surgeons use to not learn or perform the procedure, and this too is proved to be false and not a valid excuse to deny the patient the important benefits of fat grafting. If proper technique and equipment are used, lumps and irregularities are far less common than problems and complications seen after almost every other aesthetic surgery procedure we perform. In fact, we regard fat grafting as our "secret weapon" to

obtaining a smooth face. That is not to say that irregularities are not possible. Fat must be injected with meticulous care in the appropriate planes for the areas treated if contour irregularities are to be avoided. Simply put, this means injecting deep in most periorbital areas until considerable experience is obtained.

WHAT IS THE EFFECT OF WEIGHT GAIN OR LOSS?

A large weight gain will compromise any aesthetic surgery procedure, and that is arguably the case with fat grafting as well. Despite this, several anecdotal case reports are endlessly recycled at meetings and conferences regarding patients with large lips, overly full cheeks, and so on as a result of large weight gains after fat grafting. In reality, this is seldom a problem in the periorbital area.

CASE EXAMPLES

Patient example 1 (**Fig. 30**)
A. Preoperative view of a man, aged 51 years, requesting blepharoplasty. He feels he has excess skin and hooding of his lateral upper eyelid palpebral skin folds that needs to be raised and removed. The patient has had no previous plastic surgery.
B. Same patient 1 year and 4 months after fat transfer to the temples, upper and lower orbits, cheeks, and midface. Note periorbital fullness more consistent with a youthful, healthy, and masculine appearance. The upper lid palpebral skin fold has been reconstituted by filling the hollow upper orbit. The pseudohooding of his lateral upper eyelids remains unchanged, and correction has been made by filling the more medially situated "A-frame" hollow and reintegrating the lateral palpebral skin fold with the one

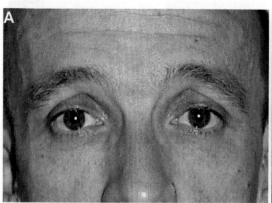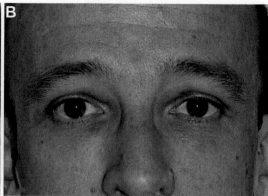

Fig. 30. Patient example 1.

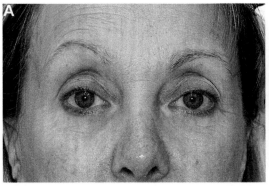
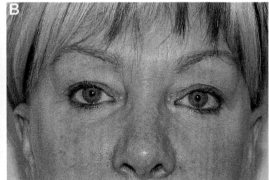

Fig. 31. Patient example 2.

reconstituted more medially. A blepharoplasty would have arguably made his orbits more hollow and aged-appearing and degraded his appearance. (Note also improvement in infraorbital, midface, and cheek areas that additionally optimizes the patient's orbital appearance).

Surgical procedure performed by Timothy Marten, MD, FACS. Courtesy of the Marten Clinic of Plastic Surgery.

Patient example 2 (**Fig. 31**)
A. Preoperative view of a woman, aged 59 years, requesting blepharoplasty. She feels she has a tired appearance and excess skin that needs to be removed on her upper and lower eyelids. The patient has had no previous plastic surgery.
B. Same patient 1 year and 3 months after fat transfer to the temples, upper and lower orbits, cheeks, and midface. She has also undergone a facelift, neck lift, and left hemiforehead lift, but no excisional eyelid surgery (blepharoplasties) was performed. A significant filling of the periorbital area can be seen and her upper eyelid palpebral skin

fold now sits in a more youthful position closer to the ciliary margin that gives her eyes a more youthful and natural appearance. A blepharoplasty would have arguably made her orbits more hollow and aged-appearing and degraded her appearance.

All surgical procedures performed by Timothy Marten, MD, FACS. Courtesy of the Marten Clinic of Plastic Surgery.

Patient example 3: previous blepharoplasty (**Fig. 32**)
A. Preoperative view of a woman, aged 53 years, who has undergone previous blepharoplasties performed by an unknown surgeon. She feels she still appears tired and that her eyes look older and changed.
B. Same patient 1 year and 3 months after fat grafting to the temples, glabella, radix, upper and lower orbits, nasojugal groove, cheeks, and midface. She has also undergone a facelift, neck lift, forehead lift, canthopexy, and laser resurfacing, but no excisional eyelid surgery (blepharoplasties) was performed. A significant filling of the periorbital area can be seen, and her upper eyelid

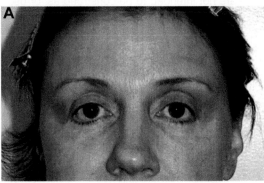
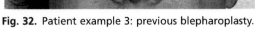
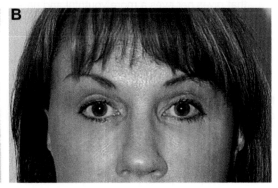

Fig. 32. Patient example 3: previous blepharoplasty.

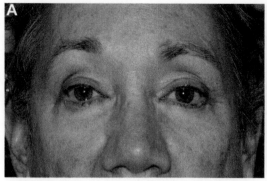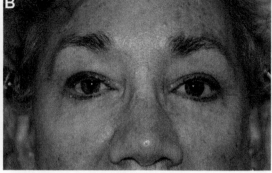

Fig. 33. Patient example 4: previous blepharoplasty.

palpebral skin fold now sits in a more youthful position closer to the ciliary margin that gives her eyes a more youthful and natural appearance. A blepharoplasty would have arguably made her orbits more hollow and aged-appearing and degraded her appearance.

All surgical procedures performed by Timothy Marten, MD, FACS. Courtesy of the Marten Clinic of Plastic Surgery.

Patient example 4: previous blepharoplasty **(Fig. 33)**

A. Preoperative view of a woman, aged 61 years, requesting secondary blepharoplasty. She feels she has a tired and appearance and excess skin that needs to be removed on her upper eyelids (previous procedures performed by an unknown surgeon).

B. Same patient 1 year and 11 months after fat transfer to the temples, upper and lower orbits, cheeks, and midface. She has also undergone a face and neck lift, but no excisional eyelid surgery (blepharoplasties) was performed. A significant filling of the periorbital area can be seen, and her upper eyelid palpebral skin fold now sits in a more youthful position closer to the ciliary margin that gives her eyes a more youthful and natural appearance. A secondary blepharoplasty would have arguably made her orbits more hollow and aged-appearing and degraded her appearance.

All surgical procedures performed by Timothy Marten, MD, FACS. Courtesy of the Marten Clinic of Plastic Surgery.

SUMMARY

Traditional blepharoplasty procedures cannot correct all aspects of the aging change occurring in the periorbital region. Fat grafting allows treatment of age-associated loss of periorbital volume not addressed by traditional blepharoplasty surgery. Fat grafting is the "missing link" in orbital and periorbital rejuvenation, and it stands as the most important addition to surgery to rejuvenate the orbital area since the introduction of the blepharoplasty technique.

Fat grafting is an artistically powerful tool to rejuvenate the periorbital area and results in a more healthy, fit, youthful, sculptural, and sensual appearance than traditional blepharoplasty alone. Fat grafting may result in an improvement in periorbital skin and tissue quality mediated through a stem cell effect. Fat grafting is often more important to rejuvenating the secondary blepharoplasty patient than the revision blepharoplasty. These benefits offset the drawbacks of increased operating time, uncertainty of graft take, and a longer period of recovery associated with the fat grafting procedure.

ACKNOWLEDGMENTS

All figures, illustrations, tables, and descriptions of concepts, methods, and technique included in this article are courtesy of the Marten Clinic of Plastic Surgery and are used with permission. Opinions expressed in this writing are those of the authors and are not intended to be construed as, or used to define, a standard of care.

REFERENCES

1. Marten T, Elyassnia D. Facial fat grafting : why, where, how, and how much. Aesthet Plast Surg 2018;42:5.
2. Marten T, Elyassnia D. Fat injection: a systemic review of injection volumes by facial subunit - discussion article aesthetic. Plast Surg 2018;42:5.
3. Marten T, Elyassnia D. Simultaneous facelift and fat grafting. In: Coleman S, Mazzola R, Pu L, editors. Fat injection from filling to regeneration. NewYork: Thieme Medical Publishers, Inc; 2018.

4. Marten T, Elyassnia D. Simultaneous facelift and fat grafting. In: Connell BF, Sundine MJ, editors. Aesthetic rejuvenation of the face and neck. New York: Thieme Medical Publishers, Inc; 2016.

5. Marten TJ. Facelift: secondary deformities and the secondary facelift. In: Neligan P, Rubin JP, editors. Plastic surgery (aesthetic),, vol. 2, 4th edition. London: Elsevier; 2018.

6. Marten T, Elyassnia D. Fat grafting in facial rejuvenation. In: Pu L, Yoshimura K, Coleman S, editors. Clinics in plastic surgery fat grafting: current concept, clinical application, and regenerative potential, part 1), vol. 42. Philadelphia: Elsevier; 2015. no 2.

7. Marten T, Elyassnia D. Simultaneous facelift and fat grafting: combined lifting and filling of the face. In: Nahai F, editor. Aesthetic plastic surgery. 3rd edition. NewYork: Thieme Medical Publishers, Inc; 2019.

8. Coleman S, Mazzola R, Pu L, editors. Fat injection from filling to regeneration. NewYork: Thieme Medical Publishers, Inc; 2018.

The Spectrum of Aesthetic Canthal Suspension

Yao Wang, MD[a,b], John B. Holds, MD[c], Raymond S. Douglas, MD, PhD[a,b], Guy G. Massry, MD[a,b,d],*

KEYWORDS

- Canthal suspension • Canthoplasty • Canthopexy • Lower blepharoplasty • Lower-eyelid retraction

KEY POINTS

- Canthal suspension can be an important adjunct to lower blepharoplasty surgery.
- Understanding canthal anatomy, nomenclature, and function is an essential element of surgical success.
- The correct canthal suspension procedure selected depends on preoperative findings and the nature of the blepharoplasty procedure performed.
- A canthoplasty is a more complex and powerful procedure, which often leads to more patient complaints than canthopexy.
- Aesthetic canthal suspension surgery has evolved into less invasive procedures, which tend to preserve canthal anatomy and integrity.

INTRODUCTION/PHILOSOPHY

Aesthetic canthal suspension (CS) is an often challenging stand-alone or adjunctive surgical procedure for the facial cosmetic surgeon. The authors believe this is because the procedure, and its variants, receives far too little detailed attention during surgical education (unless subspecialty trained), and because the literature is inconsistent in descriptions of canthal anatomy, nomenclature, and surgical interventions.[1,2] This weakness of surgical education makes operating in this very delicate area of the eyelid cumbersome and intimidating to many. The best way to develop a comfort with canthal surgery is to start at the beginning and attain a detailed and systematic understanding of these aspects of surgery.

Initial descriptions of aesthetic CS surgery surfaced in the 1960s as a means of suspending the lower eyelid as an adjunct to lower blepharoplasty.[1–4] At the time, this surgery was almost

exclusively performed via an open transcutaneous approach.[2,4] Postblepharoplasty lower eyelid retraction (PBLER) was, and still can be, a devastating complication of surgery.[5–11] One of the primary etiologic factors predisposing to PBLER after lower blepharoplasty is unaddressed lower eyelid laxity.[1,2,6,10,11] Because PBLER is a complex revisional procedure and, even in the best and most experienced of hands, often leads to ongoing functional and aesthetic issues and low patient satisfaction,[11] CS has become an important adjunct to aesthetic lower blepharoplasty.[9,12–16]

Some of the early accepted CS procedures involved complete disarticulation of the canthus, plus-minus eyelid shortening, with subsequent canthal reconstruction.[1,2,17,18] These interventions reliably aid in addressing age-related, posttraumatic, and other forms of acquired functional lower eyelid malposition.[17–22] However, whenever the canthus is "taken apart," modified, and reconstructed, it is never the same.[1,2,11] The way the

[a] Beverly Hills Ophthalmic Plastic and Reconstructive Surgery, 150 North Robertson Boulevard #314, Beverly Hills, CA 90211, USA; [b] Department of Plastic Surgery, Division of Oculoplastic Surgery, Cedars Sinai Medical Center, Los Angeles, CA, USA; [c] Ophthalmic Plastic and Cosmetic Surgery, Inc., 12990 Manchester Road, #102, St. Louis, MO 63131, USA; [d] Department of Ophthalmology, Division of Oculoplastic Surgery, Keck School of Medicine, University of Southern California, Los Angeles, CA, USA
* Corresponding author.
E-mail address: gmassry@drmassry.com

Facial Plast Surg Clin N Am 29 (2021) 275–289
https://doi.org/10.1016/j.fsc.2021.01.005
1064-7406/21/© 2021 Elsevier Inc. All rights reserved.

canthus looks, feels, and functions is usually altered.[1,2,11] In functional surgery, patient complaints related to these changes are typically buried in their satisfaction with eyelid repair as their primary problem is resolved. In aesthetic interventions, where the drive for surgery is appearance and well-being, adding a potential canthal compliant to surgery is hazardous, at best, to the surgeon. For example, the patient with an acquired involutional ectropion or entropion who needs such a procedure to relieve symptoms will often forgive a postoperative change in lower lid slant, canthal height disparity, or a minor canthal web. This is not true of the patient seeking cosmetic lower blepharoplasty. When canthal integrity is altered negatively in aesthetic surgery, an elective procedure can lead to functional and cosmetic impairment, which is not an acceptable outcome. This thinking fueled the development of various modifications of canthal surgery, which have evolved into more sophisticated and less-invasive procedures, which are less disruptive of canthal anatomy, and which often access of the canthus through smaller incisions and via distant sites.[1,2,12,23–25] The sole purpose of these modifications is to preserve canthal structure and function as much as possible to reduce the incidence of patient complaints and postoperative complications. This is where the challenge of aesthetic CS surgery surfaces. There is a delicate balance between preserving canthal architecture while performing a procedure that meets the task of supporting the lower eyelid adequately. The aesthetic eyelid surgeon must understand this and evolve in their palate of CS techniques to have success with lower blepharoplasty surgery.[1,2,7,15]

It should also be noted that good CS surgery is not about a belt-and-suspenders tightening of the lower eyelid.[1,2] This is an antiquated view of surgery, which unfortunately is still pervasive today. Eyelid malposition after lower blepharoplasty is more related to poor patient evaluation and selection, and to how the skin, muscle, and fat of the lower lid are addressed, than to the CS procedure performed. No CS procedure can overcome poorly planned and performed blepharoplasty.[1,2,11] Contemporary thought on CS surgery is that it is about creating a physiologic and tension-free degree of lower eyelid support, which acts to re-create a normal canthal angle. It is not about pulling tighter; rather, it is about support and maintaining appearance and integrity. This concept is the first and most basic concept to understand to yield reliable, consistent, and generally complication-free outcomes with aesthetic CS surgery.

In this article, the authors guide the reader through their perspective on canthal terminology, anatomy, aging changes, procedure variants, preoperative evaluation, postoperative course, and complications of surgery. Although this is just 1 view, the authors have found it to be very predictive of good surgical results.

CANTHAL ANATOMY/FUNCTION

The lateral canthal tendon (LCT) is a fibrous continuation of the terminal pretarsal and preseptal (palpebral) orbicularis fibers, which attach to the lateral orbital rim.[1,2,7,26] There is an upper and lower lid contribution to the tendon, the upper crus and the lower crus, which are collectively called crura. The LCT is approximately 1 mm thick, 3 mm wide, and 7 mm in length.[27] It is a 3-dimensional structure with both horizontal and vertical components. Horizontally, it has both an anterior and a posterior component, which attaches to the lateral orbital rim. The most critical attachment is 3 mm posterior to the lateral orbital rim at the Whitnall tubercle, which sits approximately 10 mm below the frontozygomatic suture (**Fig. 1**A).[1,2,7] This posterior horizontal attachment maintains eyelid apposition to the globe and must be re-created surgically to prevent both eyelid and ocular surface deficits. It is also attached anteriorly to the orbital rim to provide a degree of structural integrity to the tendon. The significance of this insertion is far less than the more critical posterior attachment. Vertically, the LCT sits 2 mm higher than the medial canthal tendon, giving rise to the normal canthal tilt.[7,28] If this slant is altered during CS surgery, patient satisfaction is reduced significantly.

Traditional thinking is that the LCT solely provides support to the lower eyelid to maintain its position after surgery. This thought pattern is flawed, which underscores the many facets of this very complicated anatomic structure. The LCT plays a role in upper (not just lower) eyelid position, as it is associated with the orbital septum and the lateral horn of the levator aponeurosis (**Fig. 1**B).[1,2,7] If these structures are imbricated during CS surgery, temporary or permanent ptosis can occur. Similarly, this can occur if the upper crus of the tendon is inadvertently "tucked" in surgery. The tendon plays some role in ocular motility, as the check ligament of the lateral rectus is closely associated with it, leading to a few millimeters of lateral movement of the canthus with globe abduction.[1,2,7,29] There is also a fat pad (Eisler fat pad), which is thought to be distinct from orbital/eyelid fat pads and rests in a pocket between the lateral horn of the aponeurosis and the LCT.[29] Its exact function is

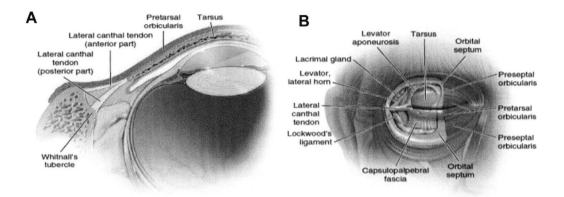

Fig. 1. (*A*) The lateral canthal tendon (LCT) has both an anterior and a posterior attachment to the lateral orbital rim. The posterior attachment is the most critical, as it maintains lower lid apposition to the globe. The posterior attachment site is the Whitnall tubercle. (*B*) Note the proximity of the LCT to other adjacent eyelid structures, including the orbital septum and Levator aponeurosis. (*From* Massry G. and Kossler A. The Spectrum of Canthal Suspension Techniques in Lower Blepharoplasty. In: Azizzadeh B, Murphy M, Johnson C, editors. Master Techniques in Facial Rejuvenation, 2nd edition. Canada: Elsevier; 2018; with permission.)

unknown.[7] The authors believe it may play a role in smooth movement of the aponeurosis over the tendon. Finally, the tendon is an active part of normal eyelid closure. The orbicularis muscle, or eyelid protractor, functions as a sphincter as it passes circumferentially around the eyelid aperture. For normal eyelid closure to occur, the muscle must be anchored medial and lateral by the canthal tendons. When the LCT dehisces or is anchored poorly, eyelid closure changes from a strong and primary vertical excursion (ie, up and down) to one that is weaker with medialization of the lateral canthus with each attempt at closure. This has been referred to as "fishmouthing" (**Fig. 2**)[30] and is presumed to reduce the biomechanical function of the orbicularis sphincter. As such, eyelid closure is deficient. Each described aspect/function of the LCT can be altered by CS surgery, and modern CS should primarily be founded on an understanding of this. Therefore, in the setting of aesthetic canthal surgery, when the correct blepharoplasty procedure

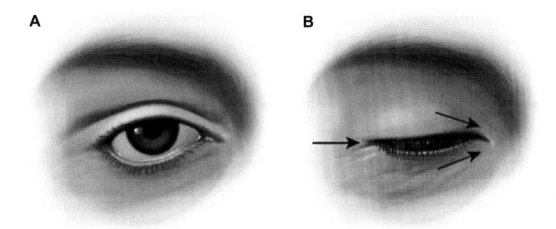

Fig. 2. (*A*) There is poor lateral canthal tendon (LCT) integrity with dehiscence. (*B*) In this scenario, the normal vertical forces applied by the sphincteric action orbicularis oculi biomechanically change as canthal support is lacking, and the lateral canthus medializes with eyelid closure (arrows). This leads to a biomechanical reduction of the strength of eyelid closure and horizontal shortening of the palpebral fissure with eyelid closure. This has been referred to as fishmouthing. (*From* Massry G. and Kossler A. The Spectrum of Canthal Suspension Techniques in Lower Blepharoplasty. In: Azizzadeh B, Murphy M, Johnson C, editors. Master Techniques in Facial Rejuvenation, 2nd edition. Canada: Elsevier; 2018; with permission.)

is performed (of primary importance), less manipulation of the canthus is prudent and typically enough.

CANTHAL AGING CHANGES

As with all areas of the face, senescence imparts functional, physiologic, and aesthetic alterations of normal anatomy. It is now widely accepted that tissue loss (both bone and fat) plays at least an equal role in facial/eyelid aging as does tissue descent.[31–35] Although historically great awareness has been placed on general facial aging changes as a whole, and on specific facial areas, such as the forehead/eyebrows, eyelids, nose, midface, and neck, little such attention has been placed on lateral canthal aging changes. However, an understanding of these changes is an essential component of mastering CS surgery. With age, the palpebral aperture changes from one that is horizontally oval (wider in that plane) to one that is rounder as the canthus migrates medially.[31] This process is a multifactorial process related to loss of integrity (laxity) of the LCT,[1,2,7] loss of orbital bone in specific areas,[36,37] loss of orbital fat (involutional enophthalmos),[38] and most likely changes in suspensory support of the globe. All these changes collectively affect the canthus, and it's many functions previously stated. This in part explains why more aggressive canthal manipulations can lead to a variety of canthal symptoms/complaints, even in the face of what appears to be excellent surgery.

CANTHAL TERMINOLOGY

One of the most confusing aspects of canthal surgery is deciphering the many names given to canthal structures and procedures.[1,2] For simplicity, the authors will designate all canthal "tightening" procedures as a form of CS. This can further be subdivided into both open and closed variants of surgery, and then into either a canthoplasty or canthopexy. Open canthal surgery involves a canthotomy (canthal incision) to suspends the lower lid,[1,2,17–22] whereas closed surgery does not.[1,2,23–25] Open surgery provides direct access and anatomic visibility to critical canthal structures and allows precision of lower lid placement. The tradeoff is that it can predispose to canthal deformity and malalignment. Conversely, in closed canthal surgery, canthal entry is from a distant site (ie, temporal upper lid crease), which can limit anatomic exposure and precision of lid placement. It does, however, more favorably preserve canthal anatomy and integrity, mitigating the chances of postoperative canthal deformity. Finally, in a canthoplasty, the LCT or terminal lower lid is cut plus-minus shortened and secured to the lateral orbital rim periosteum.[1,2] Alternatively, in a canthopexy, these lid structures are not modified, but rather the LCT or terminal lateral orbicularis muscle is secured to the lateral orbital rim with a plication suture.[1,2] Both canthoplasty and canthopexy can be performed in an open or closed fashion, with the canthoplasty variant being the more powerful and complicated procedure, which is fraught with more potential complication.

In relation to anatomic terminology, the lateral canthus is the general area where the lateral upper and lower lids meet, the commissure is their point of union, and the lateral raphe is the union of the upper and lower orbicularis fibers at and beyond the canthus.[1,2] The LCT is the connective tissue structure that connects the eyelids to the lateral orbital rim. It has also been called the lateral palpebral ligament. The lateral retinaculum is also used to describe the LCT. A retinaculum is a band around tendons to hold them in place. Because the LCT has an association with numerous other and integral canthal components, including the orbital septum, the check ligament of the lateral rectus, and lateral horn of the levator aponeurosis, the combination of these structures can be considered a structural retinaculum (**Table 1**).

PREOPERATIVE EVALUATION

Identifying the need for and type of CS is an essential element of successful lower blepharoplasty. This begins and ends with a proper preoperative assessment. First, a determination of the need for lower eyelid skin excision made. This is performed by having the patient look up and open their mouth widely. This places the lower eyelid on maximal stretch. There should not be inferior displacement of the eyelid with mouth opening. Such induced retraction suggests there is not a quantitative skin excess for excision. In this setting, skin excision predisposes to PBLER. If skin excess exists, conservative excision can be performed. When skin excision is added to lower blepharoplasty, the authors almost always add CS to surgery. Although this is not an absolute, the authors believe even minimally invasive CS is a safeguard against PBLER in these cases. The other essential element of the preoperative examination is to identify the presence of lower eyelid laxity, which is the primary factor that mandates the need for CS surgery. This can be assessed in 2 basic ways. First, the eyelid distraction test is performed (**Fig. 3**). The lower eyelid is pulled horizontally away from the lobe. If the lower eyelid can be distracted more than 8 mm from the globe, the

Table 1
Canthal nomenclature and definitions

Nomenclature	Definition
Open canthal suspension	Requires a canthal incision (canthotomy) to access the canthal tendon or terminal tarsus
Closed canthal suspension	The LCT is accessed through a distant site. The tendon can be modified and suspended, but it is done so without a canthotomy
Canthoplasty	The temporal lower lid is modified and/or shortened and secured to the lateral orbital rim, with or without surgery on the LCT
Canthopexy	The lower eyelid is suspended to the lateral orbital rim with a plication suture without modification of the LCT
Canthotomy	Lateral canthal skin incision
Lateral canthus	The general area where the upper and lower lids meet laterally
Lateral commissure	The point of union of the upper and lower lids at the lateral canthus
Lateral canthal tendon	Connective tissue structure that secures the upper and lower terminal eyelid to the lateral orbital rim
Lateral retinaculum	Another name used to describe the LCT. The confluence of several of the soft tissue structures of the lateral upper and lower eyelid that have connections with the LCT
Lateral palpebral ligament	Another synonymous name for the LCT
Lateral raphe	An area of fine fibrous bands where the terminal orbicularis muscle of the upper and lower lids meet
Orbitofacial vector	The relationship of globe projection to the lower lid and midface. When the globe and midface are aligned in a horizontal plane, the vector is neutral. When the globe projects more anterior than the midface, the vector is negative; when the globe sits posterior to the midface, the vector is positive
Ab externo	Suture passage starts outside the wound (outside in) to secure the lateral retinaculum to the Whitnall tubercle
Ab interno	Suture passage starts inside the wound to secure the lateral retinaculum to the Whitnall tubercle

LCT, lateral canthal tendon

Modified from Massry G. and Kossler A. The Spectrum of Canthal Suspension Techniques in Lower Blepharoplasty. In: Azizzadeh B, Murphy M, Johnson C, editors. Master Techniques in Facial Rejuvenation, 2nd edition. Canada: Elsevier; 2018; with permission.

test is positive and confirms lower eyelid (canthal tendon) laxity exists.[1,2] The second test is the eyelid snap-back test (**Fig. 4**). This test is performed by displacing the lower eyelid inferiorly and assessing its return to normal position without patient blink. If this is delayed, it suggests orbicularis deficit and the presence of lower eyelid laxity.[1,2] In the setting of lower blepharoplasty, it is prudent to lower one's standards for positive tests, as even subtle degrees of laxity can lead to changes on lower lid position. With the evolution

to less invasive and disruptive CS techniques, it is best to err on the side of caution when determining the need for CS and add minimally invasive surgery as needed. This is especially true (as stated) if lower lid skin excision is added, as this step increases the risk of postoperative lower eyelid malposition.

An important morphologic variant to identify when planning CS is the negative vector globe. This is present when the tip of the globe is more anterior in the vertical plane than the maximal projection of the

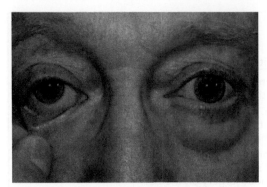

Fig. 3. The eyelid distraction test. If the lower lid can be "pulled away" more than 8 mm from globe, lower lid laxity exists. (*From* Massry G. and Kossler A. The Spectrum of Canthal Suspension Techniques in Lower Blepharoplasty. In: Azizzadeh B, Murphy M, Johnson C, editors. Master Techniques in Facial Rejuvenation, 2nd edition. Canada: Elsevier; 2018; with permission.)

midface[1,2,7,39] (**Fig. 5**). This topography predisposes the globe to bowstringing and lower lid retraction with CS. The authors call this the canthus at risk (CAR)[1] and believe such cases should be referred to a surgeon well versed in CS surgery. This can be addressed by correcting eyelid vector via midface enhancement with autologous fat,[40] synthetic filler, or alloplastic implants,[39] or by setting the globe back with custom orbital fat/bone, or combination, decompression.[40,41] The latter is reserved for specific and complicated cases, as these procedures are complex and require specialized orbital surgery training. The most common way of dealing with the CAR is by supra-placing and/or hanging back the CS suture[1,2,7] (**Fig. 6**). Hanging back the suture effectively increases the horizontal length of the lower eyelid to compensate for the increased surface area of the prominent globe. When suture

supra-placement is added, it may help mitigate lower lid malposition in these cases. Finally, in prominent globe cases, orbital rim suspension sutures can be anteriorized from the inner orbital rim, again to mitigate tension on the globe with inherent induced lower lid bowstringing and retraction.

A last comment on the evaluation for CS surgery is that one should critically observe the native lower lid tilt. As previously stated, the lateral canthus typically sits 2 mm higher than the medial canthus (normal canthal tilt). If this is not the case, it is important to document this variation and maintain it postoperatively unless the patient suggests a different desire. As a rule, however, the authors have noted patient dissatisfaction when the shape of the eyelid aperture is altered. Be very careful when altering the acuity of the canthal, angle, or slope of the lower eyelid during surgery. This can be a recipe for surgical failure.

SURGICAL PROCEDURES

Numerous variations of CS have been described to provide eyelid support during lower blepharoplasty. This spectrum of procedures involves variable degrees of canthal disarticulation and reconstruction. The following are the 3 primary CS procedures (all canthoplasties) the authors use as adjuncts to aesthetic lower blepharoplasty. A few words on canthopexy will also be included, although the authors rarely use this in approach in isolation. The procedure of choice is based on physical examination findings and surgeon clinical judgment. All surgeries are performed under general or monitored conscious sedation anesthesia depending on patient preference, and associated procedures are added. The authors have reviewed the clinical outcomes of these procedures in

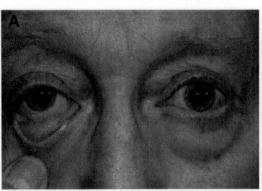
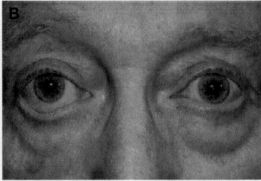

Fig. 4. The snap-back test. (*A*) If the lower lid is inferiorly displaced and (*B*) does not return to normal position without a blink, as in this example, lower lid laxity exists. (*From* Massry G. and Kossler A. The Spectrum of Canthal Suspension Techniques in Lower Blepharoplasty. In: Azizzadeh B, Murphy M, Johnson C, editors. Master Techniques in Facial Rejuvenation, 2nd edition. Canada: Elsevier; 2018; with permission.)

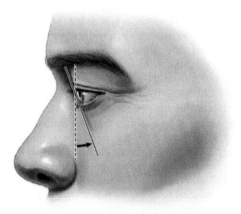

Fig. 5. A negative vector globe is demonstrated, as the tip of the globe is more anterior than the prominence of the cheek (*solid line*). The dotted lines show what would be considered a neutral vector, as the tip of the globe and cheek are in the same vertical plane. The size of the arrow correlates to the degree of negative vector. (*From* Massry G. and Kossler A. The Spectrum of Canthal Suspension Techniques in Lower Blepharoplasty. In: Azizzadeh B, Murphy M, Johnson C, editors. Master Techniques in Facial Rejuvenation, 2nd edition. Canada: Elsevier; 2018; with permission.)

depth.[42] The data collected have allowed a basis for the insights and recommendations the authors adhere to.

Open Canthal Suspension

Open canthal suspension (OCS) is the most aggressive and powerful technique. This surgery yields the most frequent postoperative complaints, and it carries the longest postoperative recovery time.[1,42]

Surgical Indication

The surgical indication is for significant lower eyelid laxity where lid shortening is typically needed. This procedure is usually performed in older patients and is the least common CS procedure the authors perform.[1,42]

The authors-preferred open CS is similar to the original description by Anderson and Gordy[17,18] of the lateral tarsal strip procedure. An 8- to 10-mm canthotomy incision is drawn with a marking pen using an existing canthal rhytid (smile line) if possible. This area is infiltrated with 1 to 2 mL of 1% Xylocaine with 1:100,000 epinephrine. An incision is made through the skin with a scalpel blade, and the underlying muscle is divided to the periosteum with the pure cutting mode of an electrocautery unit, or with a Westcott scissors. The commissure is then divided similarly to the orbital rim. The terminal eyelid is grasped with forceps and pulled anterior to the orbital rim. The traction created puts the LCT on stretch. A Westcott scissors is used to identify the inferior crus of the LCT. This is done by directing the tip of a Westcott scissors into the wound between the terminal lower eyelid and the lateral orbital rim. The scissors is moved in a side-to-side motion and will catch and then strum the inferior crus of the LCT, which is then lysed, dynamically releasing the lower eyelid. The terminal lower lid is then pulled to the lateral orbital rim at the level of the Whitnall tubercle to

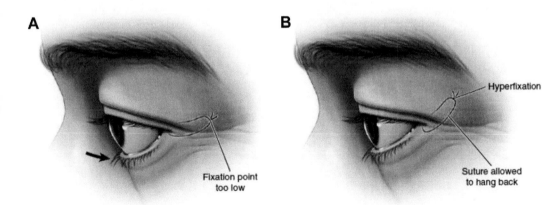

Fig. 6. (*A*) Suture fixation of the lower lid with a prominent globe. Note the bowstringing of the globe with lower eyelid retraction (*arrow*). (*B*) These changes are mitigated with supra-placement or hyperfixation and hanging back of the canthal suspension (CS) suture. (*From* Massry G. and Kossler A. The Spectrum of Canthal Suspension Techniques in Lower Blepharoplasty. In: Azizzadeh B, Murphy M, Johnson C, editors. Master Techniques in Facial Rejuvenation, 2nd edition. Canada: Elsevier; 2018; with permission.)

approximate how much eyelid tissue to excise before resecuring the eyelid to the orbital rim. Globe position must be considered with this calculation. A prominent globe requires more lid length to cover its surface area.[1,2] An overresection of eyelid in this setting can lead to bowstringing of the globe and lid retraction.[1,2,39] Conversely, if the globe is sunken (enophthalmic), more aggressive resection may be appropriate. Once the amount of lid shortening is determined, a tarsal tongue, or strip, is fashioned. The anterior and posterior lamellae are split, and the mucocutaneous junction is excised for this distance. The remaining triangle of anterior lamella overlying the tarsus is excised; the conjunctiva and lower eyelid retractors attached to the formed strip are cut from it, and the posterior surface of the tarsal tongue is deepithelialized with debriding with a scalpel blade. This is an important step, as it prevents postoperative inclusion cysts from forming. A strip of tarsus (tarsal tongue) free of surrounding tissue is now fashioned. The tarsus

is then shortened as planned. A 4-0 Vicryl suture on a P-2 half-circle needle engages the tarsus from the side facing orbicularis muscle and exits on the side facing the globe. This directionality is important to assure orientation of the eyelid (tarsus to orbital rim). The tarsus is engaged with 1 or 2 suture passes and then secured to the inner orbital rim periosteum at the level of the Whitnall tubercle. The suture is tied with a tension determined by lower eyelid position (ie, avoid bowstringing or laxity). A 5-0 Vicryl suture is then used to reform the commissure. This is a critical strep to re-create the appearance of the canthal angle. The suture is passed from the terminal lateral upper and lower lid entering external to internal wound at the gray line of both eyelids. A periosteal bite can be taken in between the eyelid bites to further sharpen the canthal angle. The canthotomy incision is then closed with interrupted 6-0 nylon suture (**Figs. 7** and **8**).

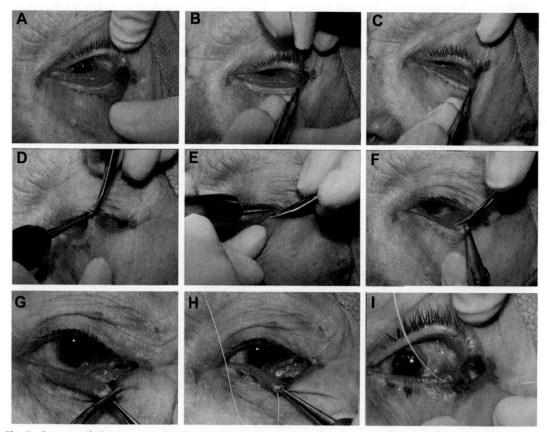

Fig. 7. Open canthal suspension (OCS) vis lateral tarsal strip procedure: (*A*) Canthotomy, (*B*) cantholysis, (*C*) dynamic release of the lower eyelid, (*D*) trimming mucocutaneous junction, (*E*) anterior lamellar excision, (*F*) tarsal release from conjunctiva and retractors, (*G*) shortening of formed tarsal strip, (*H*) tarsal strip engaged with fixation suture, (*I*) fixation suture secured to periosteum. (*From* Massry G. and Kossler A. The Spectrum of Canthal Suspension Techniques in Lower Blepharoplasty. In: Azizzadeh B, Murphy M, Johnson C, editors. Master Techniques in Facial Rejuvenation, 2nd edition. Canada: Elsevier; 2018; with permission.)

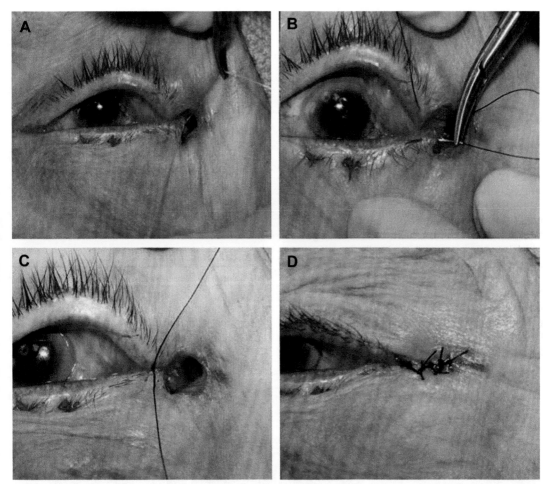

Fig. 8. (*A*) Canthal fixation suture tied, (*B*) terminal eyelid gray line (gray line placed to reform commissure), (*C*) commissure reformed, (*D*) canthotomy closed. (*From* Massry G. and Kossler A. The Spectrum of Canthal Suspension Techniques in Lower Blepharoplasty. In: Azizzadeh B, Murphy M, Johnson C, editors. Master Techniques in Facial Rejuvenation, 2ⁿᵈ edition. Canada: Elsevier; 2018; with permission.)

Closed Canthal Suspension

Closed canthal suspension (CCS) is the least aggressive and powerful technique the authors use, yet it is sufficient in most aesthetic cases. Typically, there are few postoperative complaints; it yields the quickest recovery, and by nature, is the most "aesthetic".[1,42]

Surgical Indication

The surgical indication is for the presence of eyelid laxity (minimal to slightly moderate) whereby clinical judgment dictates CS in the least invasive way. Most patients fall into this category of CS procedure.

A temporal upper eyelid crease incision is demarcated 10 mm in length. A preexisting rhytid is used if present. This area and the canthus are each infiltrated with 1 to 2 mL of 1% Xylocaine with 1:100,000 epinephrine. An incision is made

through the demarcated skin with a scalpel blade. If an upper blepharoplasty is also performed, access for CS is attained through the temporal wound. As with OCS, the remaining surgery can be performed with the pure cutting mode of an electrocautery unit or a Westcott scissors. The orbicularis muscle is divided, and a suborbicularis dissection ensues to the periosteum over the superolateral orbital rim and proceeds inferiorly until the LCT is identified. The tendon is then put on stretch and can be strummed and then lysed in a graded fashion depending on how much support of the eyelid and/or elevation of the canthus is desired. This is simplified by placing the Westcott scissors or electrocautery tip into the dissection pocket with one hand while elevating the canthus with forceps of the other hand. Most patients undergoing this variant of CS have mild laxity and only require little canthal support. In this instance, partially lysing the LCT is adequate. This creates a raw surface for re-adhession once the canthus is suspended. Because the entire inferior crus is not cut, canthal position rarely changes, which is a very important and desirable aspect of this technique. In cases whereby true minimal laxity exists, the tendon can be secured without incision, which allows plication only. The authors refer to this as a "chicken CS." In reality, it is a canthopexy plication suture. This is used when surgeons are equivocal about the need for CS but add it for mental comfort. Finally, a full release of the LCT is performed for added suspension or, rarely, to elevate the canthus. To ensure suspension to the inner orbital rim periosteum (important step) is complete, the orbital septum adjacent to the canthal tendon is incised, which often exposes the lacrimal gland (which is not an issue, as it can be displaced for suture placement). A double-armed 5-0 PDS suture on an RB-2 needle is passed both ends through the same hole in the commissure (external to internal wound), or if more support desired, through the terminal tarsus. Both ends are then passed through the exposed periosteum at the inner orbital rim. Because exposure is limited, it can be helpful to use the wooden end of a cotton-tipped applicator to identify the inner orbital rim periosteum and deflect away the lacrimal gland and adjacent

levator aponeurosis while passing the CS sutures. This ensures nonimbrication of these structures in the suspension when the sutures are tied. As with OCS, suture placement is dictated by globe position. The orbicularis muscle can then be closed with a few interrupted buried absorbable sutures and the skin with running 6-0 nylon suture (**Fig. 9**).

Commissure-Sparing Open Canthoplasty

Commissure-sparing open canthoplasty (CSOC) is a hybrid approach between the OCS and CCS. It has an intermediate level of patient complaints and recovery time between the 2 previous procedures and is more powerful than the closed surgery and less invasive than the open technique.[1,42]

Surgical Indication

The surgical indication is for intermediate eyelid laxity, and if added, midface support is needed.

A demarcation of a canthotomy incision, anesthetic infiltration, and a canthotomy with dissection to the orbital rim are performed as with the OCS variant. In this case, when the canthotomy is performed, the commissure and canthus are spared division for 3 mm. This leaves a bridge of the canthal angle intact. With direct view, septal

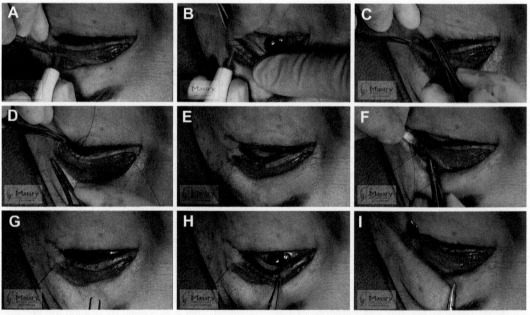

Fig. 9. Closed canthal suspension (CCS) procedure. This patient had entry through an upper blepharoplasty incision, as this was a planned procedure. (*A*) Suborbicularis/preperiosteal dissection to LCT, (*B*) cantholysis, (*C*) suture entering commissure, (*D*) suture exiting commissure, (*E*) both ends of suspension passed through commissure and exiting wound, (*F*) suspension suture engaging periosteum, (*G*) suspension suture pulled, (*H*) lower lid tension shown with upper lid elevated, (*I*) suspension suture tied. (*From* Massry G. and Kossler A. The Spectrum of Canthal Suspension Techniques in Lower Blepharoplasty. In: Azizzadeh B, Murphy M, Johnson C, editors. Master Techniques in Facial Rejuvenation, 2nd edition. Canada: Elsevier; 2018; with permission.)

attachments to the orbital rim/LCT are freed, isolating the tendon from the orbital rim periosteum. As with the CCS, the LCT is lysed in a graded fashion depending on clinical indication and degree of suspension desired. A single-armed 5-0 PDS suture on an RB-2 needle is passed through the inner orbital rim periosteum, then to-and-fro from the internal canthal wound, exiting the commissure, and then from external to internal. Terminal lower lid tarsus can be engaged as needed again per clinical judgment to control eyelid tension. The suture is then passed a second time through the periosteum and tied. Alternatively, as with the CCS, both ends of a double-armed similar suture can be passed through the same hole in the commissure external to internal wound and secured to the orbital rim periosteum. Should less vertical tension be desired on the canthus, or if a frank midface lift is needed, dissection can proceed through the canthotomy in a suborbicularis and preperiosteal plane. The orbitomalar ligament is released as needed to enter the prezygomatic space. The

terminal preseptal orbicularis can then be engaged with the same 5-0 PDS suture and secured to orbital rim periosteum or deep temporalis fascia above, depending on the lift and support desired. The canthotomy is then closed with interrupted 6-0 nylon suture (**Figs. 10** and **11**).

CANTHOPEXY

As stated, a canthopexy is a plication suture of the LCT or orbicularis muscle. In the authors subspecialty aesthetic eyelid practice (oculoplastics), they have not found this to be predictably adequate in preventing postoperative eyelid malposition after lower blepharoplasty. Their belief has been substantiated by post–lower blepharoplasty eyelid retraction cases sent to their referral practices for evaluation and management, many of which underwent canthopexy to support the lower eyelid. Again, it is typically not the CS choice, but rather the blepharoplasty performed that predisposes to retraction. However, using a plication suture in cases whereby lower lid skin

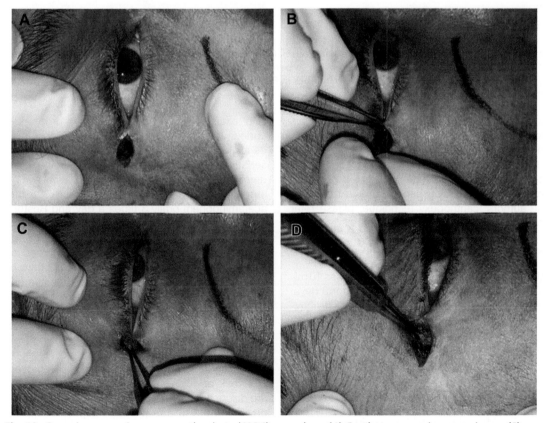

Fig. 10. Commissure-sparing open canthoplasty (CSOC) procedure. (*A*) Canthotomy-sparing commissure, (*B*) cantholysis, (*C*) grasping LCT, (*D*) grasping periosteum. (*From* Massry G. and Kossler A. The Spectrum of Canthal Suspension Techniques in Lower Blepharoplasty. In: Azizzadeh B, Murphy M, Johnson C, editors. Master Techniques in Facial Rejuvenation, 2nd edition. Canada: Elsevier; 2018; with permission.)

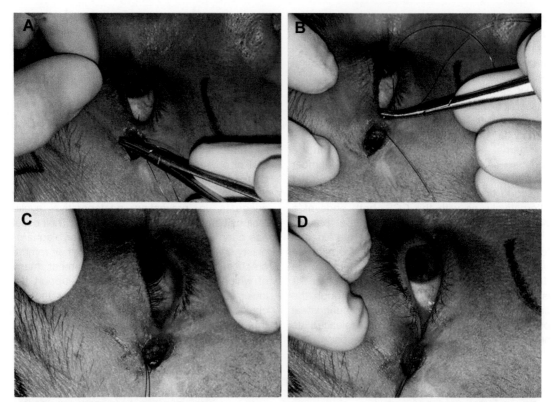

Fig. 11. Canthal suspension (CS) suture (*A*) passed internal to external at commissure, (*B*) then passed external to internal at commissure, (*C*) passed through periosteum, (*D*) placed on tension demonstrating suspension. (*From* Massry G. and Kossler A. The Spectrum of Canthal Suspension Techniques in Lower Blepharoplasty. In: Azizzadeh B, Murphy M, Johnson C, editors. Master Techniques in Facial Rejuvenation, 2nd edition. Canada: Elsevier; 2018; with permission.)

and/or muscle is excised can be a setup for this complication. Conversely, this is less frequently the case when formal canthoplasty is performed. As such, the authors rarely use a pure canthopexy for CS, except for the "chicken procedure" mentioned in the CCS section. For a review of the authors' canthopexy technique, please refer to their previous publication.[2]

POSTOPERATIVE CARE

After surgery, patients apply ice compresses 10 minutes per hour every hour while awake for 2 days. They are instructed to reduce heavy physical activity (bending, stooping, and lifting) and sleep with the head of bed elevated with 2 pillows until follow-up in 1 week. They are prescribed erythromycin ophthalmic ointment to be applied to the suture line (canthal or upper lid crease) and topical Tobradex ophthalmic drops to the eye 3 times a day for 1 week. The drops are added, as most patients have had concurrent transconjunctival lower blepharoplasty, and this is the authors' standard for this procedure. In addition, if stand-alone OCS or CSOC is performed in combination with isolated

skin excision lower blepharoplasty, drops are added, as these variants of CS have a higher incidence of chemosis. Oral narcotics and bedtime sedatives are dispensed on a case-by-case basis determined before surgery based on patient evaluation. Norco 5/325 (5 mg hydrocodone/325 mg acetaminophen) orally 3 times a day and Restoril 15 mg at bedtime are adequate. In patients with a history of postoperative nausea or motion or car sickness, or in those who are prescribed narcotics, Zofran 4 mg every 8 hours as needed for 3 days is given. Patients are evaluated just after surgery and upon discharge from the surgical center. A general visual acuity is always ascertained. Patients are also instructed to call the office should there be a noted change in vision or pain level, more than mild bleeding, significant discharge, or any constitutional symptoms. Sutures are removed at 1 week, at which time topical drops and ointment are discontinued. Unless there is concern with recovery, normal follow-up is at postoperative month 1 and month 3.

COMPLICATIONS

The discussion of complications is an important part of this article. As stated, blepharoplasty is an elective aesthetic procedure. In these cases, CS is an adjunct to enhance outcome and prevent, not cause, setbacks or complications. The authors cannot overstate the importance of "less is more" in this setting. In other words, add CS as needed but use the least invasive procedure to get the job done. This reduces the risks of complications seen with CS surgery.

The more common complications postoperatively occur within the first month of surgery. These complications include chemosis, suture reactions/infections, cysts, canthal pain/tenderness, and wound dehiscence. Chemosis can typically be managed with topical and/or oral steroids and upwards lid massage to compress and redirect the fluid. If this fails, a lateral temporary tarsorrhaphy can be added for 2 weeks. In more than 95% of cases, this resolves the issue. If chemosis persists, light conjunctival epithelial burns in a grid pattern with a low-temperature handheld cautery after lidocaine subconjunctival infiltration is highly effective. The authors believe the epithelial burns tack down the conjunctiva and prevent fluid accumulation. The external appearance of the burns typically resolves within 4 days. A conjunctival cut down can also be used in recalcitrant cases, but the authors have noted frequent recurrence and prefer the epithelial grid burn approach more. Suture reactions can be inflammatory or infectious. In either instance, a small cut down over the suture is performed, and the suture is removed. Should cellulitis be present, oral antibiotics are added. Epithelial-lined inclusion cysts are rare but can occur as with any conjunctival or cutaneous incision. These cysts are easily managed with excision. Canthal pain and tenderness are troublesome. Fortunately, they usually resolve with time and manual massage. If this fails, a cocktail of injections with wound modulators (see later discussion) can help. Should pain persist, a trial of oral tricyclic antidepressants or GABA drugs can, at times, alleviate symptoms. Finally, if permanent sutures to suspend the lid were used, their removal can be considered. The authors have only rarely noted permanent persistence of canthal pain after all measures stated for treatment are undertaken.

The most difficult complications to manage are canthal asymmetries/malalignment (dystopia), webs, and scars. Asymmetries often resolve over time with or without manual massage. If they persist, revision is warranted. As a rule, raising a lower canthus is significantly easier and more predictable than lowering a higher one. Please keep this mind, that the best way to treat this issue is prevention. Surgical intervention typically includes extensive periosteal release at the orbital rim before resecuring the canthus. Canthal webs and scars require time and massage, and chemomodulation as first-line therapy. Kenalog 5 mg/mL (0.2 mL) or 5-fluorouracil (5-FU) 50 mg/mL (0.2 mL) is helpful.[43–45] The authors prefer 5-FU, as it is not particulate (prevents rare vascular visual compromise) and tends not to cause skin dyschromia, telangiectasis, and atrophy. Injections can start as early as 2 weeks after surgery (0.2-mL aliquots) and be given every few weeks until stability is reached (typically 4 injections total).[45] Botulinum toxin A can be given in microdoses (2–4 units). This has been shown to inhibit myofibroblasts and scar formation/contraction.[44,46] The authors have anecdotally noted improvements with this form of therapy with or without added 5-FU injection. Should webs persist, surgical modification is a last option.[47] Although webs can be improved, rarely are they eliminated. Patients must be aware of this before further intervention. Finally, there is a small subgroup of patients who complain of canthal tightness and, eyelid tightness, that "my eyes feel different," and in the face of what appears as a normal appearance, that "my eyes just are not the same."[42] Fortunately, these patients are rare. Unfortunately, the authors have found no good solution in these cases. Reassurance and acknowledgment are the most helpful remedies here.

SUMMARY

CS is an integral adjunct to lower blepharoplasty, which can yield predictable and reliable outcomes when surgery is based on a detailed understanding of relevant anatomy and preoperative evaluation nuances, which dictate appropriate procedure choice. It is critical to understand that CS is about creating physiologic and tension-free lower eyelid support. CS cannot overcome the vertical traction inherent to overzealous lower blepharoplasty. In this instance, eyelid malposition can occur irrespective of how the canthus is addressed. In addition, canthal complaints and complications are more frequent when more distortion of canthal anatomy and architecture occurs. The take-home message is to add CS to support the lower lid during blepharoplasty when needed, to be familiar with the various CS procedures available to you, and to develop a comfort with these interventions. Finally, keep in mind that although CS is a critical part of successful lower blepharoplasty, when blepharoplasty is performed correctly, less is often more, and all that is needed, to achieve successful result to CS surgery.

DISCLOSURE

Dr G.G. Massry received royalties from Elsevier, Springer, Quality Medical Publishers, and Osmotica Pharmaceuticals. Dr. Holds received royalties from Springer, and is a consultant and shareholder for Horizon Pharmaceuticals, and a shareholder of Cypris Medical, Revance Thereapeutics and Panbela Therapeutics. Dr R.S. Douglas received Royalties from Springer, Osmotica Pharmaceuticals, and Horizon Pharmaceuticals.

REFERENCES

1. Massry G. Simplifying Lateral Canthal Suspension: My Approach. Presented at the Advanced Aesthetic Blepharoplasty, Midface and Contouring Meeting in St. Petersburg, Russia; October 20, 2017.
2. Kossler A, Massry G. The spectrum of canthal suspension techniques in lower blepharoplasty. In: Azizzadeh B, Murphy M, Johnson C, et al, editors. Fitzgerald. Master techniques in facial rejuvenation. New York: Elsevier; 2018. p. 152–65.
3. Tenzel RR. Treatment of lagophthalmos of the lower lid. Arch Ophthalmol 1969;81(3):366–8.
4. Webster RC, Davidson TM, Reardon EJ, et al. Suspending sutures in blepharoplasty. Arch Otolaryngol 1979;105(10):601–4.
5. Marshak H, Morrow DM, Dresner SC. Small incision preperiosteal midface lift for correction of lower eyelid retraction. Ophthalmic Plast Reconstr Surg 2010;26(3):176–81.
6. Patel BC, Patipa M, Anderson RL, et al. Management of postblepharoplasty lower eyelid retraction with hard palate grafts and lateral tarsal strip. Plast Reconstr Surg 1997;99(5):1251–60.
7. Massry GG. Managing the lateral canthus in the aesthetic patient. In: Massry GG, Murphy M, Azizzadeh B, editors. Master techniques in blepharoplasty and periorbital rejuvenation. New York: Springer; 2011. p. 185–97.
8. Rosenberg DB, Lattman J, Shah AR. Prevention of lower eyelid malposition after blepharoplasty: anatomic and technical considerations of the inside-out blepharoplasty. Arch Facial Plast Surg 2007;9(6):434–8.
9. Shorr N, Fallor MK. Madame Butterfly" procedure: combined cheek and lateral canthal suspension procedure for post-blepharoplasty, "round eye," and lower eyelid retraction. Ophthalmic Plast Reconstr Surg 1985;1(4):229–35.
10. Edgerton MT Jr. Causes and prevention of lower lid ectropion following blepharoplasty. Plast Reconstr Surg 1972;49(4):367–73.
11. Griffin G, Azizzadeh B, Massry GG. New insights into physical findings associated with postblepharoplasty lower eyelid retraction. Aesthet Surg J 2014;34(7):995–1004.
12. Carraway JH, Mellow CG. The prevention and treatment of lower lid ectropion following blepharoplasty. Plast Reconstr Surg 1990;85(6):971–81.
13. Fagien S. Algorithm for canthoplasty: the lateral retinacular suspension: a simplified suture canthopexy. Plast Reconstr Surg 1999;103(7):2042–53 [discussion: 2054–8].
14. Chong KK, Goldberg RA. Lateral canthal surgery. Facial Plast Surg 2010;26(3):193–200.
15. Massry GG. Comprehensive lower eyelid rejuvenation. Facial Plast Surg 2010;26(3):209–21.
16. Jelks GW, Glat PM, Jelks EB, et al. The inferior retinacular lateral canthoplasty: a new technique. Plast Reconstr Surg 1997;100(5):1262–70 [discussion: 1271–5].
17. Anderson RL, Gordy DD. The tarsal strip procedure. Arch Ophthalmol 1979;97(11):2192–6.
18. Anderson RL. The tarsal strip. Trans New Orleans Acad Ophthalmol 1982;30:352–63.
19. Jordan DR, Anderson RL. The lateral tarsal strip revisited. The enhanced tarsal strip. Arch Ophthalmol 1989;107(4):604–6.
20. Vagefi MR, Anderson RL. The lateral tarsal strip minitarsorrhaphy procedure. Arch Facial Plast Surg 2009;11(2):136–9.
21. Anderson RL. Tarsal strip procedure for correction of eyelid laxity and canthal malposition in the anophthalmic socket. Ophthalmology 1981;88(9):895–903.
22. Olver JM. Surgical tips on the lateral tarsal strip. Eye (Lond) 1998;12(Pt 6):1007–12.
23. Georgescu D, Anderson RL, McCann JD. Lateral canthal resuspension sine canthotomy. Ophthalmic Plast Reconstr Surg 2011;27(5):371–5.
24. Massry G. An argument for "closed canthal suspension" in aesthetic lower blepharoplasty. Ophthalmic Plast Reconstr Surg 2012;28(6):474–5.
25. Taban M, Nakra T, Hwang C, et al. Aesthetic lateral canthoplasty. Ophthalmic Plast Reconstr Surg 2010;26(3):190–4.
26. Patel A, Massry GG. Eyelid and periorbital anatomy. In: Nahai F, editor. Art of aesthetic surgery. New York: Thieme; 2019. p. 421–37.
27. Rosenstein T, Talebzadeh N, Pogrel MA. Anatomy of the lateral canthal tendon. Oral Surg Oral Med Oral Pathol Oral Radiol Endod 2000;89(1):24–8.
28. Tran KS, oh SR, Priel A, et al. Surgical anatomy of the forehead, eyelids and midface for the aesthetic surgeon. In: Massry GG, Murphy M, Azizzadeh B, editors. Master techniques in blepharoplasty and periorbital rejuvenation. New York: Springer; 2011. p. 11–24.
29. Gioia VM, Linberg JV, McCormick SA. The anatomy of the lateral canthal tendon. Arch Ophthalmol 1987;105(4):529–32.
30. McCord CD, Miotto GC. Dynamic diagnosis of "fishmouthing" syndrome, an overlooked complication of blepharoplasty. Aesthet Surg J 2013;33(4):497–504.

31. Fitzgerald R. Contemporary concepts in brow and eyelid aging. Clin Plast Surg 2013;40(1):21–42.

32. Donath AS, Glasgold RA, Glasgold MJ. Volume loss versus gravity: new concepts in facial aging. Curr Opin Otolaryngol Head Neck Surg 2007;15(4):238–43.

33. Massry GG, Hartstein ME. The lift and fill lower blepharoplasty. Ophthalmic Plast Reconstr Surg 2012;28(3):213–8.

34. Massry GG, Azizzadeh B. Periorbital fat grafting. Facial Plast Surg 2013;29(1):46–57.

35. Lambros VS. The Dynamics of Facial Aging. Presented at the Annual Meeting of the American Society for Aesthetic Plastic Surgery; April – May, 2002 Las Vegas, NV.

36. Kahn DM, Shaw RB Jr. Aging of the bony orbit: a three-dimensional computed tomographic study. Aesthet Surg J 2008;28(3):258–64.

37. Richard MJ, Morris C, Deen BF, et al. Analysis of the anatomic changes of the aging facial skeleton using computer-assisted tomography. Ophthalmic Plast Reconstr Surg 2009;25(5):382–6.

38. Kersten RC, Hammer BJ, Kulwin DR. The role of enophthalmos in involutional entropion. Ophthalmic Plast Reconstr Surg 1997;13(3):195–8.

39. Holds JBH. Management of the prominent eye. In: Massry GG, Murphy M, Azizzadeh B, editors. Master techniques in blepharoplasty and periorbital rejuvenation. New York: Springer; 2011. p. 297–306.

40. Massry GG. Commentary on: lower eyelid retraction surgery without internal spacer graft. Aesthet Surg J 2017;37(2):137–9.

41. Gupta S, Briceno C, Douglas RS. Customized minimally invasive orbital decompression for thyroid eye disease. Expert Rev Ophthalmol 2013;8:255–66.

42. Patel A, Massry G, Douglas R. Transconjunctival Blepharoplasty with Adjunctive Canthal Suspension: An Analysis of Outcomes. Presented at the Annual Meeting of the American Society for Aesthetic Plastic Surgery; October 2018 Chicago, IL.

43. Taban M, Lee S, Hoenig JA, et al. Postoperative wound modulation in aesthetic eyelid and periorbital surgery. In: Massry GG, Murphy M, Azizzadeh B, editors. Master techniques in blepharoplasty and periorbital rejuvenation. New York: Springer; 2011. p. 307–12.

44. Eftekhari K, Douglas RS, Massry GG. Scar modulation. In: Yanoff M, editor. Advances in ophthalmology and optometry. Philadelphia: Elsevier; 2016. p. 165–79.

45. Yoo DB, Azizzadeh B, Massry GG. Injectable 5-FU with or without added steroid in periorbital skin grafting: initial observations. Ophthalmic Plast Reconstr Surg 2015;31(2):122–6.

46. Jeong HS, Lee BH, Sung HM, et al. Effect of botulinum toxin type A on differentiation of fibroblasts derived from scar tissue. Plast Reconstr Surg 2015;136(2):171e–8e.

47. Massry GG. Cicatricial canthal webs. Ophthalmic Plast Reconstr Surg 2011;27(6):426–30.

The Treatment of Post-blepharoplasty Lower Eyelid Retraction

Kenneth D. Steinsapir, MD*, Samantha Steinsapir

KEYWORDS

- Post-blepharoplasty lower eyelid retraction • Hard palate graft • Canthoplasty • Vertical midface lift
- ePTFE rim implant • Drill hole canthoplasty

KEY POINTS

- Post-blepharoplasty lower eyelid retraction is caused by transcutaneous lower blepharoplasty.
- The muscular hammock of the lower eyelid is prone to injury.
- Orbital rim projection plays a critical role in post-blepharoplasty lower eyelid retraction and its correction.
- Skin grafts are aesthetically unacceptable and should be avoided.
- The best restoration results combine soft tissue advancement with autogenous grafts and alloplastic implants.

 Video content accompanies this article at http://www.facialplastic.theclinics.com

INTRODUCTION

This article surveys the post-blepharoplasty lower eyelid retraction (PBLER) literature and presents the authors' personal approach. Early investigators characterized PBLER as ectropion,[1,2] which implies the eyelid margin rotates outward off the eye surface. This is a less common post-blepharoplasty finding than a vertically short eyelid that conforms to the eye surface. After surgery, scarring in the planes of the eyelid, weakening of the lower eyelid orbicularis oculi muscle, and deficiencies of soft tissue contribute to lower eyelid malposition. Lack of projection of the inferior orbital rim contributes to a so-called negative vector lower eyelid.[3] These changes are often lumped together as lateral scleral show, or mischaracterized as ectropion.[1,2,4] Corneal exposure with dry eye symptoms is common, including foreign body sensation, contact lens intolerance, red eyes, excessive tearing, and, in more extreme cases, impairment of vision, photophobia, corneal breakdown, and ulceration.

ANATOMY

The lower eyelid is suspended by the lateral and medial canthal ligaments that insert into the orbit rim. The eyelids comprise a specialized muscular sphincter externally covered by a keratinized epithelium and internally lined by the palpebral conjunctival epithelium, a nonkeratinized squamous epithelial over a substantia propria firmly adherent to the tarsus. The lined surfaces of the eyelid glide over the bulbar conjunctiva and cornea with lubrication provided by mucin from conjunctival goblet cells and tear aqueous produced by lacrimal glands. The tarsus conforms to the eye surface, allowing the eyelid margins to act as a wiper for the cornea moving the tear film. Compared with the upper eyelid, the shape and

Orbital and Ophthalmic Plastic Surgery Division, Stein Eye Institute, David Geffen School of Medicine at UCLA, Los Angeles, CA, USA
* Corresponding author. 9001 Wilshire Blvd, Suite 305, Beverly Hills, CA 90211, USA
E-mail address: kenstein@ix.netcom.com

Facial Plast Surg Clin N Am 29 (2021) 291–300
https://doi.org/10.1016/j.fsc.2021.01.006

position of the lower eyelids are influenced significantly by tension in the canthal tendons.[5]

In the youthful face, a cushion of subcutaneous fat extends over the lateral orbital rim and zygoma, creating subtle separation between the orbital and temple aesthetic units. Medially, the nasojugal fold, or tear trough, represents the location where the inferior orbital orbicularis oculi muscle inserts medially onto the maxilla. Laterally, the palpebral-malar groove, or lid-cheek junction, is formed by the orbitomalar ligament, also called the orbicularis retaining ligament, and lateral orbital thickening.[6,7]

A solid body of work suggests branches of the facial nerve, supplying the orbicularis oculi muscle at the eyelid margin, approach perpendicularly and are at risk from an infracilliary skin/muscle incision.[8,9] A study by Choi and colleagues[10] seems to refute this, suggesting that the lateral orbicularis over the tarsus is innervated by motor nerve branches that arise medially and extend horizontally from the so-called medial orbicularis motor line. Hwang[11] has noted atonic eyelids are more common laterally. Additional research is needed to resolve this controversy.

PATHOPHYSIOLOGY

Investigators have sought to localize the injury that accounts for PBLER. Shorr and Goldberg described lid shortening from scarring in any of the eyelid planes: skin and orbicularis (anterior lamella), orbital septum (middle lamella) or conjunctiva and lower eyelid retractors (posterior lamella).[4] Other investigators similarly, attribute PBLER to scarring in any of these planes.[1]

Schwarcz and colleagues[12] investigated scarring of the middle lamella in PBLER. The investigators compared transconjunctival blepharoplasties performed in the postseptal versus the preseptal plane. This study confirms that transconjunctival lower eyelid surgery, whether preseptal or postseptal, is not associated with lower eyelid retraction. The scarring involved in transcutaneous lower blepharoplasty affects multiple layers due to direct tissue disruption and a motor nerve injury that compromises the hammock function of the lower eyelid. The surgical dissection planes inevitably are organized by dense scar tissue after transcutaneous lower blepharoplasty.

NONSURGICAL METHODS

Hyaluronic acid (HA) fillers have been used to relive PBLER. Goldberg and colleagues[13] reported on HA filler to treat lower eyelid retraction in 31 patients. The etiologies included thyroid-related orbitopathy (8/31), postsurgical (trauma repair, post-blepharoplasty, and postcancer reconstruction) (19/31), and involutional (4/31). The average case was treated with 0.9 mL per eyelid. Overall, there was a 1.04-mm reduction in inferior scleral show with treatment. Treatment effects diminished 50% over an average of 4.6 months. Complications were minor, including bruising, swelling, and contour irregularities.

Xi and colleagues[14] presented a retrospective review of 27 cases of lower eyelid retraction, including 14 post-blepharoplasty and 13 noncosmetic cases managed with HA filler. They reported 96.3% (26/27) cases that they describe as complete improvement of the retraction with no reoccurrence in 9 months of follow-up. The investigators invoked the generalized form of Hooke's law and the effect of increasing the bulk modulus of the lower eyelid with the HA filler to explain their results.

The point made by Xi and colleagues is that infiltrating a lower eyelid with HA filler increases the bulk modulus of the lower eyelid, effectively stiffening it. Under the right circumstances, injecting filler into the eyelid improves its resistance to stress and strain. The result can be an improvement in PBLER. The concept of altering the bulk modulus of the lower eyelid as the basis for improving lower eyelid retraction suggests that higher G-prime fillers should be favored over low G-prime fillers, a finding consistent with clinical experience.

SURGICAL METHODS

In 1969, Tenzel[15] described surgery for lower eyelid lagophthalmos. His repair mobilized the lateral canthal tendon from the orbital rim. The lower eyelid was de-epithelialized, and the skeletonized lower eyelid lateral tendon was accommodated into a small incision made through the exposed upper eyelid lateral canthal retinaculum and sutured in place. Anderson and Grody[16] described the "lateral tarsal strip." It consisted of a lateral canthotomy and inferior cantholysis. They split the gray line into anterior and posterior lamella, as needed. The conjunctival epithelium then was denuded to make the strip and resuspended to the orbital rim.

In 1985, Shorr and Fallor[17] reported the Madame Butterfly repair for PBLER. Their goal was functional improvement in eyelid closure and position without a skin graft. Surgery included a lateral canthotomy, cantholysis, and lateral cheek undermining. If this did not permit the eyelid to elevate, residual resistance was attributed to a midlamellar scar. An en glove lysis of the scar was performed followed by lateral canthal resuspension. The lateral cheek was resuspended to the periosteum lateral to the orbital rim. They placed the lateral canthus 4 mm above the medial canthus. Postoperatively, the lateral canthus relaxed to a more neutral position.

Baylis and colleagues[18] described a series of 30 patients with PBLER. They found scarring and contraction of the plane of the orbital septum the most common cause of retraction. Patients were managed with lateral canthotomy and en glove lysis of the scar tissue and retractors at the inferior boarder of the lower eyelid tarsus. The lower eyelid was placed on traction to the eyebrow postoperatively. When a spacer graft was needed, ear cartilage was utilized. It was inserted into the dissection tract, avoiding the need for an infracillary or transconjunctival incision. Eyelid contour irregularities due to distortion of the ear cartilage required revision in 4 of 13 cases. Their series had a very high rate of surgical revision: 58% of cases involving only scar and retraction lysis and 21% of cases when a spacer graft was used.

Siegel[19] described the use of hard palate grafts (HPGs) for eyelid reconstruction in 1985. He used HPG in 11 patients as a liner material in eyelid reconstruction. Subsequently, Kersten and colleagues[20] used HPG in managing lower eyelid retraction in 18 patients. Cohen and Shorr[21] also used HPG as part of lower eyelid retraction repair including 9 of 18 patients with PBLER in conjunction with the Madame Butterfly procedure. HPG was associated with minimal shrinkage with healing. Oral discomfort was described as acceptable and resolved in 7 days to 10 days.

Barmettler and Heo[22] found no statistical difference in the use of autologous ear cartilage, bovine acellular dermal matrix, and porcine acellular dermal matrix for the repair of lower eyelid retraction. MacIntosh and colleagues[23] studied failed cartilaginous grafts. Explanted auricular graft was enclosed by a peudoperichondial membrane. Kerfing used to improve graft flexible also left the auricular grafts susceptible to fragmentation and cracking.

Oh and colleagues[24] reported a series of 13 patients with PBLER addressed with a drill-hole canthoplasty and suborbicularis oculi fat suspension. The periosteum at the orbital rim was elevated to expose the bone and a drill hole was made 2 mm above the desired height of the lateral canthal angle. Polypropylene suture (4-0) resuspended the lateral canthal tendon to the hole. A dissection in the preperiosteal plane was used to mobilized suborbicularis oculi fat that was sutured to the drill hole. All patients were reported satisfied with their surgical results with relief of dry eye symptoms.

Taban[25] described lower eyelid retractor recession without the use of an internal spacer graft for PBLER. He excluded eyelids with midlamellar scarring, which he felt warranted a spacer graft. Success was based on subjective patient satisfaction, which was described as high with the exception of one cased described to be over corrected. This work highlights that spacer grafts are not needed in every case. A position consistent with Griffin and colleagues.[26]

Brock and colleagues[27] used autogenous dermis grafts for as a posterior eyelid spacer in 7 patients with PBLER. All eyelids demonstrated improved lower eyelid position and the patients reported improved symptoms. Other investigators have been less successful with this approach. Yoon and McCulley[28] reported a 30% complication rate in their series. Patel and colleagues[29] repaired lower eyelid retraction using HPG, midface lift, and lateral canthoplasty in 17 patients. They performed a preperiosteal midface lift via an upper or lower eyelid incision. They claimed complete correction of inferior scleral show in all cases with no major complications. However, 1 of their patients developed an oral palatal fistula.

Ben Simon and colleagues[30] reported a 5-year series of subperiosteal midface lifts with or without the use of a HPG to address lower eyelid retraction in 34 patients. They performed lateral canthotomy and cantholysis followed by a transconjunctival incision. A subperiosteal midface lift with inferior periosteotomy was performed. The mobilized midface then was sutured in multiple locations to the inferior orbital rim. Frost sutures were placed completing surgery when no midlamellar spacer was used. In total, 21% of their patients had mild residual eyelid retraction and 1 patient needed revisional surgery.

Dailey and colleagues[31] reported lower eyelid retraction repair with porcine dermal matrix (ENDURAGen, Stryker CMF, Newman, Georgia) as a spacer graft in 100 consecutive patients (160 eyelids). Complications (15% of patients) included implant exposure or rejection, irritation, inflammation, cyst formation, implant kinking, and eye pain. The implant was removed in 9 eyelids. Cosmetic results were reported as very acceptable. Grumbine and colleagues[32] also reported the use of acellular porcine dermal collagen matrix. Two of their patients were revised due to implant complications.

Taban and colleagues[33] reported on their use of "thick" acellular human dermis (AlloDerm, Allergan, Dublin, Ireland) in a consecutive series of patients presenting with lower eyelid retraction. They reported 16 of 21 eyelids had improved lower eyelid position. Five surgeries were characterized as failures. The investigators suggest that their results were comparable to HPG and that thick acellular dermis was better than thin acellular human dermis, but they did not present data to support the later conclusion.

A porous polyethylene (Medpor, Stryker, Kalamazoo, Michigan) lower eyelid spacer was introduced for the repair of lower eyelid retraction.[34] An early series using the implant was promising with a low revision and complication rate.[35] Tan and colleagues[36] found that complications, minor (26% [9/35]), and major (23% [8/35]) were common and required surgical intervention. These investigators concluded the implant should be reserved for cases where other methods have failed. Mavrikakis and colleagues[37] presented 4 cases of failed porous polyethylene lower eyelid spacers requiring explantation.

Yoo and colleagues[38] studied 5-fluorouracil with or without triamcinolone to modify postoperative healing of skin grafts in a series of 19 patients presenting with lower eyelid retraction. Patients were reported to be very satisfied with the surgical outcome and the appearance of the graft in 17 of 19 cases. The surgeon rated the eyelids as excellent in 18 of 19 cases.

McAlister and Oestreicher[39] reported that it was possible to repeat posterior lamellar grafting in cases where the initial effort was not sufficient. Most patients had a second posterior lamellar graft of hard palate mucosa (42/46 eyelids [91%]). A second procedure further reduced residual inferior scleral show, demonstrating a role for secondary posterior lamellar grafting.

Pascali and colleagues[40] reported a retrospective, 10-year study of lower eyelid retraction repair. They performed an infraciliary incision, subperiosteal midface with lower eyelid tarsal resuspension via an upper eyelid incision anchored to a drill hole at the orbital rim. Goldberg[41] noted this series reinforced the concept that vertically lifting the cheek recruits needed soft tissue and skin into these compromised eyelids. Park and colleagues[42] investigated the best graft material for reconstructing lower eyelid retraction. Many of these cases involve the use of a spacer graft combined with lateral canthoplasty, lateral tarsal strip, and midface lifting procedures. No graft material was found superior to others. The use of HPG was associated with more donor site and eyelid complications compared with other graft materials.

Galindo-Ferreiro and colleagues[43] surveyed Spanish and Brazilian oculoplastic surgeons regarding lower eyelid retraction. Respondents diagnosed lower eyelid retraction 62% of the time based on inferior scleral show and 23.5% of the time based on a limitation of lower eyelid excursion to the lower limbus. Surgeons often performed lower eyelid retraction surgery after waiting 6 or more months (54%), but correction also was performed commonly at 3 months or earlier (41.8%). Management included lateral canthoplasty, spacer graft, lower eyelid retractor recession, and cheek-lift. Among autogenous spacer grafts, auricular cartilage was most common (39.2%), followed by HPG (22.7%), and tarso-conjunctival graft (19.6%). Lower eyelid retractors were released in 84.7% of cases versus retractor dissection and excision (15.3%). In cases involving a midface lift, a preperiosteal lift was preferred (58.3%) versus subperiosteal lift (41.6%).

THE VERTICAL MIDFACE LIFT

Senior author (KDS) has developed and refined a powerful and versatile method for PBLER using a vertical midface lift method.[44] One aspect missing from all of the methods, discussed previously, is the absence of a flexible method to augment the orbital rim to help provide support for the lower eyelid. These eyelids are commonly vertically short of soft tissue in all planes, including skin. There typically is a motor injury to the muscular hammock function of the lower eyelid margin. Scarring effectively tethers the lower eyelid to the cheek. Some investigators use a drill hole placed in the lateral orbital wall in order to permanently suture recruited skin and cheek soft tissue into the lower eyelid. Although such methods do augment missing skin and soft tissue in the eyelid, they do little to correct the projection of the cheek along the lower orbital rim, which often is the fundamental reason for lower eyelid soft tissue deficiency. This is recognized as the basis for the negative vector lower eyelid.[3] The approach developed by the senior author (KDS) uses a hand-carved expanded polytetrafluoroethylene (ePTFE) orbital rim implant to both augment the orbital rim projection and also function as a felting material so that vertically lifted cheek soft tissue can be permanently fixed to the orbital rim. This allows the lifted cheek to permanently contribute skin and soft tissue volume to the lower eyelid. An HPG also is used in these reconstructions to control the shape of the lower eyelid contour. Readers are referred to the surgical video that accompanies this article to supplement the description that follows (Video 1).

Prior to surgery, the patient is sent to a dentist for a clear acrylic stent to cover the hard palate for use after the graft is harvested. The stent has retention at the base of the teeth and initially assists to control bleeding after harvesting the graft. After surgery it protects the donor site and contributes to postoperative comfort.

Surgery is performed under intravenous sedation so the patient can cooperate during surgery. General anesthesia precludes this cooperation. During surgery, the patient is sat up to judge the placement of the reconstructed lateral canthal angle. It is beneficial to immobilize the eyelids on Frost sutures after surgery for a week. Patients do not tolerate having both eyes patched simultaneously. For that reason, bilateral surgery is staged. The Frost sutures are removed on postoperative day 6 and the second side is performed as early as the next day. One side of the hard palate is anesthetized where the graft will be harvested. The lower eyelid, cheek to the gingival sulcus, and soft tissue to the zygomatic arch and temporal fossa also are anesthetized.

A methylene blue marking pen and a cotton tip applicator are used to outline a template to fabricate an ePTFE rim implant (**Fig. 1**). These markings are transferred to sterile paper and then to a block of carveable ePTFE measuring 3 cm × 7 cm × 5 mm (Surgiform, Surgiform Technology, Lugoff, South Carolina) (**Fig. 2**). The implant is carved on a nylon board with a series of #10 and #11 blades to desired shape and thickness. Caution and experience are needed to best judge implant size and thickness. As a rule, smaller implants are better accepted than over-sized implants. Commonly the finished implant may be only 2.5 mm in thickness along the orbital rim and rapidly taper to the edges with overall dimensions of 6 cm by 3 cm (**Fig. 3**). It is soaked in a solution of gentamycin (80 mg in 100 mL of injectable saline) for use later in the case.

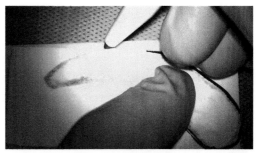

Fig. 2. The template shape is outlined on a carvable block of ePTFE that measures 3 cm by 7 cm by 5 mm. The finished implant generally is comma-shaped, with a width that extends from the lateral orbital rim to the medial canthus. The finished implants generally are less than 3-mm thick. (*Courtesy of* Kenneth D. Steinsapir, MD, Los Angeles, California).

Surgery is initiated by harvesting the HPG. It is marked with a methylene blue pen and incised with a #15 blade. The dimensions vary with the indication. Commonly a 28-mm wide, pendant-shaped HPG is harvested tapering from 6 mm posteriorly to 2 mm anteriorly (**Fig. 4**). Hemostasis is obtained and a hemostatic agent is placed in the donor site and the rinsed palate stent is snapped in place over this. The graft is set aside for later use.

A lateral canthotomy and cantholysis are performed. The lower eyelid is retracted and a trans-conjunctival/lower eyelid retractor incision is made from the lateral canthus to the caruncle (**Fig. 5**). Dissection is carried out bluntly posterior to the orbicularis oculi muscle and anterior to the orbital septum, to the orbital rim. The periosteum is opened along the orbital rim from medial to lateral. A subperiosteal dissection is performed as far inferior as the gingival sulcus, lateral over the zygomatic arch onto the masseteric fascia, and superiolaterally into the temporalis fossa

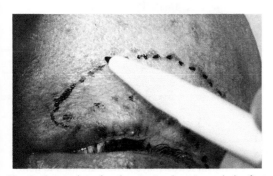

Fig. 1. A template for the rim implant is made by first outlining the orbital rim and the inferior extent of the planned implant. These marks are transferred to sterile glove wrapper paper. (*Courtesy of* Kenneth D. Steinsapir, MD, Los Angeles, California).

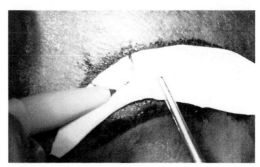

Fig. 3. The ePTFE rim implant is marked for a notch to accommodate the inferior neurovascular bundle. (*Courtesy of* Kenneth D. Steinsapir, MD, Los Angeles, California).

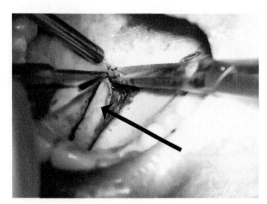

Fig. 4. Hard palate is harvested from the roof of the mouth (*arrow*). The graft needs to span the width of the eyelid and is pendant shaped. The size depends on what the individual patient needs. Commonly these are 28-mm long, tapering from 2 mm to 6 mm. (*Courtesy of* Kenneth D. Steinsapir, MD, Los Angeles, California).

(**Fig. 6**). The infraorbital neurovascular bundle is preserved carefully. The zygomaticofacial and zygomaticotemporal nerves are sacrificed to facilitate exposure. Nasally, the dissection is carried medial to the infraorbital neurovascular bundle. A long, insulated, cautery needle is used to perform a periosteotomy in the subperiosteal pocket and the soft tissue is released with gentle blunt dissection using an elevator (**Fig. 7**). The orbital rim implant is inserted into the dissected pocket after cutting a notch to accommodate the inferior neurovascular bundle. The implant is fixed to the orbital rim using 3, self-drilling, self-tapping, 5-mm long by 1.5-mm titanium microscrews: laterally, centrally, and medially (**Fig. 8**). The head of the microscrews are tightened to counter-sink

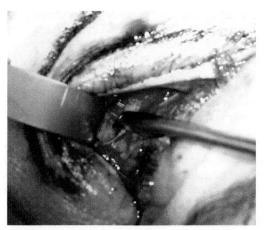

Fig. 6. Scar tissue present in the lower eyelid planes is dissected. At the orbital rim, the periosteum is incised with cautery and a subperiosteal dissection is continues inferiorly to the gingival sulcus inferiorly. Care is taken to preserve the infraorbital neurovascular bundle. Laterally, the subperiosteal dissection is carried onto the zygomatic arch and into the temporal fossa. (*Courtesy of* Kenneth D. Steinsapir, MD, Los Angeles, California).

into the ePTFE implant. These microscrews also serve as the points of suspension for the lifted cheek.

Horizontal mattress sutures (4–0 Supramid, S. Jackson, Alexandria, Virginia) are placed around each of the microscrews and passed into the cheek soft tissue and periosteum in 3 locations, vertically lifting the cheek soft tissue to the orbital

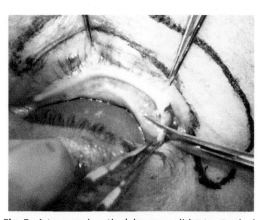

Fig. 5. A transconjunctival, lower eyelid retractor incision is made from that lateral canthus to the caruncle medially. (*Courtesy of* Kenneth D. Steinsapir, MD, Los Angeles, California).

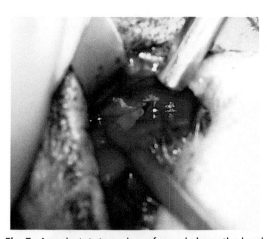

Fig. 7. A periostetotomy is performed above the level of the gingival sulcus. Mayo scissors are used to gently mobilize the malar fat pad. Next the orbital rim implant is inserted through the transconjunctival dissection and positioned on the orbital rim. (*Courtesy of* Kenneth D. Steinsapir, MD, Los Angeles, California).

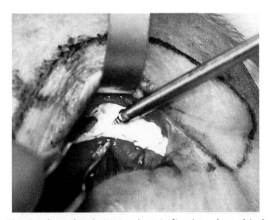

Fig. 8. The orbital rim implant is fixed to the orbital rim medially, centrally, and laterally using self-drilling, self-tapping microscrews. Horizontal mattress sutures placed at each microscrew are used to elevate the cheek vertically. (*Courtesy of* Kenneth D. Steinsapir, MD, Los Angeles, California).

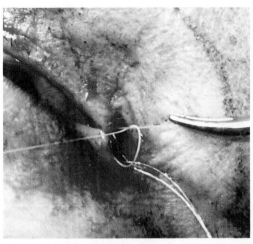

Fig. 10. The gray lines at the lateral canthus are reapproximated before tying up the deep suture that supports that lateral tarsal strip to the orbital rim. (*Courtesy of* Kenneth D. Steinsapir, MD, Los Angeles, California).

rim implant. These are tied permanently. A small lateral tarsal strip is made and the lower eyelid is resuspended to the orbital rim at the desired position. The patient always is sat up to judge the placement. The resuspension suture is not tied permanently. The patient is returned to the supine position. The eyelid is everted with forceps and the HPG is sutured into the lower eyelid with the mucosal side sutured to the conjunctival (**Fig. 9**). Once this is done, the lateral canthal resuspension suture is tied, the lateral canthal angle soft tissue is reapproximated, and the skin is sutured closed (**Fig. 10**). A therapeutic contact lens is placed when there is the potential for a corneal abrasion from the sutures used to fasten the HPG (**Fig. 11**). Frost sutures are passed in a horizontal mattress fashion in 3 locations to suture the eyelid

closed. A light pressure dressing is applied. The Frost sutures are removed at 1 week. These eyelids tend to be stiff at first and over the course of 8 weeks to 12 weeks they soften and pick the natural parabolic shape of the lower eyelid. **Figs. 12** and **13** show representative before and after images of typical cases. The senior author (KDS) has performed more than 1000 of these reconstructions since the late 1990s, with few

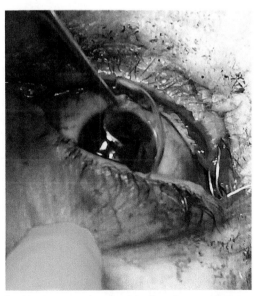

Fig. 11. A contact lens is placed on the cornea to protect the corneal surface while the eyelids are healing. *Courtesy of* Kenneth D. Steinsapir, MD, Los Angeles, California.

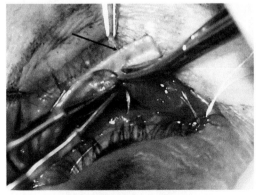

Fig. 9. The HPG is sutured in place. The arrow indicates the HPG. (*Courtesy of* Kenneth D. Steinsapir, MD, Los Angeles, California).

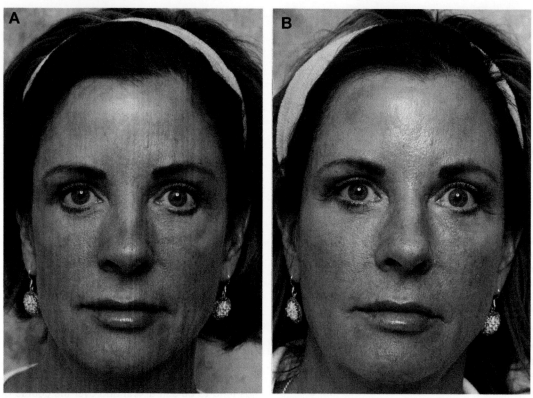

Fig. 12. (*A*). A 57-year-old woman after quadrilateral blepharoplasty with PBLER. (*B*). Six months status post–bilateral midface lift with ePTFE rim implant and HPG. (*Courtesy of* Kenneth D. Steinsapir, MD, Los Angeles, California).

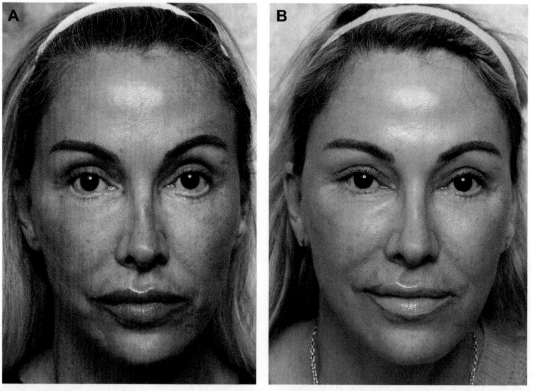

Fig. 13. (*A*). A 53-year-old, woman with PBLER following a quadralateral blepharoplasty. Note the PBLER. (*B*). One-year status post–bilateral midface lift with ePTFE rim implant and HPG. (*Courtesy of* Kenneth D. Steinsapir, MD, Los Angeles, California.)

complications. The vertical midface lift combined with the hand carved ePTFE rim implant and HPG has proved a robust, versatile, and comprehensive approach to addressing PBLER, even when other methods have failed.

SUMMARY

There are many approaches to addressing PBLER. What is critical is a detailed assessment of the individual patient. Locating the exact plane of eyelid scarring is a fool's errand. Most of these compromised eyelids have multiple issues, including a deficiency of skin, lack of normal motor tone, compromised lower eyelid length from overaggressive or repetitive lateral canthal resuspensions, internal eyelid scarring in multiple planes, and weak projection of the orbital rim. Occasionally, a patient presents with isolated lower eyelid laxity as the basis for their lower eyelid retraction, but that is exceptional. Generally, these eyelids need recruitment of skin and soft tissue, augmentation of the orbital rim, posterior eyelid grafting to shape and support the lower eyelid margin, and lateral canthal reconstruction. In addressing an eyelid with previously unsuccessful repair(s) for PBLER, the surgeon must ask how their approach will be different from the past surgeries. New resources and thinking are needed to ensure a successful outcome not achieved by the prior surgeon.

SUPPLEMENTARY DATA

Supplementary data related to this article can be found online at https://doi.org/10.1016/j.fsc.2021.01.006.

REFERENCES

1. Edgerton MT. Causes and prevention of lower lid ectropion following blepharoplasty. Plast Reconstr Surg 1972;49:367–73.
2. Hamako C, Baylis HI. Lower eyelid retractionafter blepharoplasty. Am J Ophthalmol 1980;89: 517–21.
3. Jelks GW, Jelks EB. Preoperative evaluation of the blepharoplasty patient. Bypassing the pitfalls. Clin Plast Surg 1993;20(2):213–23.
4. Shorr N, Golberg RA. Lower eyelid retraction following blepharoplasty. Am J Cosmet Surg 1989; 6:77–83.
5. Malbouisson JM, Beccega A, Cruz AA. The geometrical basis of the eyelid contour. Ophthal Plast Reconstr Surg 2000;16:427–31.
6. Kikkawa DO, Lemke BN, Dortzbach RK. Relations of the superficial musculoaponeurotic system to the orbit and characterization of the orbitomalar ligament. Ophthal Plast Reconstr Surg 1996;12:77–88.
7. Muzaffar AR, Mendelson BC, Adams WP. Surgical anatomy of the ligamentous attachment of the lower lid and the lateral canthus. Plast Reconstr Surg 2002;110:873–84.
8. Ramirez OM, Santamarina R. Spatial orientation of motor innervation to the lower orbicularis oculi muscle. Aesthet Surg J 2000;20:107–13.
9. Hwang K, Lee DK, Lee EJ, et al. Innervation of the lower eyelid in relation to blepharoplasty and midface lift: clinical observation and cadaveric study. Ann Plast Surg 2001;47:1–5.
10. Choi Y, Kang HG, Nam YS, et al. Facial nerve supply to the orbicularis oculi around the lower eyelid: anatomy and its clinical implications. Plast Reconstr Surg 2017;140:261–71.
11. Hwang K. Facia nerve supply to the orbitularis oculi around the lower eyelid: anatomy and its clinical implications. (letter). Plast Reconstr Surg 2018;141: 449e–50e.
12. Schwarcz R, Fezza JP, Jacono A, et al. Stop blaming the septum. Ophthal Plast Reconstr Surg 2016;32: 49–52.
13. Goldberg RA, Lee S, Jayasundera T, et al. Treatment of lower eyelid retraction by expansion of the lower eyelid with hyaluronic acid gel. Ophthal Plast Reconstr Surg 2007;23:343–8.
14. Xi W, Han S, Feng S, et al. The injection for the lower eyelid retraction: a mechnanical analysis of the lifting effect of the hyaluronic acid. Aesthetic Plast Surg 2019;43:1310–7.
15. Tenzel RR. Treatment of lagophthalmos of the lower lid. Arch Ophthalmol 1969;81:366–8.
16. Anderson RL, Grody DD. The tarsal strip prodcedure. Arch Ophthalmol 1979;97:2192–6.
17. Shorr N, Fallor MK. "Madame butterfly" procedure: combined cheek and lateral canthal suspension procedure for post-blepharoplasty, "round-eye,"and lower eyelid retraction. Ophthal Plast Reconstr Surg 1985;1:229–35.
18. Baylis HI, Nelson ER, Goldberg RA. Lower eyelid retraction following blepharoplasty. Ophthal Plast Reconstr Surg 1992;3:170–5.
19. Siegel RJ. Palatal grafts for eyelid reconstruction. Plast Reconstr Surg 1985;76:411–4.
20. Kersten RC, Kulwin DR, Levartovsky S, et al. Management of lower-lid retraction with hard-palate mucosa grafting. Arch Ophthalmol 1990;108: 1339–43.
21. Cohen MS, Shorr N. Eyelid reconstruction with hard palate mucosa grafts. Ophthal Plast Reconstr Surg 1992;8(3):183–95.
22. Barmettler A, Heo M. Prospective, randomized comparison of lower eyelid retraction repair with autologous auricular cartilage, bovine acellular dermal matrix (Surgimend), and porcine acellular dermal

matrix (Enduragen) spacer grafts. Ophthal Plast Reconstr Surg 2018;34:266–73.

23. MacIntosh PW, Jakobiec FA, Stagner A, et al. Failed cartilaginous grafts in the eyelid: a retrospective clinicopathological analysis of 5 cases. Ophthal Plast Reconstr Surg 2016;32:347–53.

24. Oh SR, Korn BS, Kikkawa DO. Oribitomalar suspension with combined single drill hole canthoplasty. Ophthal Plast Reconstr Surg 2013;29:357–60.

25. Taban MR. Lower eyelid retraction surgery without internal spacer graft. Aesthet Surg J 2017;37:133–6.

26. Griffin G, Azizzadeh B, Massry GG. New insights into physical finding associated with postblepharoplasty lower eyelid retraction. Aesthet Surg J 2014;34:995–1004.

27. Brock WD, Bearden W, Tann T, et al. Autogenous dermis skin grafts in lower eyelid reconstruction. Ophthal Plast Reconstr Surg 2003;19:394–7.

28. Yoon MK, McCulley TJ. Autologous dermal greafts as posterior lamellar spacers in the management of lower eyelid retraction. Ophthal Plast Reconstr Surg 2014;30:64–8.

29. Patel MP, Shapiro MD, Spinelli HM. Combined hard palate spacer graft, midface suspension, and lateral canthoplasty for lower eyelid retraction: a tripartite approach. Plast Reconstr Surg 2005;115:2105–14.

30. Ben Simon GJ, Lee S, Schwarcz RM, et al. Subperiosteal midface lift with or without a hard palate mucosal graft for correction of lower eyelid retraction. Ophthalmology 2006;113:1869–73.

31. Dailey RA, Marx DP, Ahn ES. Porcine dermal collagen in lower eyelid retraction repair. Ophthal Plast Reconstr Surg 2015;31:233–41.

32. Grumbine FL, Idowu O, Kersten RC, et al. Correction of lower eyelid retraction with englove placement of porcine dermal collagen matrix implant. Plast Reconstr Surg 2019;143:743–6.

33. Taban M, Douglas R, Li T, et al. Efficacy of "thick" acellular human dermis (AlloDerm) for lower eyelid reconstruction. Arch Facial Plast Surg 2005;7:38–44.

34. Morton AD, Nelson C, Yoshito I, et al. Porous polyethylene as a spacer graft in the treatment of lower eyelid retraction. Ophthal Plast Reconstr Surg 2000;16:146–55.

35. Wong JF, Soparkar CNS, Patrinely JR. Correction of lower eyelid retraction with high density porous polyethylene: The Medpor® lower eyelid spacer. Orbit 2001;20:217–25.

36. Tan J, Olver J, Wright M, et al. The use of porous polyethylene (Medpor) lower eyelid spacers in lid heightening and stabilization. Br J Ophthalmol 2004;88:1197–200.

37. Mavrikakis I, Poitelea C, Parkin B, et al. Medpor lower eyelid spacer: does it biointegrate? Orbit 2009;28:58–62.

38. Yoo DB, Azizzadeh B, Massry GG. Injectable 5-FU with or without added steroid in periorbital skin grafting: Initial observation. Ophthal Plast Reconstr Surg 2015;31:122–6.

39. McAlister CN, Oestreicher JH. Repeat posterior lamellar grafting for recalcitrant lower eyelid retraction is effective. Orbit 2012;31:307–12.

40. Pascali M, Botti C, Cervelli V, et al. Lower eyelid retraction: a 10-year clinical retrospective study. Plast Reconstr Surg 2017;140:33–45.

41. Goldberg RA. Discussion: vertical midface lifting with periorbital anchoring in the management of lower eyelid retraction: a 10-year clinical retrospective study. Plast Reconstr Surg 2017;140:46–8.

42. Park E, Lweis K, Alghoul SA. Comparison of efficacy and complications among various spacer grafts in the treatment of lower eyelid retraction: A systematic review. Aesthet Surg J 2017;37:743–54.

43. Galindo-Ferreiro A, Fernandez E, Weill D, et al. A web-based survey of oculoplastic surgeons regarding the management of lower lid retraction. Semin Ophthalmol 2019;34(3):125–30.

44. Steinsapir KD. Aesthetic and restorative midface lifting with hand-carved, expanded polytetrafluroethylene orbital rim implants. Plast Reconstr Surg 2003;22:1727–37.

Treatment Options for Lower Eyelid Festoons

Brian H. Chon, MD, Catherine J. Hwang, MD, Julian D. Perry, MD*

KEYWORDS

- Festoons • Malar mounds • Malar edema • Malar bags • Lower eyelid • Tetracycline • Doxycycline

KEY POINTS

- Festoons are also referred to as malar mounds and malar edema. No clear nomenclature exists to describe these lesions.
- Nonsurgical options for treating festoons include fillers, laser and trichloroacetic peels, radiofrequency thermoplasty and microneedling, and sclerosing therapies such as deoxycholic acid, tetracycline, and doxycycline injections.
- Surgical options include direct excision, skin muscle flap, extended blepharoplasty and midface lift.
- Although a variety of treatments options exist, festoons remain frustrating to the patient and challenging for the surgeon.

INTRODUCTION

The lack of clear nomenclature to describe the deficit in the superolateral cheek beneath the eyelid/cheek junction termed a "festoon" parallels our lack of understanding of this condition, yet the phenotype of this crescentic triangular sagging, with or without fluid accumulation, is as unmistakable as it is frustrating to both the patient and the surgeon. This article aims to present our current understanding and treatment of the conditions widely known as "festoons."

FESTOONS BACKGROUND, ETIOLOGY, AND ANATOMY

The clinicopathology of festoons and malar mounds is not well understood. These lesions may appear with age as tissues gradually descend in a redundant fashion over the malar eminence; however, they can also occur early in life. Some patients may not notice a festoon until it is pointed out to them, or in unfortunate cases, only after blepharoplasty has hollowed the lower eyelids to unmask it (**Fig. 1**).

A combination of tissue laxity (skin and orbicularis oculi), a weakened orbital retaining ligament, and weakening of the firm attachment of the inferiorly located zygomaticocutaneous ligament (ZCL) can lead to inferior displacement of the skin and orbicularis, forming a bulge over the prezygomatic region.[1,2] Fluid buildup in this region can accompany the redundant anterior tissues.

Terminology

Several terms are used to describe festoons, including malar mounds, malar edema, saddle bags, fluid bags, palpebral bags, and lower eyelid bags. Kpodzo and colleagues[3] suggest using 3 distinct terms: malar edema, malar mound, and festoons. Malar edema refers to fluid over the malar eminence. Malar mound refers to soft tissue prominence, usually orbicularis muscle or fat, over the malar eminence. Finally, festoons refer to the "cascading hammocks of lax skin and orbicularis muscle that hang between the medial and lateral canthi." Although these 3 terms may represent distinct entities, they may represent points on the spectrum of the same pathophysiologic condition. In this article the term "festoon" is used to encompass the entire spectrum of fluid-associated mounds over the malar eminence (**Fig. 2**).

Oculofacial Plastic Surgery, Department of Ophthalmology, Cole Eye Institute, Cleveland Clinic Foundation, 9500 Euclid Avenue, Cleveland, OH 44195, USA
* Corresponding author.
E-mail address: perryj1@ccf.org

Facial Plast Surg Clin N Am 29 (2021) 301–309
https://doi.org/10.1016/j.fsc.2021.02.005
1064-7406/21/© 2021 Elsevier Inc. All rights reserved.

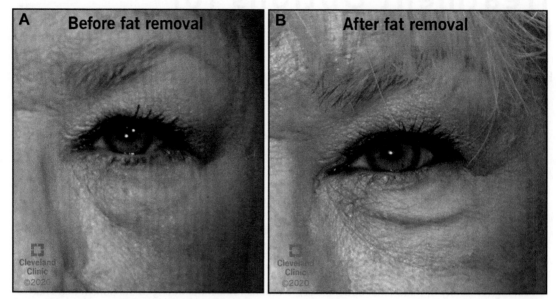

Fig. 1. This patient with festoons underwent fat removal blepharoplasty (*A*). The festoon is more visible after removing the surrounding camouflaging fat (*B*). (Reprinted with permission, Cleveland Clinic Center for Medical Art & Photography © 2020. All Rights Reserved.)

Anatomy

To understand festoons, a brief description of the anatomy is instructive. The prezygomatic space or festoon space is marked superiorly and inferiorly at the lid–cheek junction and the midcheek, respectively.[3] The upper border is marked by the orbitomalar ligament (OML), the lower border by the ZCL.

Malar bags/festoons are consistently found approximately 2.5 to 3.0 cm below the lateral canthus.[4]

The upper border of a festoon is at the lateral lid–cheek junction. The OML, described by Kikkawa and colleagues,[5] coincides with the boundary. The OML is a soft tissue structure which originates at the inferior orbital rim/arcus marginalis and courses through the orbicularis oculi muscle, and

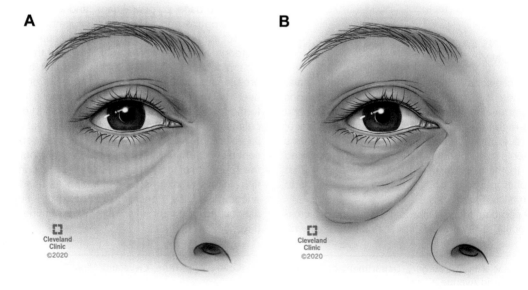

Fig. 2. Diagram (*A*) depicts a common mild festoon phenotype. Diagram (*B*) depicts a more prominent festoon with lax skin and orbicularis muscle hanging in a triangular shape beneath the eyelid/cheek junction. (Reprinted with permission, Cleveland Clinic Center for Medical Art & Photography © 2020. All Rights Reserved.)

inserts into the dermis, at the level of the lid–lower eyelid cheek transition. The insertion corresponds with both the lid–cheek junction laterally and the and nasojugal groove medially. The OML has connective tissue components (collagen and elastin) that undergo involutional change with age (Kikkawa and colleagues[5]) and elongate, which allows tissue ptosis and contribute to the appearance of festoons. The OML is also important in the appearance of lower eyelid orbital fat prolapse. The OML acts as the inferior boundary of orbital fat prolapse and thus can enhance the appearance of eyelid bags.[4,6] Orbital fat prolapse is a commonly encountered age-related change that occurs superior to the OML. This characteristic distinguishes it from festoons, which are located below the OML (**Fig. 3**).

Medially, the upper and lower boundaries of the festoon converge, approximately at the mid-pupil line. In this area, there is a convergence of the palpebromalar groove superiorly, the tear trough medially, and the midcheek groove or nasojugal fold inferiorly, giving a Y-shaped appearance.[7]

The malar septum originates at the inferior orbital rim, descends inferiorly through the suborbicularis oculi fat (SOOF), penetrates the orbicularis oculi before inserting into the mid-cheek dermis. It is thought that the interdigitation of the malar septum with the fibrous septa of the SOOF fat creates an impermeable barrier from the orbital rim to the cheek skin. The function of the malar septum is postulated to partition the eye from the lower face.[4]

The inferior border of the festoon is at the ZCL. Mendelson and colleagues described the inferior border of the prezygomatic space as the ZCL. The zygomatic ligaments are stronger than the OML.[2] The zygomatic ligaments originate from the periosteum of the zygoma near the origins of the zygomaticus major, zygomaticus minor, and levator labii superioris (**Fig. 4**). The ZCL extends anteriorly into the overlying soft tissue and dermis, forming the midcheek furrow.[8]

Characteristics of Festoons

Festoons act as a fluid sponge. Patients with malar mounds tend to be predisposed to prolonged postoperative swelling, suggesting a lymphatic origin for festoons.[2] Shoukath and colleagues[9] evaluated the lymphatic drainage of the lower eyelid region. The lymphatic drainage of the eyelid is composed of both a superficial and deep lymphatic system. Relevant to festoons, the deep lymphatic vessels travel within the roof of the prezygomatic space traveling deep to the preseptal orbicularis oculi, travel within the SOOF space, and then eventually drain into the preauricular lymph nodes and submandibular lymph nodes.[9]

Periocular edema can present both as generalized eyelid puffiness as well as festoons, and both can be caused or aggravated by a variety of inflammatory conditions, such as postoperative edema and systemic malignancies, such as angiosarcoma or lymphoma.[10,11] Specific systemic inflammatory causes of facial edema and/or festoons include acne rosacea, acne vulgaris, systemic lupus erythematosus, sarcoidosis, allergic dermatitis, dermatomyositis, and angioedema.[12] Periocular topical medications causing blepharitis and

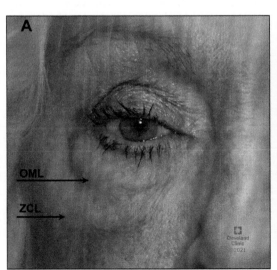
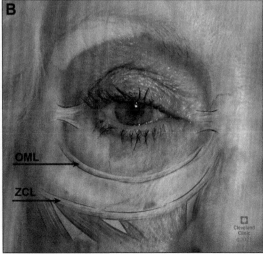

Fig. 3. This clinical photograph demonstrates a typical festoon (*A*), bounded by the OML and the ZCL (*B*). ORL, orbital retaining ligament. (Reprinted with permission, Cleveland Clinic Center for Medical Art & Photography © 2020. All Rights Reserved.)

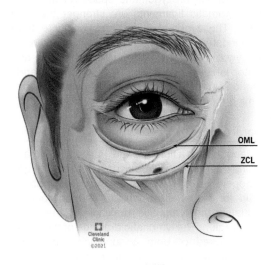

Fig. 4. This illustration demonstrates the ligamentous attachments that surround the festoon. ORL, orbital retaining ligament. (Reprinted with permission, Cleveland Clinic Center for Medical Art & Photography © 2020. All Rights Reserved.)

conjunctivitis can also produce eyelid edema and festoons, including drops such as apraclonidine, brimonidine, dorzolamide, and pilocarpine, and ointments such as bacitracin and erythromycin. Allergies may include drug-related blepharoconjunctivitis, as well as vernal keratoconjunctivitis and contact dermatitis. Some additional causes of contact dermatitis that might produce eyelid edema and festoons include cosmetics, occupational allergens, hair dyes, nail polishes, and sunscreens.

The most common inflammatory condition associated with festoons is ocular rosacea. Ocular rosacea is a chronic inflammation of the periocular skin associated with erythematous and thickened skin and telangiectasias, papules, and pustules. This condition may lead to conjunctival chemosis and hyperemia, erythema, and thickening of the eyelid margin from meibomitis and blepharitis, as well as periocular skin telangiectasias, erythema, and eyelid swelling. Chronic eyelid lymphedema and festoons can result from chronic rosacea.[11,13,14] In severe cases, rosacea can be associated with lymphedema of the eyelids, known as Morbihan disease.[13] Chronic inflammation from acne rosacea may cause fibrosis, loss or destruction of elastin around lymphatic vessels, and cause the obstruction of lymphatic vessels leading to lymphedema that presents in the periocular region.[11,13–15]

Eyelid and cheek tissue laxity contribute to the appearance of festoons. In 1 study,[16] the appearance of festoons and malar bags were compared in participants between upright position and supine positioning. Tear trough, cheek volume, steatoblepharon, malar bags, and nasolabial folds were all significantly decreased in supine positioning. Malar bags and festoons were less prominent with supine positioning in 84% of cases.[16]

Festoons can occur without tissue laxity as well. Some individuals present with festoons at an early age, before significant aging changes appear in the lower eyelid and cheek regions. Occasionally, festoons can occur in early childhood or at birth and are known as congenital festoons. It is unclear whether festoons that present earlier in life possess a different pathophysiology from festoons that occur later in life. Acquired festoons are improved with forceful closure of the eyes, improve with laterally pulling of the lower eyelid upwards and laterally, and worsen with botulinum toxin. In patients with congenital festoons, forceful closure and lateral pulling improve but do not resolve the festoon, and the festoon does not change with botulinum toxin injections.[17]

Festoons can worsen in a variety of clinical settings. Malar mounds or festoons may be prominent in patients with thyroid disorders and those with allergies,[18] as well as postoperatively with infraorbital incisions.[19] Other causes of malar bags include patients with systemic disease such as chronic renal disease, allergy, or hepatic cirrhosis.[20] Postoperative edema is thought to be a combination of postoperative inflammation and lymphatic dysfunction.[9] Eyelid lymphedema has also been noted to occur after neck dissection and radiotherapy for metastatic squamous cell carcinoma to cervical lymph nodes. It is thought that submandibular and deep cervical lymph node removal can lead to chronic lymphedema.[21]

Case reports have noted festoon formation after botulinum toxin injections. In 1 case study, botulinum toxin was injected into the lateral canthus and infraorbital region. One theory for the formation of the festoon was weakening of the orbicularis oculi pumping mechanism, leading to localized lymphedema.[22] Asaadi[17] refer to this as a "positive botox test" in acquired festoons, because a weakening and laxity of the orbicularis oculi can contribute to the formation of festoons, with worsening of festoons with botulinum toxin noted in acquired festoons, although not seen with congenital festoons.

Hyaluronic acid gel (HAG) fillers can worsen or possibly even cause festoons. Owing to the hydrophilic nature and isovolemic degradation of HAG fillers, these products when injected in the periocular region can worsen or potentially even cause festoons. Fillers injected into the periorbital hollows may result in malar edema in as many as 15% of patients.[23] Improvement can occur after injection of hyaluronidase, but some festoons persist even after multiple hyaluronidase injections.[24–26] HAG filler treatment in the tear trough and midface area is an increasing and troublesome cause, as well as an aggravating factor, in patients presenting with festoons.

EVALUATION
Relevant Medical History

Before considering treatment options, it is important to evaluate for treatable or modifiable contributing factors to eyelid edema. A significant number of medications can cause eyelid edema, some including acetaminophen, aspirin, nonsteroidal anti-inflammatory drugs, hormonal supplements, and prednisone, among many other medications. In addition to oral medications, a variety of topical ophthalmic eyedrops and ointments can cause either blepharoconjunctivitis or medication allergy that can contribute to eyelid edema. In suspected medications, if possible the medication should be held for at least 2 weeks to evaluate for causation.[10]

Medical conditions that can contribute to eyelid edema include ocular rosacea, thyroid eye disease, floppy eyelid syndrome, obstructive sleep apnea, and blepharochalasis. Conditions leading to systemic edema such as cardiac, renal hepatic disease, low protein states, lymphatic obstruction, and hypothyroidism can contribute to eyelid edema. Allergic conditions can also worsen festoons, whether environmental, drug related, or other causes of hypersensitivity reactions. Signs of allergy include itching, vertical eyelid rhytids, eyelid erythema, and thickening.[10]

Clinical Evaluation

It is important to differentiate between causes of lower eyelid bags. Festoons should be differentiated from lower eyelid fat prolapse, or steatoblepharon. Lower eyelid fat prolapse is located above the location of a festoon. Fat prolapse presents as fullness in the lower eyelid, above the OML. Although orbital fat in a young individual is located with the orbital space above the inferior orbital rim, with aging changes the fat can drape over and below the inferior orbital rim. Festoons present as a triangular shape below the OML and inferior orbital rim, in the area of the cheek. A festoon will always be located inferior to prolapsed orbital fat.

Once correctly identified, the festoon can then be further evaluated. The pinch test is 1 method of evaluating festoons. The clinician pinches the festoon skin at various sites to assess for the degree of orbicularis oculi bulk contributing to the festoon.[27] This test can be used to differentiate

between a predominantly fluid-filled structure from a predominantly soft tissue one.

An additional test, the squinch test, evaluates the orbicularis oculi muscle as the patient squeezes their eyelids tightly closed. This maneuver demonstrates the maximum contraction of the orbicularis oculi and highlights the degree of muscle involvement in the appearance of the festoon. In orbicularis laxity, the squinch test should significantly improve the appearance of festoons. If orbital fat is a contributing factor then the fat portion will not be effaced by the maneuver, but rather dislocated.[27]

Because some of the surgical options for festoon management incorporate lower eyelid tightening, lower eyelid laxity should be evaluated using the snapback test and/or the eyelid distraction test.

FESTOONS MANAGEMENT: NONSURGICAL

A variety of nonsurgical treatments have been attempted to improve festoons.

Although HAG fillers can worsen festoons, they can be used carefully to try to conceal them[28] The filler material can be injected into the surrounding areas of volume loss. High viscosity filler material may also cause a "posterior girdle" effect to improve the appearance of festoons.[29] Overcorrection can lead to worsening distension of weak ligaments in the area (such as the OML) and even cause postinjection edema that worsens festoons, particularly if there are already disrupted lymphatics.[23] The pros and cons of this approach must be carefully weighed with the patient because some filler-related worsening of festoons may not be reversible with hyaluronidase.

Hyaluronidase has been used for non–filler-related festoons. Some patients with idiopathic edema and no known history of filler use had some improvement in their festoons with hyaluronidase injection.[24] However, in our practice, this effect seems to be temporary at best. Oral diuretics are also another option, but again we have not noticed predictable improvement in our patients who have tried this option. Spironolactone (Aldactone) in doses of 25 to 100 mg/d are generally used.

Laser treatment with CO_2 and Er:YAG ablative lasers have been described for the treatment of malar bags. Because there is no repositioning of soft tissue, the treatment is best served for mild festoons or with mild excess skin laxity. Risks include pigmentary changes, scarring, ectropion, and eyelid retraction.[30–32]

Radiofrequency microneedling has been attempted for festoons.[33,34] Jeon and Geronemus[34]

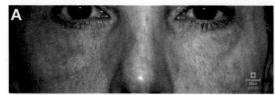
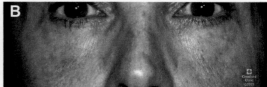

Fig. 5. The patient (*A*) shows improvement in festoons after intralesional tetracycline injection (*B*). (Reprinted with permission, Cleveland Clinic Center for Medical Art & Photography © 2020. All Rights Reserved.)

published a report of 2 patients who had improvement of festoons using microneedle radiofrequency technology. The procedure benefits from being noninvasive can be repeated.[34] Bipolar radiofrequency microneedling works by delivering thermal injury to the dermis and fat and is thought to improve rhytids by increasing collagen and elastic fibers.[35] Other nonsurgical treatment options include radiofrequency thermoplasty and trichloroacetic acid or other chemical peels.[36]

Tetracycline injections have been used for the reduction of festoons (**Fig. 5**). Tetracycline has been used in other areas of the body for its sclerosing properties. The exact mechanism of action is not known, although it is thought that the ability of tetracycline to inhibit matrix metalloproteinases and growth factor–like activity to stimulate fibroblast proliferation contribute to the ability of sclerodesis of the festoon space. Complications including ischemia, necrosis, persistent postinjection pain, and nerve palsies were not seen.[37,38] The authors inject tetracycline 2%, 0.2 to 0.5 mL per lesion (**Fig. 6**). It may take weeks to see the effect, and we have injected some festoons more than once, at least 90 days apart. Festoons that are not related to hyaluronic acid filler injection seem to respond best to the injection.

Doxycycline has also been used as a sclerosing agent.[39] Doxycycline is a member of the tetracycline family and has been used as sclerosing agent in other areas of the body. The mechanism of sclerosing is thought to be due to inhibition of matrix metalloproteinases, cell proliferation, and inhibition of vascular endothelial growth factor.[40] Doxycycline is more available for direct use, and may provide a treatment alternative that seems to have similar results to tetracycline. However, it is a more potent sclerosant than tetracycline, and we are awaiting more data regarding its safety before trying this option.

In congenital festoons, because subcutaneous fat seems to be a significant factor in the appearance of festoons, some investigators have considered the use of deoxycholic acid (Kybella, Allergan, Irvine, CA) if surgical excision is deferred.[17] However, this product may produce significant periocular side effects, and we have not tried this method.

No nonsurgical treatment predictably improves festoons, so excellent communication between surgeon and patient is of paramount importance. Communication includes discussing the risks, possible lack of improvement, and the off-label use of these nonsurgical festoon treatments. The surgeon should ensure that patients understand these issues thoroughly before proceeding with treatment. It may take several visits to vet these options as well as the surgical options with a patient.

FESTOONS MANAGEMENT: SURGICAL

A variety of surgical treatments have been used for festoons, with varying degrees of success. The variety of techniques advocated should clue the reader in to the variability of results, and inability of any one technique to consistently achieve superior results.

Direct Festoon Excision

Direct festoon excision represents one option for surgical treatment,[41,42] typically when skin excess or laxity represents a major component of the lesion, as opposed to orbicularis laxity or redundancy or soft tissue ptosis. This technique obviously results in a visible scar, so patient selection is important in choosing this technique. Additional lateral canthal resuspension should be considered

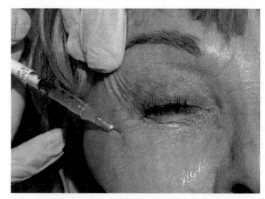

Fig. 6. This patient is receiving 0.3 mL of tetracycline 2% solution for the treatment of a mild festoon. The medication is injected intralesionally in aliquots of 0.1 to 0.2 mL.

in cases with any amount of horizontal eyelid laxity to decrease the likelihood of iatrogenic lower eyelid retraction. Recurrence is common with direct excision because the ligamentous boundaries of the lesion are largely unaltered.

Skin Muscle Flap or Extended Blepharoplasty

A skin muscle flap may be performed when skin excess exists, with an effort to conceal the scar in the subciliary area. The excess tissue is excised and the remaining flap redraped and tightened across the festoon to lessen its appearance. This technique does not affect the underlying ligaments or septum. The orbicularis may be suspended to orbital rim periosteum to stabilize the eyelid and decrease the chance of postoperative eyelid retraction.[1,43–45] Lateral canthal resuspension can also be performed to decrease this risk. However, redraping does not address the primary pathophysiology, and by trying to treat a problem 2 cm inferior to the incision, it risks lower eyelid retraction, undercorrection, and recurrence regardless of techniques to stabilize horizontal eyelid laxity and prevent retraction.

Midface Lift

A midface lift allows for release of the OML and malar septum. Important considerations in tightening of the orbicularis include complete release of restraining ligaments, such as the OML and lateral orbital thickening, and a vertical lift of SMAS tissue.[2]

Anastassov and St Hilaire[46] noted that their technique of midface lift can treat malar descent, lateral festoons, tear trough deformity, melojugal sulcus, buccal fat pad, and muscle descent. In their technique, either through a lower eyelid blepharoplasty incision or transconjunctivally, a subperiosteal dissection is performed to the maxillary alveolus, piriform rim, and zygomatic buttress. The midface is then resuspended to the deep temporal fascia.

Hoenig and colleagues[47] noted improvement in the appearance of malar festoons with a subperiosteal vertical midface lift. A temporal incision is made down to the deep temporalis fascia, and dissection continues subperiosteally over the midface under the orbicularis oculi muscle. Through a buccal incision, cheek soft tissue is further released. Sutures are passed through the midface soft tissues, traveling subperiosteally to the deep temporal fascia. An orbicularis flap is sutured to the orbital rim and excess skin is excised.

In a case report, Krakauer and colleagues[36] described a surgical technique for treatment of festoons using a midface lift. The technique uses a subciliary incision, a subperiosteal midface lift, lower eyelid tarsal strip operation, and skin-orbicularis flap sutured to the lateral orbital rim periosteum.[36]

Stevens and coworkers[48] described a triple-layer midface for the midface lift. The 3 layers for the lift are the postseptal fat, SOOF, and musculo-cutaneous layer of skin and orbicularis oculi.[48] A subciliary incision is made with supraperiosteal dissection. The postseptal fat layer is made by releasing the arcus marginalis, allowing the fat to herniate and is then sutured below the inferior orbital rim. The SOOF layer is lifted and fixed to the lateral orbital rim periosteum. The myocutaneous flap is elevated to the periosteum as well, superior to the SOOF fixation suture. The benefits of the triple layer midface lift include filling the tear trough with redraping of orbital fat and a vertical lift of the SOOF and myocutaneous tissue. A benefit of the myocutaneous flap over a purely skin flap is decreased postoperative swelling by preserving the superficial lymphatic system, thought to be from 20% to 30% with skin flap, to less than 2% with a myocutaneous flap.

Owsley and Zweifler[49] note that, in performing a midface lift, eyelid swelling is decreased if the dissection of the malar septum is avoided.

Liposuction and Fat Excision

Rosenberg[50] described the use of superficial suction lipectomy in the treatment of malar bags. The theory was that the fat, which lies in between the dermis and orbicularis muscle, is the significant factor in malar bags. A 3-mm incision is made at the lateral canthus, a 2.3 mm cannula is inserted into the subdermal plane, and suction of the subcutaneous fat is then undertaken until the bulging tissue has been removed and is no longer palpable.[50] However, this technique does not address the orbicularis muscle, skin excess, or lid edema. Risks with this are skin perforation with cannulation, as well as bruising and swelling. No hematomas, seromas, weakness of the lower eyelid or infections were seen.

Liapakis and Paschali[20]s described combining liposuction and orbicularis oculi suspension for the treatment of malar bags. Liposuction was completed through an incision in the lateral alar area, using a blunt 0.3-cm tip cannula. The midface was mobilized in the subperiosteal plane, which addresses the OML and malar septum, and the lift made by a suture connecting the deep temporal fascia underneath a temporal incision to the lateral fibers of the orbicularis oculi.

Asaadi[17] noted that, for the treatment of congenital festoons, lipectomy is a critical step in any surgical treatment because the etiology of congenital and acquired festoons are different. Congenital festoons, in their study, consistently involve supraorbicularis fat in the prezygomatic space. Asaadi[17] also noted that, for congenital festoons, in addition to a midface lift with OML and ZCL ligament release, subcutaneous fat removal is needed for sufficient treatment. A midface lift alone or subcutaneous fat removal alone was not felt to be sufficient, because often congenital festoons, in adults, can have both laxity and subcutaneous fat as factors in their appearance of festoons.

SUMMARY

Festoons represent a frustration to the patient and a challenge to the surgeon. They often limit the overall results of blepharoplasty, and may lead to patient dissatisfaction with surgery unless the patient is properly educated about our limitations in treating this condition. Nonsurgical treatment options are improving, and the results of tetracycline family compounds are encouraging. A variety of surgical treatments may conceal the appearance of festoons or even modestly improve the underlying pathophysiology. As our understanding of this condition improves, so too will our treatments.

DISCLOSURE

Unrestricted grant award from Research to Prevent Blindness to the Department of Ophthalmology at Cole Eye Institute (RPB1508DM).

REFERENCES

1. Furnas DW. Festoons of orbicularis muscle as a cause of baggy eyelids. Plast Reconstr Surg 1978; 61(4):540–6.
2. Mendelson BC, Muzaffar AR, Adams WP Jr. Surgical anatomy of the midcheek and malar mounds. Plast Reconstr Surg 2002;110(3):885–96 [discussion 897–911].
3. Kpodzo DS, Nahai F, McCord CD. Malar mounds and festoons: review of current management. Aesthet Surg J 2014;34(2):235–48.
4. Pessa JE, Garza JR. The malar septum: the anatomic basis of malar mounds and malar edema. Aesthet Surg J 1997;17(1):11–7.
5. Kikkawa DO, Lemke BN, Dortzbach RK. Relations of the superficial musculoaponeurotic system to the orbit and characterization of the orbitomalar ligament. Ophthal Plast Reconstr Surg 1996;12(2):77–88.
6. Goldberg RA, McCann JD, Fiaschetti D, et al. What causes eyelid bags? Analysis of 114 consecutive patients. Plast Reconstr Surg 2005;115(5): 1395–402 [discussion 1403–394].
7. Wong CH, Mendelson B. Facial soft-tissue spaces and retaining ligaments of the midcheek: defining the premaxillary space. Plast Reconstr Surg 2013; 132(1):49–56.
8. Mendelson BC, Hartley W, Scott M, et al. Age-related changes of the orbit and midcheek and the implications for facial rejuvenation. Aesthetic Plast Surg 2007;31(5):419–23.
9. Shoukath S, Taylor GI, Mendelson BC, et al. The lymphatic anatomy of the lower eyelid and conjunctiva and correlation with postoperative chemosis and edema. Plast Reconstr Surg 2017;139(3):628e–37e.
10. Sami MS, Soparkar CN, Patrinely JR, et al. Eyelid edema. Semin Plast Surg 2007;21(1):24–31.
11. Bernardini FP, Kersten RC, Khouri LM, et al. Chronic eyelid lymphedema and acne rosacea. Report of two cases. Ophthalmology 2000;107(12):2220–3.
12. Harvey DT, Fenske NA, Glass LF. Rosaceous lymphedema: a rare variant of a common disorder. Cutis 1998;61(6):321–4.
13. Carruth BP, Meyer DR, Wladis EJ, et al. Extreme eyelid lymphedema associated with rosacea (Morbihan Disease): case series, literature review, and therapeutic considerations. Ophthal Plast Reconstr Surg 2017;33(3S Suppl 1):S34–8.
14. Marzano AV, Vezzoli P, Alessi E. Elephantoid oedema of the eyelids. J Eur Acad Dermatol Venereol 2004;18(4):459–62.
15. Wilkin JK. Rosacea. Pathophysiology and treatment. Arch Dermatol 1994;130(3):359–62.
16. Mally P, Czyz CN, Wulc AE. The role of gravity in periorbital and midfacial aging. Aesthet Surg J 2014;34(6):809–22.
17. Asaadi M. Etiology and treatment of congenital festoons. Aesthetic Plast Surg 2018;42(4):1024–32.
18. Naik MN. Hills and valleys: understanding the undereye. J Cutan Aesthet Surg 2016;9(2):61–4.
19. McCord CD, Kreymerman P, Nahai F, et al. Management of postblepharoplasty chemosis. Aesthet Surg J 2013;33(5):654–61.
20. Liapakis IE, Paschalis EI. Liposuction and suspension of the orbicularis oculi for the correction of persistent malar bags: description of technique and report of a case. Aesthetic Plast Surg 2012;36(3):546–9.
21. Sagili S, Selva D, Malhotra R. Eyelid lymphedema following neck dissection and radiotherapy. Ophthal Plast Reconstr Surg 2013;29(6):e146–9.
22. Goldman MP. Festoon formation after infraorbital botulinum A toxin: a case report. Dermatol Surg 2003;29(5):560–1 [discussion 561].
23. Goldberg RA, Fiaschetti D. Filling the periorbital hollows with hyaluronic acid gel: initial experience with 244 injections. Ophthal Plast Reconstr Surg 2006; 22(5):335–41 [discussion 341–33].
24. Iverson SM, Patel RM. Dermal filler-associated malar edema: treatment of a persistent adverse effect. Orbit 2017;36(6):473–5.

25. Hilton S, Schrumpf H, Buhren BA, et al. Hyaluronidase injection for the treatment of eyelid edema: a retrospective analysis of 20 patients. Eur J Med Res 2014;19:30.

26. Zoumalan CI. Managing periocular filler-related syndrome prior to lower blepharoplasty. Aesthetic Plast Surg 2019;43(1):115–22.

27. Furnas DW. Festoons, mounds, and bags of the eyelids and cheek. Clin Plast Surg 1993;20(2):367–85.

28. Braz AV, Black JM, Pirmez R, et al. Treatment of malar mounds with hyaluronic acid fillers: an anatomical approach. Dermatol Surg 2018;44(Suppl 1): S56–60.

29. Papageorgiou K, Chang HS, Isaacs D, et al. Refining the goals of oculofacial rejuvenation with dynamic ultrasonography. Aesthet Surg J 2012; 32(2):207–19.

30. Roberts TL 3rd. Laser blepharoplasty and laser resurfacing of the periorbital area. Clin Plast Surg 1998;25(1):95–108.

31. Roberts TL, Yokoo KM. In pursuit of optimal periorbital rejuvenation: laser resurfacing with or without blepharoplasty and brow lift. Aesthet Surg J 1998; 18(5):321–32.

32. Hunzeker CM, Weiss ET, Geronemus RG. Fractionated CO_2 laser resurfacing: our experience with more than 2000 treatments. Aesthet Surg J 2009; 29(4):317–22.

33. Ramesh S, Wulc A. Combination radiofrequency microneedling for festoons. San Francisco, CA: ASOPRS Fall Scientific Symposium.; 2019.

34. Jeon H, Geronemus RG. Successful noninvasive treatment of festoons. Plast Reconstr Surg 2018; 141(6):977e–8e.

35. Huang J, Yu W, Zhang Z, et al. Clinical and histological studies of suborbital wrinkles treated with fractional bipolar radiofrequency. Rejuvenation Res 2018;21(2):117–22.

36. Krakauer M, Aakalu VK, Putterman AM. Treatment of malar festoon using modified subperiosteal midface lift. Ophthal Plast Reconstr Surg 2012;28(6):459–62.

37. Perry JD, Mehta VJ, Costin BR. Intralesional tetracycline injection for treatment of lower eyelid festoons: a preliminary report. Ophthal Plast Reconstr Surg 2015;31(1):50–2.

38. Chon B, Hwang C, Perry J. Long term patient experience with tetracycline injections for festoons. Plast Reconstr Surg 2020;146(6):737e–43e.

39. Godfrey KJ, Kally P, Dunbar KE, et al. Doxycycline injection for sclerotherapy of lower eyelid festoons and malar edema: preliminary results. Ophthal Plast Reconstr Surg 2019;35(5):474–7.

40. Han L, Su W, Huang J, et al. Doxycycline inhibits inflammation-induced lymphangiogenesis in mouse cornea by multiple mechanisms. PLoS One 2014; 9(9):e108931.

41. Bellinvia P, Klinger F, Bellinvia G. Lower blepharoplasty with direct excision of skin excess: a five-year experience. Aesthet Surg J 2010;30(5):665–70.

42. Einan-Lifshitz A, Hartstein ME. Treatment of festoons by direct excision. Orbit 2012;31(5):303–6.

43. Farrior RT, Kassir RR. Management of malar folds in blepharoplasty. Laryngoscope 1998;108(11 Pt 1): 1659–63.

44. Carriquiry CE, Seoane OJ, Londinsky M. Orbicularis transposition flap for muscle suspension in lower blepharoplasty. Ann Plast Surg 2006;57(2):138–41.

45. Lassus C. Benefits from lifting of the lower eyelid. Aesthetic Plast Surg 2000;24(6):424–8.

46. Anastassov GE, St Hilaire H. Periorbital and midfacial rejuvenation via blepharoplasty and sub-periosteal midface rhytidectomy. Int J Oral Maxillofac Surg 2006;35(4):301–11.

47. Hoenig JF, Knutti D, de la Fuente A. Vertical subperiosteal mid-face-lift for treatment of malar festoons. Aesthetic Plast Surg 2011;35(4):522–9.

48. Stevens HP, Willemsen JC, Durani P, et al. Triple-layer midface lifting: long-term follow-up of an effective approach to aesthetic surgery of the lower eyelid and the midface. Aesthetic Plast Surg 2014; 38(4):632–40.

49. Owsley JQ, Zweifler M. Midface lift of the malar fat pad: technical advances. Plast Reconstr Surg 2002;110(2):674–85 [discussion 686–77].

50. Rosenberg GJ. Correction of saddlebag deformity of the lower eyelids by superficial suction lipectomy. Plast Reconstr Surg 1995;96(5):1061–5.

The Prominent Eye—What to Watch Out For

Hannah Landsberger[a], Yao Wang, MD[b,1], Raymond S. Douglas, MD, PhD[c],*

KEYWORDS

- Proptosis • Thyroid eye disease • Globe prominence

KEY POINTS

- Proptosis may be caused various congenital or acquired conditions, with thyroid eye disease being the most common acquired etiology.
- Untreated globe prominence can lead to a variety of complications due to the potential for diminished mechanical function of the eyelid.
- Globe prominence and its associated features may be managed conservatively with injectable fillers and/or botulinum toxin type A or surgically via orbital decompression, blepharoplasties, and facial contouring procedures.
- Familiarity with eyelid and orbital anatomy and surgical treatment options is imperative in producing a good aesthetic and functional result.

INTRODUCTION

The prominent globe (proptosis) poses a unique set of challenges to the surgeon attempting aesthetic or reconstructive surgery.[1] Physicians must pay special attention to avoid poor outcomes or worsening aesthetic appearance or causing ocular or visual disturbances.[2] Patients are at risk for a variety of complications, due to potential diminished mechanical function of the eyelid, such as scleral show, lagophthalmos, strabismus, eyelid retraction, exposure keratopathy, and ulceration.[3,4]

Globe prominence can be associated with a variety of congenital conditions, such as a shallow orbit, hypoplasia of the maxilla and zygoma, or craniofacial syndromes (Crouzon or Pfeiffer syndromes).[1,2] Additionally, a prominent globe may be seen with increased axial length of the globe, such as in moderate to high myopia.[2] Most commonly, a prominent globe is due to an acquired disease state, such as thyroid eye disease (TED).[2,4]

It is imperative that patients with prominent globes are diagnosed and managed before aesthetic interventions. For example, patients with TED can experience a variety of clinical manifestations that lead to changes in their facial anatomy. These manifestations can include eyelid swelling, eyelid retraction, proptosis, strabismus, brow fat expansion, preaponeurotic fat expansion, glabellar rhytids, and expansion of the soft tissues in the cheeks, buccal fat, and eyebrows.[2,4] Attempting to correct patients' cosmetic concerns with subtractive upper and lower blepharoplasty without addressing the position of the globe or orbital rim results in suboptimal outcomes and has the potential to cause debilitating exposure symptoms, tearing, and unfavorable cosmetic results.[1,2] Due to these potential complications, it sometimes is necessary first to perform surgery aimed at altering globe position and orbit architecture before performing cosmetic periocular procedures.

This article reviews the various treatment options that should be considered when evaluating

[a] Nova Southeastern University Dr. Kiran C. Patel College of Allopathic Medicine, 11766 Wilshire Blvd, Suite 325, Los Angeles, CA 90025, USA; [b] Department of Surgery, Division of Ophthalmology, Cedars-Sinai Medical Center, Los Angeles, CA, USA; [c] State Key Laboratory of Ophthalmology, Zhongshan Ophthalmic Center, Sun Yat-sen University, Guangzhou, China
[1] Present address: 150 North Robertson Boulevard, Suite 314, Beverly Hills, CA 90211.
* Corresponding author. Cedars Sinai Medical Center, West Medical Office Towers, 8635 West Third Street, Suite 650West, Los Angeles, CA 90048.
E-mail address: raymonddouglasmd@gmail.com

Facial Plast Surg Clin N Am 29 (2021) 311–321
https://doi.org/10.1016/j.fsc.2021.02.004

a patient with a prominent globe. Although TED is the primary etiology of globe prominence that this article focuses on, these treatment modalities can be utilized in treating any cause of a prominent globe. No matter the etiology, the underlying cause of a prominent globe should be identified and addressed as needed before cosmetic procedures are attempted.

ANATOMIC ASSOCIATIONS

The normal position of the lower eyelid is maintained by a balance of tendons, ligaments, muscle, and orbital volume. The medial and lateral canthal tendons function as a sling to maintain the eyelid height and anatomic position along the undersurface of the globe. Ligaments keep the soft tissue of the eyelid and cheek attached the facial bones. Of primary concern to eyelid surgeons is the orbicularis muscle, which tonically contracts in a sphincteric fashion to maintain lower eyelid position. Finally, the fat and bone that maintain the orbital volume provide stability to the face and the lower eyelid. This delicate balance easily can be disrupted and lead to lower lid retraction, particularly in patients with globe prominence.

Globe prominence may be due to an increase in the volume of fat and/or ocular muscles, such as in TED, nonsyndromic exorbitism, midface hypoplasia, soft tissue or bony lesions, or a congenitally enlarged globe.[5,6] All these conditions create a negative vector eyelid, in which the cornea protrudes past the malar eminence.[2,7,8] Patients with negative vector eyelids are at greater risk of experiencing lower lid malposition after aesthetic surgery due to the force exerted by the prominent globe on the lower eyelid, which forces the eyelid to support itself against the upward slope of the globe (**Fig. 1**).[7,9] For example, when patients have globe prominence with a negative vector eyelid, special care must be taken in the canthal suspension of lower eyelid blepharoplasty in order to avoid bowstringing of the globe.[9]

Patients with prominent globes, including those patients with TED, tend to have eyelid retraction, a high upper eyelid crease, increased periorbital volume/fat prolapse, and increased prominence of tear trough (**Fig. 2**). Each of these physical findings requires recognition and thoughtful evaluation and surgical planning because patients with prominent eyes require more complex techniques to avoid unnecessary complications.

SURGICAL TREATMENT OPTIONS

Surgical treatment options for globe prominence and eyelid retraction have evolved over the years to become less invasive, produce better cosmetic results, and provide greater patient satisfaction.[10] Because TED is the most frequent etiology of globe prominence or proptosis, we are using TED as an example to frame this discussion.

The traditional surgical management of non–vision-threatening TED included a 4-staged surgical approach of orbital decompression, eye muscle surgery, correction of eyelid malposition, and blepharoplasty.[11] This approach was believed to increase predictability because each step would affect the planning of the subsequent procedures, ultimately producing the best result in the fewest procedures.[11] The multistaged approach, however, has disadvantages, such as a lengthy patient time commitment due to the need for a healing interval between surgeries, increased patient cost, high patient anxiety, and added incisions and healing leading, to the formation of more scar tissue, all of which can factor into decreased patient satisfaction.[12–14] Recently, studies have shown that orbital decompression surgery produces predictable changes in eyelid position and contour.[12–14] Furthermore, a single-staged facial reconstruction, including bilateral orbital, aesthetic eyelid, and facial surgery, produces safe, efficacious, and predictable aesthetic results that are comparable to those from a multistaged approach with fewer disadvantages and less downtime (**Figs. 3** and **4**).[12–14] These studies clearly demonstrate how globe prominence affects the eyelid contour and relative height (**Fig. 5**).

The authors recommend a customized approach to aesthetic reconstructive surgery based on an individual's facial characteristics and changes that have occurred due to eye prominence. There is great individual variability in the facial anatomy, including periorbital bone

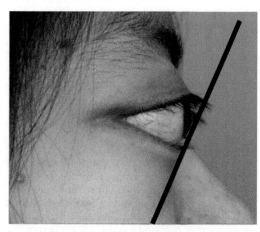

Fig. 1. A female patient with cornea protruding past the malar eminence, creating a negative vector eyelid.

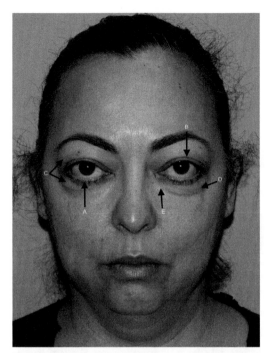

Fig. 2. A patient with bilaterally symmetric prominent globes. Note the presence of A, lower eyelid retraction; B, high upper eyelid crease; C, increased periorbital volume; and D, lower eyelid fat herniation with E, increased prominence of tear trough.

projection and soft tissue expansion in the cheeks, buccal fat, and eyebrow. It is imperative that the surgeon considers the patient's inherent facial structure as well as the changes due to TED, rather than limiting the surgical goal to globe positioning, when planning surgery. Furthermore, the surgeon should evaluate each patient thoroughly and discuss the orbital and periorbital changes within the context of their facial morphology and aging process so that realistic surgical plans and goals that reduce the effects of TED can be established.[15] discuss the orbital and periorbital changes within the context of the facial morphology and aging process so that realistic surgical plans and goals.[15] With TED, the surgeon should stress that the goal of surgery is to improve their function and appearance as closely as possible to their predisease state, but that complete rehabilitation not always is possible. Predisease photographs help the surgeon and patient develop realistic expectations for the surgery.[15]

ORBITAL DECOMPRESSION

Although orbital decompression initially was performed only in vision-threatening cases due to optic neuropathy or uncontrollable ocular exposure,

improved and minimally invasive techniques have led to expanded indications for purely cosmetic purposes. Orbital decompression surgery should be customized to each patient, taking into account the type and magnitude of decompression necessary, all of which likely reduce the need for additional eyelid or periorbital procedures.[15] It is imperative that the physician considers each patient's clinical characteristics, such as compressive optic neuropathy, eyelid retraction, fat versus muscle predominant disease, and nonaxial globe displacement, when surgical planning.[16,17]

Planning for aesthetic reconstruction for patients with prominent globes begins with an evaluation of the 3-dimensional (3-D) globe position, which helps guide the type and magnitude of potential orbital decompression (**Fig. 6** has a flow diagram). It is important that preoperative computed tomography (CT) scan be performed so that the bony anatomy can be assessed, including the diploe of the lateral wall, to plan the amount of bone decompression. The most common anatomic targets for decompression are the deep lateral orbital wall, medial wall, and orbital floor. The authors prefer a deep lateral orbital decompression demarcated by decompression posterior to the course of the zygomaticotemporal nerve to achieve significant axial reduction from the zygomatic basin (inferolateral orbit adjacent to the inferior orbital fissure), superior lateral, and deep sphenoid (**Fig. 7**).[3] Orbital fat removal is the initial step in orbital decompression not only in fat predominant fat-predominate TED but also muscle-predominant and mixed disease.[18] Fat decompression can be the initial step in the management of prominent eyes in patients without TED. Decompression in the region of the zygomatic basin can help reduce relative hyperglobus as well as improve the relationship of the lower eyelid and globe, reducing lower eyelid retraction in a highly predictable manner.[3] This method potentially eliminates the need for lower eyelid retraction repair in mild to moderate TED and in cases of eyelid retraction without TED. The most severe cases of TED may require lower eyelid retraction repair, performed via recession of the lower eyelid retractors or placement of hard palate grafts, although in the authors' practice these circumstances are rare. Further reduction in axial proptosis also may be achieved as needed with fat decompression, which is especially effective in fat predominant disease.[3,10,17–20] redundant.

In cases that require additional proptosis reduction, or in patients with thin diploe of the lateral wall, the authors can perform a medial wall decompression with removal of the medial strut based on the degree of reduction needed, based on the surgeon's clinical judgment. This addition

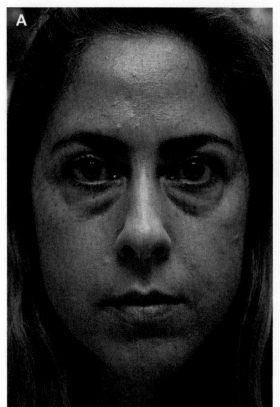
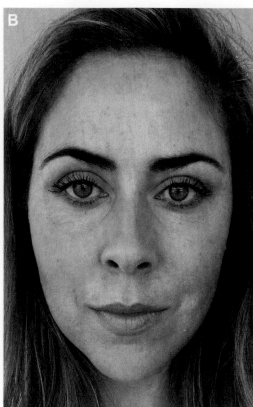

Fig. 3. A 32-year-old woman with history of TED and displeased with eye bulging, increased periorbital fat expansion, and buccal fat expansion. She underwent a bilateral upper eyelid blepharoplasty, bilateral lateral wall decompression, bilateral lower eyelid blepharoplasty with fat repositioning, and bilateral buccal fat removal. (*A*) Shows preoperative photo and (*B*) shows postoperative photograph at 4 months. (Reproduced with permission from Douglas RS. Commentary on: Simultaneous Aesthetic Eyelid Surgery and Orbital Decompression for Rehabilitation of Thyroid Eye Disease: The One-Stage Approach. Aesthet Surg J. 2018;38(10): 1062-1064).

can provide up to 3 mm of additional axial reduction.

EYELID RETRACTION REPAIR

Upper and lower eyelid retraction enhance the appearance of a prominent globe, contributing the a staring appearance.[21] Bartley[22] proposed the classification of causes of eyelid retraction as neurogenic (eg, dorsal midbrain syndrome), myogenic (eg, TED), mechanistic (eg, eyelid malposition or globe prominence), and miscellaneous (eg, optic nerve hypoplasia). Although both upper and lower eyelid retraction are related most commonly to TED, upper eyelid retraction is the most common clinical sign of TED.[4,21] Upper eyelid retraction also may occur iatrogenically, as a primary condition, or in association with other medical conditions that fall within the 4 categories. Lower eyelid retraction also may be caused by a wide variety of conditions but is less likely to be due to neurogenic causes.[21]

Lower eyelid retraction may be related to globe prominence, a shallow orbit, poor malar projection, lower eyelid flaccidity, iatrogenic causes, and intrinsic factors to the soft tissues of the eyelid and cheek.[21,22] Both upper and lower eyelid retraction can be potential complications from a variety of procedures, such as overly aggressive blepharoplasty or extraocular muscle surgery.[21] Having prior surgery is a complicating factor in eyelid retraction repair because it may require scar release, full-thickness skin grafting, and other additional treatments.[2,21,23]

Upper Eyelid Retraction Repair

It has been shown that there is minimal change in upper eyelid position after axial orbital decompression.[24] Therefore, it is imperative to evaluate the upper eyelid position during preoperative planning since the final positioning of the upper eyelid, with symmetric eyelid platform show, plays a critical

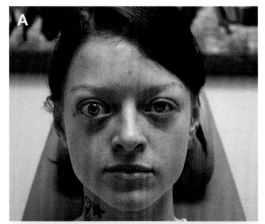

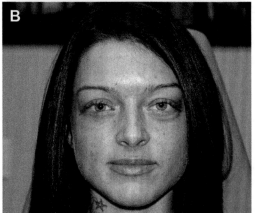

Fig. 4. (*A*) Presurgical and (*B*) 2 months postsurgical photographs of a 26-year-old woman who suffered from TED with right-sided proptosis much worse than left (exophthalmometry 27 mm on the right and 24 mm on the left), right upper and lower eyelid retraction, and bilateral midface volume deficiency. She underwent bilateral lateral wall and fat decompression, right-sided medial wall decompression, right upper eyelid posterior approach blepharotomy, and bilateral fat grafting to cheeks and nasal midface.

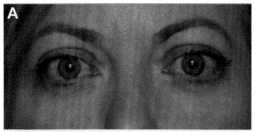

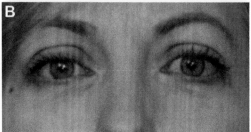

Fig. 5. Normal eyelid contour restored following proptosis reduction via orbital decompression. (*A*) Patient with proptosis and eyelid retraction due to TED, leading to greater vertical eyelid contour. (*B*) Patient postoperative after orbital decompression demonstrating return to normal eyelid contour.

role in patient satisfaction. Upper eyelid retraction repair may be performed via an anterior or posterior approach, depending on the amount of upper eyelid retraction determined preoperatively.[14] If the upper eyelid retraction is less than 3 mm, the authors typically perform a posterior Müller extirpation with the patient under general anesthesia after orbital decompression because intraoperative adjustment usually is not required.[12,14] If the upper eyelid retraction is greater than or equal to 3 mm, the authors prefer an anterior full-thickness blepharotomy performed under monitored anesthesia care prior to induction of general anesthesia for the subsequent orbital decompression.[25] This allows the surgeon to assess eyelid position intraoperatively and surgically modify as needed. It is important to release the lateral horn of the levator aponeurosis to avoid lateral flare in patients with TED. When there is expected to be significant proptosis reduction (5 mm or more), the upper eyelid should be left slightly elevated (1 mm) because the eyelid position can lower postoperatively in such cases (**Fig. 8**).[15]

Lower Eyelid Retraction Repair

Lower eyelid retraction can have a multifactorial cause, typically related to instability of the lower eyelid due to horizontal laxity of the tarsoligamentous sling or orbicularis muscle.[23] Other causes may involve scarring or tethering of the middle lamellae from trauma or previous surgery or weakened vertical support of the lower eyelid because of midface descent.[23,26] Globe prominence, due to TED or nonthyroid causes, also is a common cause of lower eyelid retraction.[23] As a general rule, lateral tarsal strip with canthoplasty by itself is an ineffective way to treat lower eyelid retraction patients because it can worsen lower eyelid retraction via bowstringing effect.[2] The techniques used to treat lower eyelid retraction in TED are applicable to patients with lower eyelid retraction of any other etiology.

As discussed previously, it has been shown that there is a statistically significant correlation between orbital decompression and improving lower eyelid positioning.[24] The authors have demonstrated that for every 3 mm to 4 mm of proptosis

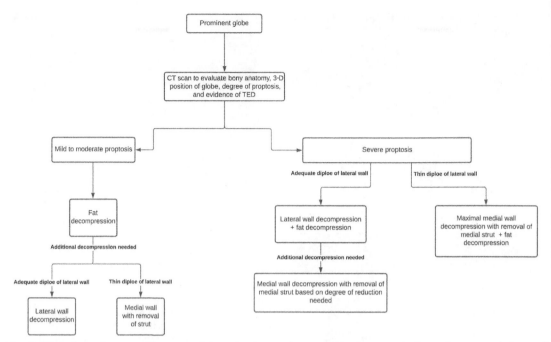

Fig. 6. Flow chart demonstrating steps for evaluation and treatment of proptosis depending on severity and anatomy.

reduction, a reduction of 1 mm of lower eyelid retraction can be expected.[3] Decompression targeting the deep lateral orbit surrounding the inferior orbital fissure can improve lower eyelid positioning further. When bone is removed from this area, it appears that the globe is able to move inferior relative to the eyelid, thus reducing eyelid retraction.[3] Customized decompression surgery alone may not be enough to sufficiently correct lower eyelid retraction in patients with

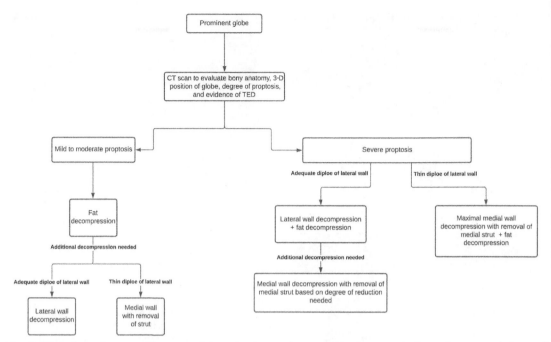

Fig. 7. Orbital model showing the anatomic targets for orbital bony decompression. DS, deep sphenoid bone; MW, medial orbital wall; OF, orbital floor; SL, superior lateral; ZB, zygomatic basin.

severe lower eyelid retraction.[13] In such cases, retraction repair can be performed under general anesthesia after decompression, with lower eyelid retractors released via a transconjunctival approach.[27] Lower eyelid retractor release may be performed with or without subperiosteal midface-suborbicularis oculi fat lifting and scar lysis or internal eyelid spacer graft.[13] Midface lifting may be performed in cases in which additional lower eyelid anterior lamella (skin) is needed.[13] If there is significant anterior lamellar deficiency, a skin graft or flap may be required. In the authors' experience, a spacer graft rarely is needed but should be considered in cases where it is not possible to achieve adequate decompression, orbicularis weakness and/or cicatricial changes are present, or lateral contour of the eyelid is rounded. The authors prefer to use a hard palate graft if a spacer graft is deemed necessary. Frequently, the authors place a temporary lateral tarsorrhaphy to maintain the upward pull in the immediate postoperative period for 1 week.

In patients with TED, it is imperative to assess the presence of vertical strabismus as well as a patient's risk of developing vertical strabismus after decompression surgery before considering lower eyelid retraction repair. In patients who already have vertical strabismus, it usually is warranted to defer lower eyelid surgery because strabismus surgery involving the inferior rectus often has unexpected effects on the position of the lower

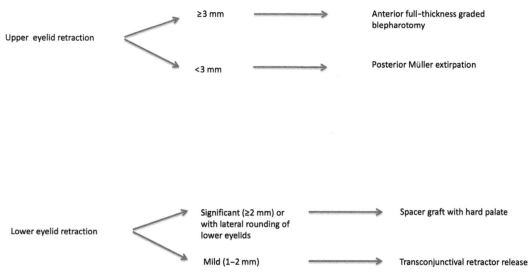

Fig. 8. Flow diagram of upper and lower eyelid retraction repair for patients undergoing simultaneous decompression surgery. (*Top*) Note that blepharotomies typically are performed with the patients under monitored anesthesia, to allow surgeons to assess the height, shape, and contour of the upper eyelids. It is important to release the lateral horn of the levator aponeurosis to avoid lateral flare. In cases of 5 mm or more of proptosis reduction, the eyelid positioning should be left slightly elevated (1 mm). (*Bottom*) Lower eyelid retraction repair is typically performed after decompression (under general anesthesia). Note that every 3 mm to 4 mm of orbital decompression reduces the lower eyelid retraction by 1 mm. If additional retraction repair is needed (and mild), release the lower eyelid retractors (transconjunctivally). If significant lower eyelid retraction present, consider placement of hard palate. This rarely is needed but used in cases where lateral lower eyelid rounding in present.

eyelid.[15] In patients who do not have strabismus present at their presentation, their risk of developing strabismus is dependent on the surgeon's personal rates of post-decompression strabismus.[15] The senior author (RS) has reported that his rates of strabismus are most dependent on the type of decompression and the preoperative muscle size. Patients with fat predominant disease and normal size extraocular muscles have a very low risk of diplopia after lateral and/or medial wall decompression (<2%). Patients with large extraocular muscles have approximately 3% risk of developing new-onset diplopia after lateral wall decompression. The risk of developing new-onset double vision in these patients increases to approximately 10% with the addition of medial wall decompression. Inferior rectus manipulation can affect lower eyelid position in cases with preexisting strabismus where surgery is indicated, which is why it is advisable to defer lower eyelid retraction repair until after strabismus surgery. Such cases where there is preexisting vertical misalignment are instances in which a staged procedure may be more beneficial.

Overall, the authors believe it is safe and reasonable to perform lower eyelid retraction repair and decompression surgery in a single stage due to the relatively low rates of diplopia after decompression surgery. It is crucial to preoperatively counsel patients about the risk of developing diplopia and/or their potential need for additional surgery.

UPPER AND LOWER BLEPHAROPLASTY

In patients with prominent eyes who are not undergoing simultaneous orbital decompression, upper eyelid blepharoplasty (including upper eyelid fat excision) should be conservative in nature to avoid lagophthalmos and worsening appearance of globe protuberance. Additionally, surgeons should not aggressive debulk the orbicularis muscle, because removal results in orbicularis weakness and poor closure.

In patients with prominent eyes, the eyelid crease tends to be higher compared with nonprominent globes. In such patients, marking the crease below the anatomic crease is recommended to avoid the appearance of a high lid crease. Upper eyelid blepharoplasty in patients with TED can be performed with various modifications, such as preaponeurotic fat sculpting versus repositioning and debulking of the brow fat pad. This subtractive technique is often necessary in patients with TED because the entire eyelid/brow complex expands, causing significant volume expansion.[14] If necessary, the lacrimal gland should be repositioned by expanding the bony fossa during decompression and suturing the gland posteriorly, tucking it within the fossa. This step is important in creating an aesthetically pleasing upper eyebrow contour. The authors have found that adding a brow fat suspension suture to upper eyelid blepharoplasty improve the transition between the eyebrow and eyelid. In this procedure, the free ends of the orbicularis muscle at the upper and lower edges of the blepharoplasty incision are secured to the superior arcus marginalis periosteum. Joining these structures mechanically elevates and repositions the ptotic brow fat pad to create a more youthful appearance.[28]

A transconjunctival lower lid blepharoplasty with orbicularis retaining ligament release and fat excision versus repositioning can be performed in the standard fashion as well. Great care should be taken when performing these procedures because the fat from TED patients tends to be highly vascular.[29]

Lower eyelid skin excision must be conservative because aggressive skin excision causes lower eyelid retraction. Chemical/laser resurfacing can be performed to tighten the skin in a conservative manner. Canthal suspension, as discussed previously, can be difficult. A hang back modification may be necessary to prevent bowstringing of the globe. The suture also can be secured on a higher position along the lateral orbital rim. Additionally, midface suspension with orbicularis plication helps support the lower eyelid and canthus.

FACIAL CONTOURING PROCEDURES

The surgeon should assess the entire face during the preoperative evaluation. This includes evaluation of the tear trough, degree of cheek projection, temporal hollowing, contour and height of the eyebrow, and any other contour deficits or abnormal projection. In TED, there are unnatural soft tissue changes to the upper eyelid/brow unit. There also could be relative nasal midface deficiency. Facial fat grafting can be performed to the nasal midface and/or cheek to increase projection and reduce the appearance of proptosis. Fat grafting to the tear trough also can reduce the appearance of the hollow and proptosis.

Orbital rim augmentation via placement of implant or osteotomy and bone advancement can also be used to augment the midface and lessen the prominence of the eye. These can be done in conjunction with orbital decompression to further reduce relative proptosis may allow to less aggressive decompression in certain cases.[1] Onlay grafts or implants is less invasive that has the added benefits of less operative time and lower morbidity.[1] The implant can be placed through a variety of incisions based on the patient's needs as well as the other surgical aspects being performed. Osteotomy with rim advancements has the advantage of not introducing materials that may later lead to infection but is not easily reversible. Further, it is invasive, has the risk of temporalis muscle atrophy, and may have less predictable outcomes due to variable resorption.[1] Lower eyelid blepharoplasty with fat repositioning can also augment the nasal midface in the appropriate patient. This avoids the risks and complications of a foreign implant.[2]

NONSURGICAL TREATMENT OPTIONS
Fillers

Although surgery is the definitive treatment of globe prominence and eyelid retraction found in TED, injectable fillers are a precise and minimally invasive method to augment along the orbital rim and tear trough for patients wanting noninvasive approach or as a postoperative adjunct.[2] The use of hyaluronic acid (HA) gel has expanded from its use as a cosmetic filler to being used for more functional treatments, such as eyelid retraction and lagophthalmos.[4] Studies have shown that HA injections are an effective temporary treatment for both upper and lower eyelid retraction.[30,31] HA fillers provide volume enhancement and relief of ocular exposure symptoms and allow for adjustment of eyelid position in patients awaiting definitive surgery for eyelid retraction or who prefer a minimally invasive treatment.[30,31]

The two main injection techniques for HA filler are transcutaneous and transconjunctival approaches, with the aim of placing the filler at the level of the eyelid retractors to lengthen them in both the upper and lower eyelids.[32] For upper eyelid retraction, placement of HA filler at this level has the additional benefit of adding weight to the eyelid (liquid lid weight), whereas, in the lower lid, HA fillers provide scaffolding support to the lower eyelid so that it is elevated against the inferior orbital rim.[32] Kohn and colleagues[30] found that subconjunctival injection of HA fillers into the levator plane was effective in both the active and inactive stages of TED, with those treated in the active phase having more prolonged effects from the HA gel injections. They believe that these findings suggest that HA may play a role in preventing the fibrosis that occurs in the active stage of TED.[30]

Although HA is a temporary treatment option for eyelid retraction with benefits that decrease over time, the effects can be prolonged with maintenance injections.[30] Furthermore, HA is titratable, is reversible, and typically has low complication rates, making it a desirable option to ameliorate ocular exposure symptoms.[30] Hyaluronidase also may be used to reverse an undesirable result after HA injection, immediately reducing the fullness or contour abnormality and continuing to work over the next 24 hours.[30,33] HA, however, does not directly release extensive cicatrix, which may occur in some patients, rendering it an ineffective treatment modality for those patients.[34] Patients may experience self-limited and typically transient complications, such as erythema, edema, ecchymoses, tenderness, and pain.[4,30,31] Patients also must be made aware of the rare, but severe, complications of HA injection, which include tissue necrosis and embolization to the orbital circulation.[30,31]

Botulinum Toxin Type A

Although the exact mechanism of upper eyelid retraction in TED still is unclear, many proposed theories involve overactivation of the levator palpebrae superioris (LPS) or Müller muscles.[35] Surgery still is the gold standard treatment of upper eyelid retraction in the inactive phase of TED, but there is a need for treatment modalities during the active phase when patients are not considered surgical candidates. Botulinum toxin type A (BTA) has proved an effective temporary treatment method for upper eyelid retraction, particularly during the active phase of TED when surgery typically is not an option.[35] Patients with upper eyelid retraction who have not yet reached the inactive phase of TED may experience symptoms due to corneal exposure or may be displeased with their cosmetic appearance, all of which may be ameliorated temporarily with the use of BTA injections.

Studies on the effects of BTA injection have used transcutaneous or transconjunctival injections to target the LPS, often adjusting the amount of BTA injected based on the severity of upper eyelid retraction.[32] Morgenstern and colleagues[35] reported that transconjunctival BTA injection was more effective when given in the inflammatory phase of TED as opposed to the postinflammatory phase associated with fibrosis. They proposed that BTA injection may release inflammatory contracture, prevent fibrosis caused by muscle shortening and tethering from restricted motion, or allow for a more symmetric appearance.[35] In contrast, Costa and colleagues[36] found that there was significant improvement in upper eyelid retraction in patients with both active and inactive TED, but that the effects were significantly longer in the TED patients with inactive disease. These results are temporary, however, and vary between patients, making the resulting appearance somewhat unpredictable.[4,35,37,38] Studies utilized varying dosages, injection sites, follow-up periods, and outcome criteria, which make it difficult to determine a consensus guideline. Furthermore, there are potential side effects of BTA injection, such as ptosis, diplopia, and new onset or worsening of preexisting strabismus.[4,35] These side effects and variability in outcome occurred regardless of injection method—transconjunctival or transcutaneous. A transconjunctival injection approach, however, may yield more predictable results than a percutaneous approach due to the increased effect on the Müller muscle and the decreased undesirable effect of orbicularis muscle weakening.[35]

SUMMARY

Globe prominence has a variety of medical associations, including syndromic craniosynostosis, high myopia, midface hypoplasia, and TED. Proptosis is a notable and common complicating factor when performing cosmetic periocular surgery. It is important to determine and consider the cause of globe prominence in order to avoid surgical complications when performing eyelid surgery on patients with proptosis. Understanding the nuances of these patients' orbit and periorbital tissue helps avoid complications and subpar aesthetic results.

There are a variety of corrective and cosmetic techniques that can be combined to prevent the underlying problem from worsening and provide safe and cosmetically appropriate surgery to this challenging patient population. Treating surgical complications in these patients requires more complex reconstructive techniques than are needed for patients without prominent eyes. This article hopefully provides readers with a new appreciation for the intricacies involved in treating globe prominence, performing eyelid surgery in this patient population, and the potential to produce suboptimal results due to the nuances of tailoring these procedures to the prominent globe.

DISCLOSURE

Dr R.S. Douglas reports receiving consulting fees from Horizon Therapeutics and Osmotica Pharmaceuticals.

REFERENCES

1. Goldberg RA, Soroudi AE, McCann JD. Treatment of prominent eyes with orbital rim onlay implants: four-year experience. Ophthal Plast Reconstr Surg 2003; 19(1):38–45.
2. Holds JB. Management of the prominent eye. In: Massry GG, Murphy MR, Azizzadeh B, editors. Master techniques in blepharoplasty and periorbital rejuvenation. New York (NY): Springer; 2011. p. 297–306.

3. Pieroni Goncalves AC, Gupta S, Monteiro MLR, et al. Customized minimally invasive orbital decompression surgery improves lower eyelid retraction and contour in thyroid eye disease. Ophthal Plast Reconstr Surg 2017;33(6):446–51.

4. Wang Y, Tooley AA, Mehta VJ, et al. Thyroid orbitopathy. Int Ophthalmol Clin 2018;58(2):137–79.

5. Krastinova-Lolov D, Bach CA, Hartl DM, et al. Surgical strategy in the treatment of globe protrusion depending on its mechanism (Graves' disease, nonsyndromic exorbitism, or high myopia). Plast Reconstr Surg 2006;117(2):553–64.

6. Baujat B, Krastinova D, Bach CA, et al. Orbital morphology in exophthalmos and exorbitism. Plast Reconstr Surg 2006;117(2):542–50 [discussion 551–2].

7. Codner MA, McCord CD. Eyelid and periorbital surgery. 2nd edition. New York: CRC Press; 2016.

8. Mommaerts MY. Definitive treatment of the negative vector orbit. J Craniomaxillofac Surg 2018;46(7):1065–8.

9. Massry GG. Comprehensive lower eyelid rejuvenation. Facial Plast Surg 2010;26(3):209–21.

10. Goldberg RA. Advances in surgical rehabilitation in thyroid eye disease. Thyroid 2008;18(9):989–95.

11. Shorr N, Seiff SR. The four stages of surgical rehabilitation of the patient with dysthyroid ophthalmopathy. Ophthalmology 1986;93(4):476–83.

12. Ben Simon GJ, Mansury AM, Schwarcz RM, et al. Simultaneous orbital decompression and correction of upper eyelid retraction versus staged procedures in thyroid-related orbitopathy. Ophthalmology 2005;112(5):923–32.

13. Taban MR. Combined orbital decompression and lower eyelid retraction surgery. J Curr Ophthalmol 2018;30(2):169–73.

14. Bernardini FP, Skippen B, Zambelli A, et al. Simultaneous aesthetic eyelid surgery and orbital decompression for rehabilitation of thyroid eye disease: the one-stage approach. Aesthet Surg J 2018;38(10):1052–61.

15. Douglas RS. Commentary on: simultaneous aesthetic eyelid surgery and orbital decompression for rehabilitation of thyroid eye disease: the one-stage approach. Aesthet Surg J 2018;38(10):1062–4.

16. Gillespie EF, Smith TJ, Douglas RS. Thyroid eye disease: towards an evidence base for treatment in the 21st century. Curr Neurol Neurosci Rep 2012;12(3):318–24.

17. Bothun ED, Scheurer RA, Harrison AR, et al. Update on thyroid eye disease and management. Clin Ophthalmol 2009;3:543–51.

18. Gupta S, Briceño CA, Douglas RS. Customized minimally invasive orbital decompression for thyroid eye disease. Expert Rev Ophthalmol 2013;8(3):255–66.

19. Kingdom TT, Davies BW, Durairaj VD. Orbital decompression for the management of thyroid eye disease: an analysis of outcomes and complications. Laryngoscope 2015;125(9):2034–40.

20. Palmero MO, Lucarelli MJ. Evolving techniques in orbital decompression of thyroid orbitopathy. Philipp J Ophthalmol 2007;32(1):28–31.

21. Chang EL, Rubin PA. Upper and lower eyelid retraction. Int Ophthalmol Clin 2002;42(2):45–59.

22. Bartley GB. The differential diagnosis and classification of eyelid retraction. Ophthalmology 1996;103(1):168–76.

23. Hahn S, Desai SC. Lower lid malposition: causes and correction. Facial Plast Surg Clin North Am 2016;24(2):163–71.

24. Cho RI, Elner VM, Nelson CC, et al. The effect of orbital decompression surgery on lid retraction in thyroid eye disease. Ophthal Plast Reconstr Surg 2011;27(6):436–8.

25. Demirci H, Hassan AS, Reck SD, et al. Graded full-thickness anterior blepharotomy for correction of upper eyelid retraction not associated with thyroid eye disease. Ophthal Plast Reconstr Surg 2007;23(1):39–45.

26. Ben Simon GJ, Lee S, Schwarcz RM, et al. Subperiosteal midface lift with or without a hard palate mucosal graft for correction of lower eyelid retraction. Ophthalmology 2006;113(10):1869–73.

27. Yoo DB, Griffin GR, Azizzadeh B, et al. The minimally invasive, orbicularis-sparing, lower eyelid recession for mild to moderate lower eyelid retraction with reduced orbicularis strength. JAMA Facial Plast Surg 2014;16(2):140–6.

28. Eftekhari K, Peng GL, Landsberger H, et al. The brow fat pad suspension suture: safety profile and clinical observations. Ophthal Plast Reconstr Surg 2018;34(1):7–12.

29. Naik MN, Nair AG, Gupta A, et al. Minimally invasive surgery for thyroid eye disease. Indian J Ophthalmol 2015;63(11):847–53.

30. Kohn JC, Rootman DB, Liu W, et al. Hyaluronic acid gel injection for upper eyelid retraction in thyroid eye disease: functional and dynamic high-resolution ultrasound evaluation. Ophthal Plast Reconstr Surg 2014;30(5):400–4.

31. Goldberg RA, Lee S, Jayasundera T, et al. Treatment of lower eyelid retraction by expansion of the lower eyelid with hyaluronic Acid gel. Ophthal Plast Reconstr Surg 2007;23(5):343–8.

32. Grisolia ABD, Couso RC, Matayoshi S, et al. Nonsurgical treatment for eyelid retraction in thyroid eye disease (TED). Br J Ophthalmol 2017. https://doi.org/10.1136/bjophthalmol-2017-310695.

33. Zamani M, Thyagarajan S, Olver JM. Functional use of hyaluronic acid gel in lower eyelid retraction. Arch Ophthalmol 2008;126(8):1157–9.

34. Chang HS, Lee D, Taban M, et al. En-glove" lysis of lower eyelid retractors with AlloDerm and dermis-fat grafts in lower eyelid retraction surgery. Ophthal Plast Reconstr Surg 2011;27(2):137–41.

35. Morgenstern KE, Evanchan J, Foster JA, et al. Botulinum toxin type a for dysthyroid upper eyelid retraction. Ophthal Plast Reconstr Surg 2004;20(3):181–5.

36. Costa PG, Saraiva FP, Pereira IC, et al. Comparative study of Botox injection treatment for upper eyelid retraction with 6-month follow-up in patients with thyroid eye disease in the congestive or fibrotic stage. Eye (Lond) 2009;23(4):767–73.

37. Träisk F, Tallstedt L. Thyroid associated ophthalmopathy: Botulinum toxin A in the treatment of upper eyelid retraction - A pilot study. Acta ophthalmol Scand 2002;79:585–8.

38. Uddin JM, Davies PD. Treatment of upper eyelid retraction associated with thyroid eye disease with subconjunctival botulinum toxin injection. Ophthalmol 2002;109(6):1183–7.

Nonsurgical Light and Energy–Based Devices
Utility in Eyelid and Periorbital Surgery

Kerry Heitmiller, MD[a], Christina Ring, MD[a], Nazanin Saedi, MD[a,*], Brian Biesman, MD[b]

KEYWORDS

- Periorbital rejuvenation • Skin tightening • Periorbital rhytides
- Radiofrequency microfocused ultrasound

KEY POINTS

- Various light and energy–based devices are utilized successfully for nonsurgical periorbital rejuvenation.
- Ablative laser resurfacing achieves significant clinical improvement, although associated with a longer recovery period and increased risk of adverse effects.
- Nonablative modalities are alternatives for periorbital rejuvenation associated with shorter recovery times and a more favorable side-effect profile.
- The specific modality selected should be tailored to the individual patient, patient preferences, and patient goals of treatment.

INTRODUCTION

The eyes play an important role in human interaction and overall facial appearance. The periorbital region is one of the first areas to show signs of aging.[1] These changes include rhytides, dyschromia, skin laxity, textural changes, and telangiectasia.[2] As such, patients commonly seek cosmetic treatment of periorbital rejuvenation to achieve a more youthful appearance. Traditional surgical interventions, including blepharoplasty, remain the gold standard for periorbital rejuvenation. Downtime and risk, however, associated with surgery, make nonsurgical light and energy–based methods increasingly popular, even though the objectives are somewhat different. The goal with these treatments is to achieve a natural aesthetic appearance while minimizing patient recovery times and associated adverse events. This article discusses the various nonsurgical light and energy–based devices available for periorbital rejuvenation.

PERIORBITAL RHYTIDES

The development of periorbital rhytides is multifactorial, with photoaging and movement of the orbicularis oculi both playing a role. Neuromodulators and soft tissue augmentation are used in treatment, but the focus of this article is on lasers and energy-based devices. Periorbital rhytides are common reasons patients seek cosmetic treatment, and both ablative resurfacing lasers and nonablative lasers successfully are used to treat periocular rhytides.

Ablative laser resurfacing was one of the earliest nonsurgical modalities utilized for periorbital rejuvenation. Ablative laser resurfacing devices include the carbon dioxide (CO_2) laser and the 2940-nm Er:YAG laser. Fully ablative laser resurfacing involves vaporization of the entire epidermis as well as part of the dermis, leading to collagen shrinkage, increased collagen production, and tissue remodeling, resulting in clinical improvement.[3,4] These devices are used in conjunction

[a] Department of Dermatology and Cutaneous Biology, Thomas Jefferson University, Philadelphia, PA, USA;
[b] Ophthalmology, Dermatology, Otolaryngology, Vanderbilt University Medical Center, Nashville, TN, USA
* Corresponding author. Department of Dermatology, 833 Chestnut Street, Suite 740, Philadelphia, PA 19107.
E-mail address: nsaedi@gmail.com

Facial Plast Surg Clin N Am 29 (2021) 323–334
https://doi.org/10.1016/j.fsc.2021.01.007

with blepharoplasty but also are shown to be effective for the treatment of periorbital wrinkles when used as monotherapy.[4–13]

Fully ablative CO_2 laser demonstrates consistent efficacy for the treatment of periorbital rhytides with significant clinical improvement.[4,7–13] In 2004, Alster and Bellew[13] performed a retrospective study of 67 patients, evaluating the safety and efficacy of high-energy pulsed CO_2 laser as monotherapy for the treatment of dermatochalasis and periorbital wrinkles. All patients demonstrated significant improvement in dermatochalasis and periorbital rhytides; however, those with more severe dermatochalasis and rhytides at baseline demonstrated greater improvement than those with mild to moderate findings at baseline.[13] Fully ablative treatment with CO_2 resurfacing lasers is accompanied by long recovery periods, most commonly prolonged erythema that can persist for 3 months to 4 months.[14,15] Other adverse effects include postprocedural hyperpigmentation, hypopigmentation, milia, infection, scarring, and ectropion.[14–21] Lower lid ectropion is considered a rare but severe complication, with the greatest risk in those who have undergone previous blepharoplasty.[14,20,22] The medial one-third of the lower lid is the highest-risk area for developing ectropion. In the authors' experience, patients with flat cheeks and prominent eyes also are at higher risk for lower lid ectropion. Prior to treatment with CO_2 laser resurfacing, patients are counseled appropriately on these potential adverse effects,

and realistic expectations of outcomes should be established (**Fig. 1**). The authors believe that full ablative laser skin resurfacing remains the gold standard in the treatment of moderate to severe eyelid and periorbital photoaging changes.

An effort to achieve a favorable result with fewer adverse events led to the application of fractional laser resurfacing. Fractional ablative resurfacing delivers ablative injury to microscopic columns of tissue in regularly spaced arrays, leaving parts of the intervening skin intact. This allows for more rapid epithelialization and decreased postprocedural recovery time. Rates of adverse effects also are reduced, including dyschromia due to decreased melanin absorption.[23,24] Kotlus[25] evaluated the efficacy and safety of dual-depth fractional CO_2 laser ablation (Lumenis, Santa Clara, California) for the treatment of periorbital rhytides and observed a 53% improvement in periocular rhytides and 42% improvement in skin laxity. The recovery profile was favorable without prolonged erythema or serious complications, and only 2 patients experienced postinflammatory hyperpigmentation that resolved in 3 months with topical hydroquinone 4% cream.[25] Similarly, Bonan and colleagues[26] observed significant improvement, rated as moderate, marked, or excellent response, in skin tightening and periorbital rhytides in 69% of patients 1 year after treatment with the fractional CO_2 laser. Notably, 82% of patients demonstrated measurable eyebrow elevation 1 year after treatment.[26] In practice, the degree of brow elevation

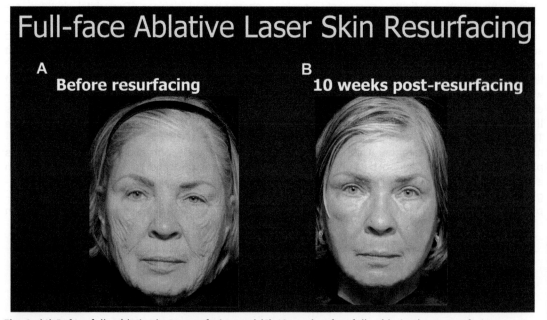

Fig. 1. (*A*) Before fully ablative laser resurfacing and (*B*) 10 weeks after fully ablative laser resurfacing.

after treatments often is clinically irrelevant. Clinical results with ablative fractional lasers are comparable to the standard ablative CO_2 resurfacing lasers but with more rapid recovery times and a better risk profile. Multiple treatments may be required, however, with ablative fractional lasers for optimal outcomes.[4] Although the recovery time after ablative fractional resurfacing is shorter than after full ablative resurfacing, it still is not insignificant for most patients.

The 2940-nm Er:YAG laser is another ablative laser that clinically improves periorbital wrinkles.[27–30] When compared with the CO_2 laser, the traditional short-pulsed Er:YAG laser has a more superficial depth of ablation with little coagulation and is considered less effective for deeper or severe rhytides, requiring more passes to achieve the same degree of tissue ablation.[29,30] Given the superficial energy absorption, the Er:YAG laser is associated with faster recovery times and decreased risk of scarring or adverse effects compared with the CO_2 laser. In a comparative, randomized, split-face trial of the fractional CO_2 laser and the fractional Er:YAG long-pulsed laser for the treatment of periorbital wrinkles, they demonstrated comparable efficacy.[31] A recent review of the literature argued that the Er:YAG laser should be considered the treatment of choice for fine lines and superficial rhytides, whereas the CO_2 laser was better for deeper, severe rhytides and moderate to severe dermatochalasis.[32] Newer long-pulsed Er:YAG systems have been developed that allow for increased depth of ablation and better coagulation, yielding results comparable to the CO_2 laser.[33–35] These devices have 2 Er:YAG laser heads that combine short ablative and long sublative coagulative pulses, allowing for greater modification of optimal ablation depth and coagulation. Studies evaluating the efficacy of these newer Er:YAG systems demonstrate significant improvement in rhytides, including moderate to severe rhytides.[33–35]

In order to maximize the results of laser therapy, pretreatment of periorbital rhytids with botulinum toxin 1 week to 6 weeks prior to laser therapy is shown to enhance and prolong the effects of ablative laser resurfacing.[36,37] Therefore, pretreatment with neuromodulators should be offered and discussed with patients prior to performing any ablative laser resurfacing procedure to maximize potential clinical improvements. Although the authors encourage pretreatment with neuromodulators, this is not an absolute requirement for treatment.

Nonablative fractional lasers (NAFLs), including the 1540-nm and 1550-nm erbium-doped mid-infrared lasers, the 1540-nm Er:GLASS laser, the 1440-nm NAFL, and the 1410-nm NAFL, demonstrate significant clinical improvement in periorbital wrinkles with minimal adverse effects.[1,38–40] In the authors' experience, the 1550-nm NAFL yields superior results compared with other nonablative therapies. In the original split-face study, 30 patients with periorbital wrinkles were treated using the 1550-nm NAFL with the handheld scanning device.[41] At 1 month after the last treatment, 54% demonstrated moderate to significant improvement in periocular wrinkles and 53% had moderate improvement in skin texture. At 3 months' follow-up, 34% and 47%, respectively, had at least moderate improvement in wrinkles and skin texture.[41] Long-term studies are needed to determine the sustainability of these effects in comparison to those seen with ablative procedures. In a study evaluating the long-term benefits of the 1540-nm Er:GLASS laser for the treatment of perioral and periocular rhytides, up to 30% of patients demonstrated sustained improvement at 35 months' follow-up.[42] All patients underwent 5 treatments at 6-week intervals, with 5 patients receiving 2 maintenance treatments at 14 weeks and 20 weeks. Therefore, although resurfacing with NAFLs may provide long-term clinical results, multiple treatments or maintenance treatments may be required to sustain these results, in contrast to ablative fractional resurfacing that provides significant improvement following a single treatment. Although these nonablative devices often are not used solely for periorbital rejuvenation, they are popular full-face treatments and are done more commonly than ablative procedures.

When discussing nonablative lasers for improving rhytides, NAFLs have been the most effective; however, other nonablative devices have been studied. Treatment with these devices produces dermal thermal injury while preserving the integrity of the epidermis, leading to less risk for adverse effects and shorter postprocedural downtimes. Although intense pulsed light (IPL) commonly is used to treat dyschromia and vascular lesions, it has demonstrated minimal effectiveness in improving periorbital rhytides.[43–45] Based on the current literature and the authors' experience, IPL offers no significant improvement in periorbital rhytides but does improve the appearance of some vascular lesions and dyschromia. Although studies suggest IPL is relatively safe in darker-skinned patients, caution should be taken, and appropriate preprocedural counseling performed.

IPL has demonstrated efficacy in the treatment of dry eye disease and increasingly is used in the periocular area for this indication. Dry eye disease is a multifactorial condition due to abnormalities of tear production, gland function, and the ocular surface. There appears to be an association with meibomian gland dysfunction and inflammatory skin conditions that occur in close proximity to the periocular area, including rosacea. Initially, IPL was noted to be helpful for symptoms of dry eye while patients were receiving treatment of facial rosacea.[46] Studies demonstrate consistent improvements in signs and symptoms of dry eye disease after IPL treatment with and without adjunctive meibomian gland expression.[46–52] Typically, treatments involve several IPL sessions, each consisting of IPL pulses from tragus to tragus just below the lower eyelids, although recent studies have demonstrated safety and efficacy with a unique handpiece treating the upper eyelids as well.[46] Postulated explanations for the effectiveness of IPL in treating dry eye disease secondary to meibomian gland dysfunction include heating and softening of the abnormal meibum, reduction of epithelial turnover, decreased risk of gland obstruction, modulation of proinflammatory and anti-inflammatory molecules, suppression of matrix metalloproteinases, thrombosis of local vessels delivering secreted inflammatory markers involved in the inflammatory response, decreased *Demodex* species and local bacterial load contributing to chronic inflammation, and photomodulation.[46,53] Ultimately, these effects result in a diminished local inflammatory response and promote normal meibomian gland function, alleviating the signs and symptoms of dry eye disease.

The 595-nm pulsed dye laser (PDL) traditionally has been utilized for vascular lesions but also has been shown to improve periorbital rhytides, although results are inconsistent and often not clinically relevant. Zelickson and colleagues evaluated the safety and efficacy of the 585-nm PDL in 20 patients with mild to moderate or moderate to severe periorbital rhytides.[54] After a single treatment, 9/10 patients with mild to moderate rhytides demonstrated greater than 50% improvement and 3/10 of these patients demonstrated greater than 75% improvement, which was maintained at 6 months' follow-up. Those with moderate to severe rhytides demonstrated less clinical improvement. Significant postprocedural purpura and edema lasting for 1 week to 2 weeks were noted in a majority of patients.[55] Although these devices commonly are used to treat vascular lesions, these studies show improvement in skin texture with a series of treatments. From a practical clinical perspective, the PDL treatment does not produce meaningful improvement in wrinkling. When PDL is used to treat dark circles caused by vascular changes within the eyelid skin, improvement in overall skin quality can be noted.

Based on current data, the Nd:YAG laser at various pulse durations is effective in the treatment of periorbital wrinkles. In a split-face study, Chang and colleagues[56] evaluated the efficacy of the 1064-nm long-pulsed Nd:YAG laser for periorbital wrinkles in 20 Korean patients and found that all patients demonstrated modest improvement after 3 treatments. Mean wrinkle score on the laser-treated side decreased by approximately 35%, whereas no change was observed on the control side. These clinical improvements were not maintained at 6 months' follow-up. No serious adverse effects were observed during the study. This suggests that the long-pulsed Nd:YAG may be a safe and effective option for treating periorbital wrinkles, even in patients of darker skin types. More than 3 treatment sessions likely are needed to maintain long-term clinical improvement.

Although ablative resurfacing produces the most consistent and significant improvement in periorbital rhytides, nonablative lasers are potential alternatives that offer less risk of erythema, pigmentary changes, or scarring and shorter recovery periods. Given that nonablative devices produce less injury and damage to the skin, these modalities require several treatment sessions to achieve desirable cosmetic outcomes, and the degree of clinical improvement often is less than with ablative resurfacing, even with multiple treatments.

PERIORBITAL SKIN TIGHTENING

Periorbital skin laxity and dermatochalasis are additional components of photoaging that often are troublesome to patients, prompting them to seek aesthetic treatment. Similar to periorbital rhytides, ablative and nonablative laser devices have demonstrated efficacy in improving periorbital skin laxity and dermatochalasis. Studies also demonstrate the efficacy of other light and energy-based devices including radiofrequency (RF) devices and microfocused ultrasound (MFUS) devices in promoting periorbital skin tightening and improving dermatochalasis, achieving tissue tightening by dermal heating.

Ablative laser resurfacing and fractional ablative laser resurfacing are efficacious in treating rhytides and improving periorbital skin laxity, with the latter modality having a more favorable risk profile.[13,25,26] NAFL devices also are effective in the treatment of periorbital skin laxity. Sukal and colleagues[54] evaluated the effects of the 1550-nm NAFL device on eyelid tightening and eye aperture opening in 31 patients who underwent 3 to 7 treatments at 3-week to 4-week intervals. One month after the last treatment, all patients exhibited some eyelid tightening, with 55% having greater than 50% tightening. An increase in eyelid aperture was observed in 56% of patients.[54] Patients experienced mild to no edema postoperatively and there were no reports of dyschromia, persistent erythema, or scarring.[54] Although the results of this study suggest NAFL devices are safe and effective options to improve periorbital skin laxity, in clinical practice, NAFL devices are not used for skin tightening.

RF devices are another modality that demonstrate efficacy for periorbital rejuvenation. These devices generate heat deep in the dermis and hypodermis, with limited effects on the epidermis, via a rapidly alternating electric current. The current is delivered by 1 or more skin electrodes. The thermal injury stimulates immediate collagen contraction and promotes progressive tissue remodeling and collagen and elastin production, resulting in skin tightening. The number of treatment electrodes characterizes the RF device as monopolar, bipolar, or multipolar. Monopolar RF devices have a single treatment handpiece or paddle, whereas bipolar and multipolar devices have multiple electrodes against the skin with current flowing between them. In addition, RF devices with microneedling are available that invasively deliver current through a needle or array of needles into the skin.

The first monopolar RF device (Thermage, Solta, Hayward, California) was approved by the United States Food and Drug Administration for the treatment of periorbital rhytides in 2002.[57] It currently is the only device cleared for use on the eyelid itself. Fitzpatrick and colleagues[58] performed a multicenter study of 86 patients who received a single treatment and observed Fitzpatrick wrinkle scale score improvements of at least 1 point in 83% of subjects 6 months after treatment; 62% of patients also demonstrated an eyebrow lift of at least 0.5 mm. Associated adverse effects were minimal, including transient erythema and edema.[58] In a prospective, multicenter trial, Biesman and colleagues[59] treated the eyelids of 72 patients with a single session using a monopolar RF device (Thermage). A shallow treatment tip was developed and utilized to deliver heat more superficially compared with existing treatment tips to decreasing the risk of injury to vital structures within the eye or eyelid. Six months after treatment, upper eyelid tightening and lower eyelid tightening were noted in 88% and 71% to 74% of patients, respectively. No serious adverse events were reported.[59] Similar results with improvement in periorbital skin tightness following treatment with monopolar RF devices is reported.[60–64] This particular monopolar RF device

remains the only skin tightening device with a specific indication for use on the eyelids.

Transcutaneous, temperature-controlled, monopolar RF devices have been developed for treatment in the periorbital area to maximize safety by ensuring treatment temperatures remain within an appropriate range[65] (**Fig. 2**).

Studies evaluating bipolar RF devices similarly demonstrate efficacy in promoting periorbital skin tightening. Lolis and Goldberg[66] evaluated the safety and efficacy of a bipolar fractional RF device (eMatrix, Syneron Medical, Irvine, California) in 20 patients with periorbital rhytides and laxity. Each patient underwent 3 treatments at 4-week intervals. At 6 months after the last treatment, 50% of patients demonstrated moderate to marked improvement. Treatments were well tolerated, with only 3 patients experiencing postinflammatory hyperpigmentation that resolved with hydroquinone cream.[66] Later studies similarly demonstrate improvement in facial wrinkles and laxity with various treatment protocols utilizing fractional bipolar RF devices[67] or fractional multipolar RF devices[68] with a favorable safety profile. In all of these studies, patients of varying skin types demonstrated improvement with only occasional, mild side effects observed, including transient discomfort, erythema, and edema. Most patients were able to return to their daily routines almost immediately after treatment.

Microneedling RF devices were developed to enhance dermal heating by delivering energy directly through needles that penetrate the skin to a predetermined depth. Greater collagen remodeling is stimulated by both the dermal heating and the physical stimulation. In 2009, Hantash and colleagues[69,70] performed the initial studies evaluating the effects of a novel bipolar microneedling RF device, revealing the associated with neocollagenesis and neoelastogenesis. Kim and colleagues[71] evaluated the efficacy of a fractional RF microneedling device for the treatment of periorbital rhytides in 11 Asian women undergoing 3 treatments at 3-week intervals. Three months after the last treatment, significant improvement in periorbital rhytides was observed. All patients tolerated the treatment, and no adverse events were reported.[71]

RF devices appear to be an effective nonsurgical modality for the treatment of periorbital laxity, safe in patients of all skin types with no downtime with proper energy and a favorable side-effect profile. Response to treatment may be more gradual with effects seen in 4 weeks to 6 weeks or even 6 months after treatment.[56] These devices are becoming increasingly popular, with a wide discrepancy between devices. These devices can be effective for skin tightening; however, it is

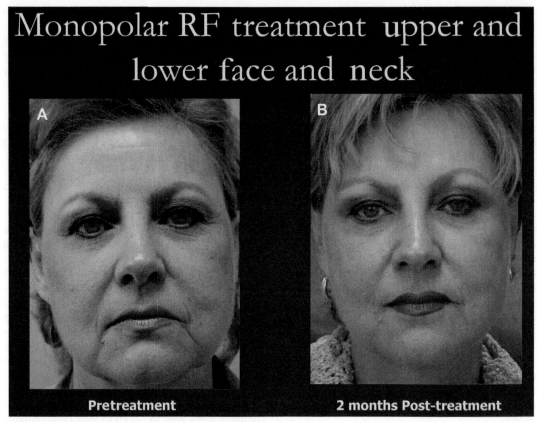

Fig. 2. (*A*) Before treatment with monopolar RF to upper face, lower face, and neck, and (*B*) 2 months after treatment with monopolar RF to upper face, lower face, and neck.

treatment and technique dependent. There is a need for more standardized treatments and a way to compare the different available devices. Fractionated RF and microneedling with RF are invasive, and these devices have a depth of penetration, which is why there is a potential risk of postinflammatory hyperpigmentation. These devices should be used with great care on the eyelid skin. Treatment of eyelid skin with RF microneedling currently is off-label from a regulatory perspective.

MFUS is another noninvasive modality utilized for periorbital rejuvenation. MFUS acts by depositing points of microthermocoagulation at specific depths into the dermis, creating discrete points of skin contraction, promoting skin tightening and improvement in skin laxity.[1] The MFUS device (Ultherapy, Ulthera, Mesa, Arizona) is the first and only energy-based device Food and Drug Administration approved for aesthetic lift of the brow, neck, and submental area.[72,73] The device is applied to the periorbital region (outside of the eyelids) and forehead to promote eyebrow lift and should not be used on the eyelids or within the orbital rim, because the eye cannot be shielded safely during treatment. Pak and colleagues[74] evaluated the safety and efficacy of an MFUS device (Ulthera System, Ulthera) for periorbital rejuvenation and observed skin tightening and improvement in infraorbital laxity in all treated patients. Patients tolerated the procedure well with minimal pain during treatment and no adverse effects were reported.[74] Although patients are reported to have minimal pain, in the authors' experience, there is pain associated with the procedure that should be managed. Because the user is able to visualize the depth being targeted during treatment with ultrasound, only a certain zone is targeted, leaving remaining depths unaffected similar to a fractionated device, resulting in faster postprocedural recovery times. Newer devices on the market (Sofwave, Israel) deliver the ultrasound energy to a fixed depth (1.5 mm) within the skin (Sofwave), removing the need to precisely visualize the depth during treatment.[75] Given that MFUS spares the epidermis, it is a favorable modality to use in patients prone to postinflammatory hyperpigmentation.[76] MFUS appears to be a safe and effective alternative for nonsurgical eyebrow lift and periorbital rejuvenation.

RF devices and MFUS are effective treatment modalities for improving periorbital skin laxity with minimal down time, depending on the device, and decreased risk of associated adverse effects. The authors' clinical experience is that there is variability in the results depending on the patient. Those patients with severe laxity and atrophic skin are not good candidates for these treatments and do not have optimal outcomes. These devices are effective, but, as discussed previously, they are not a replacement for surgery.

PERIORBITAL HYPERPIGMENTATION

Periorbital hyperpigmentation is another aspect of photoaging that occurs in the periorbital region. Periorbital hyperpigmentation may be secondary to dyschromia, translucency of the thin periorbital skin, or underlying cutaneous vasculature,[77] which can manifest as a brown or purple-red discoloration infraorbitally. Patients frequently seek cosmetic therapy for periorbital hyperpigmentation, or dark circles, under the eyes, because this has been associated with a tired or older appearance. Currently, the literature evaluating the efficacy of medical treatment of periorbital hyperpigmentation is mixed, without real data to confirm consistent benefit. Periorbital hyperpigmentation is treated successfully with various laser and light devices targeting vascularity and pigment.

Studies have shown significant improvement in infraorbital hyperpigmentation with CO_2 laser resurfacing.[78] A risk of postprocedural dyschromia, especially in those with darker skin types, may limit use of ablative laser resurfacing in this patient population. The daily use of a bleaching cream for several weeks prior to and after the procedure can decrease the risk of subsequent pigmentary alteration.[79]

IPL demonstrates efficacy in the treatment of periorbital pigmentation when used for periorbital rejuvenation.[43] Negishi and colleagues[45] treated 97 Asian patients with 3 to 6 sessions of IPL and observed good or excellent improvement in periorbital pigmentation in 90% of patients. In addition, these patients had improvement in periorbital telangiectasias and skin texture. Subsequent studies confirm improvement in pigmentation with IPL.[80,81] IPL effectively treats periorbital hyperpigmentation, even in darker-skinned individuals, with the additional benefit of treating associated vascular lesions and improving skin texture.

Several studies have established the efficacy of the 1064-nm Q-switched and long-pulsed Nd:YAG laser in treating periorbital hyperpigmentation, especially when associated with underlying vasculature.[82–86] Several studies also support the use of the 694-nm QS ruby laser for periorbital hyperpigmentation.[87–89] Following treatment, 80% to 93% of patients demonstrated good to excellent results, with up to 89% of patients experiencing greater than 50% improvement.[87,88] Most patients experienced only mild pain and erythema.[87,88]

Newer technologies, such as the picosecond laser, are shown to be effective for periorbital dyschromia. In a study evaluating the picosecond 755-nm alexandrite laser, a significant improvement of periorbital hyperpigmentation was noted without any reports of postinflammatory hyperpigmentation at 3 months' follow-up.[82]

These nonablative lasers appear to have a relatively favorable side-effect profile with decreased risk of dyschromia and minimal postprocedural downtime. Selection of a specific modality for the treatment of periorbital hyperpigmentation is based on individual patient characteristics, patient preferences, and goals of cosmetic treatment to ensure optimal results, similar to when approaching treatment of periorbital rhytides or laxity.

PERIORBITAL TELANGIECTASIAS AND VASCULAR LESIONS

Telangiectasias and prominent vasculature, commonly seen in other areas of the face, are particularly bothersome in the periorbital area.[90] The efficacy of laser treatment depends on several factors, including target chromophore, vessel size, vessel depth, and vascular flow rate. Many laser and light systems, such as the 532-nm potassium titanyl phosphate (KTP) laser, PDL, and IPL, represent treatment options, with PDL and long-pulsed 532-nm laser treatment of choice for superficial telangiectasias.[91–93]

Treatment of facial reticular veins in the periocular area frequently is a requested cosmetic procedure. Patients may have a genetic predisposition or develop reticular veins after cosmetic surgery. Invasive therapies, including cautery, sclerotherapy, and phlebectomy, rarely are used due to side effects, including ulceration and blindness.[94,95] Due to these serious side effects, use of the 1064-nm Nd:YAG lasers has increased, which penetrate deeper into the dermal blood vessels, thereby decreasing the risk of epidermal damage. The treatment endpoint is disappearance of blue, which is achieved by increasing the fluence slowly, if needed. Warning endpoints include graying or whitening of the skin, which can result in blistering and scarring.[96] Smaller veins on the lower eyelids may require higher fluences, whereas veins on the upper eyelids may be treated with lower fluences. Small arterioles near the eyelashes, despite their high-pressure flow, also may respond to laser therapy[97] (**Fig. 3**).

The treatment of periocular reticular veins with the 1064-nm laser can lead to safety issues given the close proximity to the eyes. Ocular complications, including macular holes, uveitis, pupillary abnormalities, vitreous hemorrhage, and conjunctival burns, have been reported after use of the 1064-nm Nd:YAG laser for cosmetic treatment.[97–105] There also is a potential risk of permanent loss of the eyelashes with treatment. Therefore, eye protection, as discussed later, is paramount during treatment to decrease the risk of these complications.

PERIORBITAL REJUVENATION TREATMENT SAFETY

Prior to operating any of the Light and energy based devices, discussed previously, it is important to be aware of potential risks of treatment and to discuss these risks with patients. Treatment with laser devices is associated with several ocular complications, including corneal damage, anterior uveitis, iris or pupillary abnormalities, retinal burns, vitreous hemorrhages, and conjunctival burns.[100–105] Laser hair removal of the periorbital area has caused many ocular injuries, and it is not recommended due to the associated risk.

Prior to treatment, regardless of the body location being treated, the patient is given wraparound goggles to be worn throughout the procedure, with the appropriate optical density and wavelength ranges of protection. Laser aids (disposable adhesive eye protectors) alternatively are utilized during treatment with NAFLs, covering the upper eyelid while allowing access to the brow and infraorbital region. Additional precautions are taken if treatment of the periorbital area near the eyelid margins or on the eyelid itself is anticipated for NAFL treatments. A metal or plastic corneoscleral protective lens shield is placed prior to these treatments. Metal shields are used with any laser device. When using an RF device, opaque plastic eye shields are utilized because these are shown to provide adequate protection of the eye during RF procedures. Metal shields cannot be used during RF treatment.

Ocular protection devices do not eliminate the risk of injury. A recent review reported that eye injury occurred in 33% of cases in which eye protection, including metal corneal shields, were provided,[105] likely associated with overheating of the metal corneal shields during the procedure. Therefore, other preventative measures, including pulling the infraorbital skin away from the orbit during treatment and directing the laser away

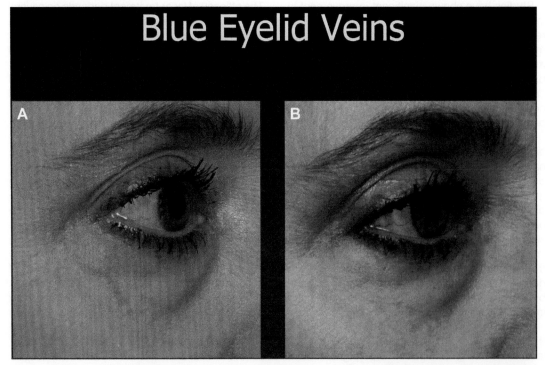

Fig. 3. (A) Before treatment with long-pulsed Nd:YAG and (B) 1 week after treatment with long-pulsed Nd:YAG.

from the eye, also should be employed to minimize complication risk. Sufficient cooling of the treated area between pulses during treatment to prevent overheating of the metal corneal shields and thermal injury is important.

SUMMARY

Periorbital rejuvenation is a common reason for patients to seek cosmetic treatment. There are several nonsurgical light and energy–based devices available that are used to effectively treat the various aspects of periorbital rejuvenation without the risks of an invasive, surgical procedure. Although ablative laser resurfacing appears to offer the most impressive clinical improvements, nonablative devices result in noticeable cosmetic improvement with a more favorable side-effect profile and shorter recovery times. The specific modality selected for periorbital rejuvenation is tailored to a patient's individual characteristics, preferences, and aesthetic goals. Patients with prominent vascular lesions may benefit more from treatment with vascular lasers, whereas patients with predominantly periorbital hyperpigmentation may achieve optimal outcomes with the Nd:YAG or alexandrite lasers. Patients with skin textural changes, skin laxity, and rhytides may see the most benefit with an NAFL, RF device, or MFUS. It is likely, with continued advancements, that additional effective nonsurgical light and energybased devices will become available in the future for periorbital rejuvenation.

REFERENCES

1. Fathi R, Pfeiffer MD, Tsoukas M. Minimally invasive eyelid care in dermatology: medical, laser, and cosmetic therapies. Clin Dermatol 2015;33:207–16.
2. Glaser DA, Patel U. Enhancing the eyes: use of minimally invasive techniques for periorbital rejuvenation. J Drugs Dermatol 2010;9(8):s118–28.
3. Alster TS, Rosenbach A, Huband L. Improvement in dermatochalasis with high-energy, pulsed CO2 laser cutaneous resurfacing. Dermatol Surg 1999; 25:1299–302.
4. Glaser DA, Kurta A. Periorbital rejuvenation: overview of nonsurgical treatment options. Facial Plast Surg Clin North Am 2016;24:145–52.
5. Carter SR, Seiff SR, Choo PH, et al. Lower eyelid CO2 laser rejuvenation. Ophthalmology 2001;108:437–41.
6. Roberts TL, Yokoo KM. In pursuit of optimal periorbital rejuvenation: laser resurfacing with or without blepharoplasty and brow lift. Aesthet Surg J 1998;18(5):321–32.
7. Fitzpatrick R, Goldman M, Satur N, et al. Pulsed carbon dioxide laser resurfacing of photoaged skin. Arch Dermatol 1996;132:395–402.
8. Alster T. Comparison of two high-energy, pulsed carbon dioxide lasers in the treatment of periorbital rhytides. Dermatol Surg 1996;22:541–5.
9. Waldorf HA, Kauvar ANB, Geronemus RG. Skin resurfacing of fine to deep rhytides using char- free carbon dioxide laser in 47 patients. Dermatol Surg 1995;11:940–6.
10. Manaloto RMP, Alster TS. Periorbital rejuvenation: a review of dermatologic treatments. Dermatol Surg 1999;25:1–9.
11. West TB, Alster TS. Effect of botulinum toxin type A on movement-associated rhytides following CO2 laser resurfacing. Dermatol Surg 1999;25(4):259–61.
12. Alster TS, Garg S. Treatments of facial rhytides with a high-energy pulsed carbon dioxide laser. Plast Reconstr Surg 1996;98:791–4.
13. Alster TS, Bellew SG. Improvement of dermatochalasis and periorbital rhytides with a high-energy pulsed CO2 laser: a retrospective study. Dermatol Surg 2004;30:483–7.
14. Nanni CA, Alster TS. Complications of cutaneous laser surgery: a review. Dermatol Surg 1998;24:209–19.
15. Blanco G, Clavero A, Soparkar CNS, et al. Periocular laser complications. Semin Plast Surg 2007;21:74–9.
16. Bernstein LJ, Kauvar ANB, Grossman MC, et al. The short- and long-term side effects of carbon dioxide laser resurfacing. Dermatol Surg 1997;23:519–25.
17. Ho C, Nguyen Q, Lowe NJ, et al. Laser resurfacing in pigmented skin. Dermatol Surg 1995;21:1035–7.
18. Monheit GD. Facial resurfacing may trigger the herpes simplex virus. Cosmet Dermatol 1995;8:9–16.
19. Sriprachya-Anunt S, Fitzpatrick RE, Goldman MP, et al. Infections complicating pulsed carbon dioxide laser resurfacing for photoaged facial skin. Dermatol Surg 1997;23:527–36.
20. Weinstein C. Ultrapulse carbon dioxide laser removal of periocular wrinkles in association with laser blepharoplasty. J Clin Laser Med Surg 1994;12:205–9.
21. Moran ML. Office-based periorbital rejuvenation. Facial Plast Surg 2013;29:58–63.
22. Alster TS. Laser resurfacing of rhytides. In: Alster TS, editor. Manual of cutaneous laser techniques. Philadelphia: Lippincott-Raven; 1997. p. 103–22.
23. Alexiades-Armenakas MR, Dover JS, Arndt KA. The spectrum of laser skin resurfacing: nonablative, fractional, and ablative laser resurfacing. Dermatology 2008;58(5):719–37.
24. Carniol PJ, Hamilton MM, Carniol ET. Current status of fractional laser resurfacing. JAMA Facial Plast Surg 2015;17(5):360–6.

25. Kotlus BS. Dual-depth fractional carbon dioxide laser resurfacing for periocular rhytidosis. Dermatol Surg 2010;36:623–8.

26. Bonan P, Campolmi P, Cannarozzo G, et al. Eyelid skin tightening: a novel 'Niche' for fractional CO2 rejuvenation. J Eur Acad Dermatol Venereol 2012; 26:186–93.

27. Teikemeier G, Goldberg DJ. Skin resurfacing with the erbium:YAG laser. Dermatol Surg 1997;23: 685–7.

28. Ross VE. The erbium laser in skin resurfacing. In: Alster TS, Apfel- berg DG, editors. Cosmetic laser surgery. New York: John Wiley; 1998. p. 57–84.

29. Alster TS. Comparison of six erbium:YAG lasers for cutaneous re- surfacing: a clinical and histopatho- logical evaluation. Lasers Surg Med 1999;24(2): 87–92.

30. Alster TS. Extended clinical experience with erbium:YAG cutaneous laser resurfacing. Lasers Surg Med 1998;23(Suppl. 10):34.

31. Karsai S, Czarnecka A, Junger M, et al. Ablative fractional lasers (CO2 and Er:YAG): a randomized controlled double-blind split-face trial of the treat- ment of peri-orbital rhytides. Lasers Surg Med 2010;42:160–7.

32. Papadavid E, Katsambas A. Lasers for facial reju- venation: a review. Int J Dermatol 2003;42:480–7.

33. Caniglia RJ. Erbium:YAG laser skin resurfacing. Facial Plast Surg Clin North Am 2004;12:373–7.

34. Avram DK, Goldman MP. The safety and effective- ness of single-pass erbium:YAG laser in the treat- ment of mild to moderate photodamage. Dermatol Surg 2004;30:1073–6.

35. Farshidi D, Hovenic W, Zachary C. Erbium:yttrium aluminum garnet ablative laser resurfacing for skin tightening. Dermatol Surg 2014;40:S152–6.

36. Zimbler MS, Holds JB, Kokoska MS, et al. Effect of botulinum toxin pretreatment on laser resurfacing results: a prospective, randomized, blinded trial. Arch Facial Plast Surg 2001;3:165–9.

37. Yamauchi P, Lask G, Lowe N. Botulinum toxin type A gives adjunctive benefit to periorbital laser resur- facing. J Cosmet Laser Ther 2004;6(3):145–8.

38. Augustyniak A, Rotsztejn H. Fractional non-ablative laser treatment at 1410 nm wavelength for periorbi- tal wrinkles-reviscometrical and clinical evaluation. J Cosmet Laser Ther 2016;18(5):275–9.

39. Lupton JR, Williams CM, Alster TS. Nonablative laser skin resurfacing using a 1540 nm erbium glass laser: a clinical and histologic analysis. Der- matol Surg 2002;28:833–5.

40. Fournier N, Dahan S, Barnean G, et al. Nonablative remodeling: Clinical, histologic, ultrasound imag- ery and profilometric evaluation of a 1540 nm Er: Glass laser. Dermatol Surg 2001;27:799–806.

41. Manstein D, Herron GS, Sink RK, et al. Fractional resurfacing: a new concept for cutaneous remodeling using microscopic patterns of thermal injury. Lasers Surg Med 2004;34:426–38.

42. Fournier N, Lagarde JM, Turlier V, et al. A 35-month profilometric and clinical evaluation of non-ablative remodeling using a 1540-nm Er:glass laser. J Cosmet Laser Ther 2004;6:126–30.

43. Kim KH, Geronemus RG. Nonablative laser and light therapies for skin rejuvenation. Arch Facial Plast Surg 2004;6:398–409.

44. DiBernardo BE, Pozner JN. Intense pulsed light therapy for skin rejuvenation. Clin Plast Surg 2016;43(3):535–40.

45. Negishi K, Tezuka Y, Kushikata N, et al. Photoreju- venation for Asian skin by intense pulsed light. Der- matol Surg 2001;27(7):627–31.

46. Toyos R, Toyos M, Wilcox J, et al. Evaluation of the safety and efficacy of intense pulsed light treat- ment with meibomian gland expression of the up- per eyelids for dry eye disease. Photomodul Photomed Laser Surg 2019;37:527–31.

47. Dell SJ, Gaster RN, Barbarino SC, et al. Prospective evaluation of intense pulsed light and Meibomian gland expression efficacy on relieving signs and symptoms of dry eye disease due to Meibomian gland dysfunction. Clin Ophthalmol 2017;11:817–27.

48. Vegunta S, Patel D, Shen JF. Combination therapy of intense pulsed light therapy and meibomian gland expressions (IPL/MGX) can improve dry eye symptoms and meibomian gland function in patients with refractory dry eye: a retrospective analysis. Cornea 2016;35:318–22.

49. Vora GK, Gupta PK. Intense pulsed light therapy for the treatment of evaporative dry eye disease. Curr Opin Ophthalmol 2015;26:314–8.

50. Toyos R, McGill W, Briscoe D. Intense pulsed light treatment for dry eye disease due to meibomian gland dysfunction: a 3-year retrospective study. Photomed Laser Surg 2015;33(1):41–6.

51. Craig J, Chen Y, Turnbull P. Prospective trial of intense pulsed Light for the treatment of meibo- mian gland dysfunction. Invest Ophthalmol Vis Sci 2015;56(3):1965–70.

52. Jiang X, Lv H, Song H, et al. Evaluation of the Safety and Effectiveness of Intense Pulsed Light in the Treatment of Meibomian Gland Dysfunction. J Ophthalmol 2016;2016:1910694.

53. Dell SJ. Intense pulsed light for evaporative dry eye disease. Clin Ophthalmol 2017;11:1167–73.

54. Sukal SA, Chapas AM, Bernstein LJ, et al. Eyelid tightening and improved eyelid aperture through nonablative fractional resurfacing. Dermatol Surg 2008;34:1454–8.

55. Zelickson BD, Kilmer SL, Bernstein E, et al. Pulsed dye laser therapy for sun damaged skin. Lasers Surg Med 1999;25:229–36.

56. Chang SE, Choi M, Kim MS, et al. Long-pulsed Nd: YAG laser on periorbital wrinkles in Asian patients:

randomized split face study. J Dermatol Treat 2014; 24(4):283–6.

57. Sukal SA, Geronemus RG. Thermage: the nonablative radiofrequency for rejuvenation. Clin Dermatol 2008;26:602–7.

58. Fitzpatrick R, Geronemus R, Goldberg D, et al. Multicenter study of noninvasive radiofrequency for periorbital tissue tightening. Lasers Surg Med 2003;33:232–42.

59. Biesman BS, Baker SS, Carruthers J, et al. Monopolar radiofrequency treatment of human eyelids: a prospective, multicenter, efficacy trial. Lasers Surg Med 2006;38:890–8.

60. Abraham MT, Chiang SK, Keller GS, et al. Clinical evaluation of non-ablative radiofrequency facial rejuvenation. J Cosmet Laser Ther 2004;6:136–44.

61. Ruiz-Esparza J. Noninvasive lower eyelid blepharoplasty: a new technique using nonablative radiofrequency on periorbital skin. Dermatol Surg 2004; 30:125–9.

62. Nahm WK, Su TT, Rotunda AM, et al. Objective changes in brow position, superior palpebral crease, peak angle of the eyebrow, and jowl surface area after volumetric radiofrequency treatments to half of the face. Dermatol Surg 2004;30: 922–8.

63. Javate RM, Grantoza CL, Buyacan KF. Use of an imaging device after nonablative radiofrequency (Pelleve): treatment of periorbital rhytids. Ophthal Plast Reconstr Surg 2014;30(6):499–503.

64. Migliardi R, Tofani F, Donati L. Non-invasive periorbital rejuvenation: radiofrequency dual radiowave energy source (RF) and light emission diode system (LED). Orbit 2009;28(4):214–8.

65. Key DJ, Boudreaux L. A proposed method for upper eyelid and infrabrow tightening using a transcutaneous temperature controlled radiofrequency device with opaque plastic eye shields. J Drugs Dermatol 2016;15(11):1302–5.

66. Lolis MS, Goldberg DJ. Assessment of safety and efficacy of a bipolar fractionated radiofrequency device in the treatment of periorbital rhytides. J Cosmet Laser Ther 2014;16(4):161–4.

67. Gold MH, Biesman BS, Taylor M. Enhanced high-energy protocol using a fractional bipolar radiofrequency device combined with bipolar radiofrequency and infrared light for improving facial skin appearance and wrinkles. J Cosmet Dermatol 2017;16:205–9.

68. Roh NK, Yoon YM, Lee YW, et al. Treatment of periorbital wrinkles using multipolar fractional radiofrequency in Korean patients. Lasers Med Sci 2017; 32:61–6.

69. Hantash BM, Ubeid AA, Chang H, et al. Bipolar fractional radiofrequency treatment induces neoelastogenesis and neocollagenesis. Lasers Surg Med 2009;41(1):1–9.

70. Hantash BM, Renton B, Berkowitz RL, et al. Pilot clinical study of a novel minimally invasive bipolar microneedle radiofrequency device. Lasers Surg Med 2009;21(2):87–95.

71. Kim JK, Roh MR, Park G, et al. Fractionated microneedle radiofrequency for the treatment of periorbital wrinkles. J Dermatol 2013;40:172–6.

72. White WM, Makin IR, Barthe PG, et al. Selective creation of thermal injury zones in the superficial musculoaponeurotic system using intense ultrasound therapy: A new target for noninvasive facial rejuvenation. Arch Facial Plast Surg 2007;9:22–9.

73. ULTHERA® System (featuring DeepSEE® technology for Ultherapy®)[instructions for use]. Mesa, AZ: Ulthera,® Inc.; 2019.

74. Pak CS, Lee YK, Jeong JH, et al. Safety and efficacy of Ulthera in the rejuvenation of aging lower eyelids: a pivotal clinical trial. Aesthetic Plast Surg 2014;38:861–8.

75. Sofwave® medical (Sofwave®) [physician brochure]. Sofwave Medical Ltd; 2020.

76. White WM, Makin IR, Slayton MH, et al. Selective transcutaneous delivery of energy to porcine soft tissues using Intense Ultrasound (IUS). Lasers Surg Med 2008;40:67–75.

77. Momosawa A, Kurita M, Ozaki M, et al. Combined therapy using Q-switched ruby laser and bleaching treatment with tretinoin and hydroquinone for periorbital skin hyperpigmentation in Asians. Plast Reconstr Surg 2008;121(1):282–8.

78. West TB, Alster TS. Improvement of infraorbital hyperpigmentation following carbon dioxide laser resurfacing. Dermatol Surg 1998;24(6):615–6.

79. Glavas IP, Purewal BK. Noninvasive techniques in periorbital rejuvenation. Facial Plast Surg 2007; 23(3):162–7.

80. Sadick NS. Update on non-ablative light therapy for rejuvenation: a review. Lasers Surg Med 2003; 32:120–8.

81. Herne KB, Zachary CB. New facial rejuvenation techniques. Semin Cutan Med Surg 2000;19: 221–31.

82. Vanaman Wilson MJ, Jones IT, Bolton J, et al. Prospective studies of the efficacy and safety of the picosecond 755-, 1,064-, and 532-nm lasers for the treatment of infraorbital dark circles. Lasers Surg Med 2018;50(1):45–50.

83. Xu T-H, Yang Z-H, Li Y-H, et al. Treatment of infraorbital dark circles using a low-fluence Q-switched 1,064-nm laser. Dermatol Surg 2011;37(6): 797–803.

84. Ma G, Lin X-X, Hu X-J, et al. Treatment of venous infraorbital dark circles using a long-pulsed 1,064-nm neodymium-doped yttrium aluminum garnet laser. Dermatol Surg 2012;38(8):1277–82.

85. Cho S, Lee SJ, Chung WS, et al. Acquired bilateral nevus of Ota-like macules mimicking dark circles

under the eyes. J Cosmet Laser Ther 2010;12(3): 143–4.

86. Sarkar R, Ranjan R, Garg S, et al. Periorbital hyperpigmentation: a comprehensive review. J Clin Aesthet Dermatol 2016;9(1):49–55.

87. Xu T-H, Li Y-H, Chen JZS, et al. Treatment of infraorbital dark circles using 694-nm fractional Q-switched ruby laser. Lasers Med Sci 2016; 31(9):1783–7.

88. Lowe NJ, Wieder JM, Shorr N, et al. Infraorbital pigmented skin. Preliminary observations of laser therapy. Dermatol Surg 1995;21(9):767–70.

89. Watanabe S, Nakai K, Ohnishi T. Condition known as "Dark Rings under the Eyes" in the Japanese population is a kind of dermal melanocytosis which can be successfully treated by Q-switched ruby laser. Dermatol Surg 2006;32:785–9.

90. Goldman MP. Optimal management of facial telangiectasia. Am J Clin Dermatol 2004;5:423–34.

91. Sarradet DM, Hussain M, Goldberg DJ. Millisecond 1064-nm neodymium:YAG laser treatment of facial telangiectasias. Dermatol Surg 2003;29:56–8.

92. Karsai S, Roos S, Raulin C. Treatment of facial telangiectasia using a dual-wavelength laser system (595 and 1,064 nm): a randomized controlled trial with blinded response evaluation. Dermatol Surg 2008;34:702–8.

93. Rohrer T, Chatrath V, Iyengar V. Does pulse stacking improve the results of treatment with variable-pulse pulsed-dye lasers? Dermatol Surg 2004;30: 163–7.

94. Alam M, Dover J, Arndt K. Treatment of facial telangiectasia with variable-pulse high-fluence pulsed-dye laser: comparison of efficacy with fluences immediately above and below the purpura threshold. Dermatol Surg 2013;29:681–5.

95. Lai SW, Goldman MP. Treatment of facial reticular veins with dynamically cooled, variable spot-sized 1064 nm Nd:YAG laser. J Cosmet Dermatol 2007; 6:6–8.

96. Chen DL, Cohen JL. Treatment of Periorbital Veins with Long-Pulse Nd:YAG Laser. J Drugs Dermatol 2015;14:1360–2.

97. Roider J, Buesgen P, Hoerauf H, et al. Macular injury by a military range finder. Retina 1999; 19(6):531–5.

98. Sakaguchi H, Ohji M, Kubota A, et al. Amsler grid examination and optical coherence tomography of a macular hole caused by accidental Nd:YAG laser injury. Am J Ophthalmol 2000;130(3):355–6.

99. Chuang LH, Lai CC, Yang KJ, et al. A traumatic macular hole secondary to a high-energy Nd:YAG laser. Ophthal Surg Lasers 2001;32(1):73–6.

100. Hagemann LF, Costa RA, Ferreira HM, et al. Optical coherence tomography of a traumatic Neodymium: YAG laser- induced macular hole. Ophthalmic Surg Lasers Imaging 2003;34(1):57–9.

101. Harris MD, Lincoln AE, Amoroso PJ, et al. Laser eye injuries in military occupations. Aviat Space Environ Med 2003;74(9):947.

102. Lin CC, Tseng PC, Chen CC, et al. Iritis and pupillary distortion after periorbital cosmetic alexandrite laser. Graefes Arch Clin Exp Ophthalmol 2011; 249(5):783–5.

103. Hammes S, Augustin A, Raulin C, et al. Pupil damage after periorbital laser treatment of a port-wine stain. Arch Dermatol 2007;143(3):392–4.

104. Chuang GS, Farinelli W, Christiani DC, et al. Gaseous and particulate content of laser hair removal plume. JAMA Dermatol 2016;152:1320–6.

105. Huang A, Phillips A, Adar T, et al. Ocular injury in cosmetic laser treatments of the face. J Clin Aesthet Dermatol 2018;11(2):15–8.

Eyelid and Periorbital Dermal Fillers
Products, Techniques, and Outcomes

José Raúl Montes, MD[a],*, Elizabeth Santos, MPH-A, DrPH[b], Claudia Amaral, BS[c]

KEYWORDS

- Aging eyelid • Periorbital rejuvenation • Dermal fillers • Periocular anatomy • Tear trough
- Shallow orbit • Deep set eyes • Deep upper eyelid sulcus

KEY POINTS

- There are a variety of dermal fillers approved by the US Food and Drug Administration, each with unique properties that make them suitable for volume augmentation at different areas of the face.
- Injectables, particularly hyaluronic acid fillers and biostimulant agents, are a useful, minimally invasive alternative for treatment of patients with specific anatomic features.
- Negative vector topography can be corrected with tear trough and midface injections with hyaluronic acid, as well as biostimulant agent deposition at the maxilla and about the orbitomalar ligament.
- Hyaluronic acid fillers can be used to dissimulate postoperative high upper eyelid crease and volume subtraction.
- Injectables can be used to achieve an enhanced final result in patients after surgical reconstruction for trauma or prior cosmetic surgery.

 Video content accompanies this article at http://www.facialplastic.theclinics.com.

INTRODUCTION

Anatomy is essential for filler injection safety and a guiding compass for treatment design. This article focuses on 4 topics: patient assessment, dermal filler selection, anatomic findings, and injection techniques. It includes visual examples that illustrate signature features that are encountered in oculoplastic practice.

PATIENT ASSESSMENT

During patient evaluation, anatomic variations and individual factors are identified, allowing the physician to determine the most appropriate treatment approach. The facial shape must be evaluated from different angles and both at rest and during animation to correctly assess its proportion and symmetry.[1,2] It is important to determine the patient's needs and expectations, discuss the physician's evaluation with the patient, and combine both to produce an effective and satisfactory treatment plan.[1]

Dr Ava Shamban coined the concept of a "signature feature" and, in theory, we all have one.[3] Shamban highlights the importance of preserving these features during aesthetic

a Department of Ophthalmology, University of Puerto Rico School of Medicine, José Raúl Montes Eyes and Facial Rejuvenation, 735 Ponce de Leon Avenue Suite 813, San Juan, PR 00917, USA; b José Raúl Montes Eyes and Facial Rejuvenation, 735 Ponce de Leon Avenue Suite 813, San Juan, PR 00917, USA; c University of Puerto Rico School of Medicine, Medical Sciences Campus, PO BOX 365067, San Juan, PR 00936, USA
* Corresponding author.
E-mail address: jrmontes@jrmontes.com

Facial Plast Surg Clin N Am 29 (2021) 335–348
https://doi.org/10.1016/j.fsc.2021.01.003

enhancement, as they contribute to what makes an individual recognizable to others.[3] Physicians can focus on these salient features and decide whether they can be enhanced or diffused by working around them. For example, in a patient with 2 signature features, a prominent nose and full lips, injectables can be used to enhance the lips and minimize the nose prominence (**Fig. 1**). The result is the simultaneous balancing and preservation of both features.

Dr Steven Dayan proposes a 2-fold approach to patient assessment: symmetry as an objective and eyes as the focal point of facial rejuvenation.[4] Asymmetric features require asymmetric patterns of injection to achieve this goal (**Fig. 2**). A common misconception is that facial shaping with injectables is exclusively about adding volume. However, the possibility of volume reduction plays a role in patient assessment. In a patient with lower face or masseteric hypertrophy, volume can be decreased using a neurotoxin, and deficient midface and temples can be compensated using a biostimulant agent (**Fig. 3**).

Nonsurgical facial rejuvenation provides a number of advantages for the patient: it is safe, less invasive, and entails a shorter recovery period.[5]

Volume restoration is an important part of facial rejuvenation, and dermal fillers are effective methods of achieving this objective.[5] There are a series of dermal fillers that have been approved by the US Food and Drug Administration (FDA), each with unique properties that make them suitable for different procedures and facial regions (**Table 1**).[6-9]

DERMAL FILLERS
Hyaluronic Acid Fillers

Hyaluronic acid (HA) fillers are commonly used for volume restoration in different regions of the face. The available FDA-approved HA fillers can be grouped into several categories based on their characteristics and the technology used to create them (see **Table 1**). Hylacross technology produces monophasic gels, resulting in a product composed of cohesive molecules with a 24 mg/mL concentration of highly cross-linked HA.[10] These products are long lasting, soft, and easy to use.[10] Their hydrophilic properties lead to a diffuse filling effect on injected soft tissues.[11] Vycross technology combines low and high molecular weight HA.[10] It has a high G′ and low

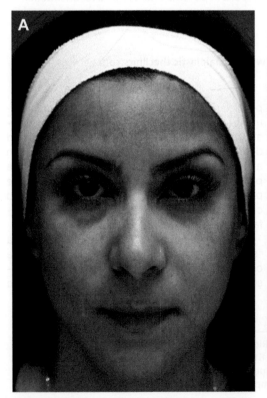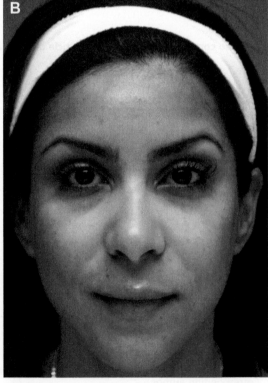

Fig. 1. Injectables were used to enhance the lips and minimize the nose prominence, thus striking a balance. (*A*) Before treatments. (*B*) After neurotoxin injection, midface (Juvéderm Voluma XC) and perioral (Restylane Silk) filler injection.

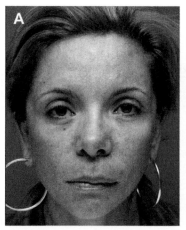
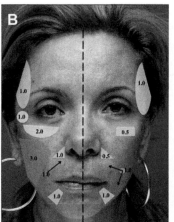
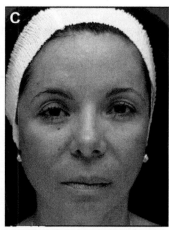

Fig. 2. Asymmetric features require asymmetric patterns of injection. (*A*) Before treatment. (*B*) Left side: 1.0 mL, 0.5 mL, 1.0 mL Deep Injection and 1.0 mL superficial injection. Right side: 1.0 mL, 1.0 mL, 2.0 mL, 1.0 mL, 1.0 mL and 3.0 mL, 1.0 mL superficial injection. (*C*) After 6 session of poly-L-lactic acid (PLLA), a total of 10 vials.

swelling capacity, resulting in the ability to produce a high lift.[10] Their concentration varies from product to product, ranging from 15 mg/mL to 20 mg/mL. Nonanimal stabilized HA (NASHA) uses a sizing technology: it breaks up the cross-linked HAs by passing them through sizing screens.[10] These products have a concentration of 20 mg/mL. Products made with XpresHAn technology have the same concentration of 20 mg/mL, but they vary in their degree of cross-linking. HA fillers made with cohesive polydensified matrix technology have the lowest G′ of the HA fillers, accounting for their lower elasticity and viscosity.[10] In cohesive polydensified matrix technology, non–cross-linked HA is added in the second

cross-linking stage, resulting in a product with a variable degree of cross-linking.[6,12]

Biostimulant Agents

Calcium hydroxyapatite (Radiesse) and poly-L-lactic acid (PLLA; Sculptra) are 2 FDA-approved biostimulant agents. Radiesse is made of calcium hydroxyapatite spheres suspended in a sodium carboxymethylcellulose gel carrier.[11] It is more substantial in consistency and has minimal hydrophilic properties in comparison with HA fillers.[8] PLLA functions by stimulating the body to produce its own collagen.[13] It does so by activating fibroblasts, resulting in gradual soft tissue augmentation.[14] Although its effects are not immediate,

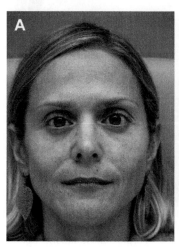
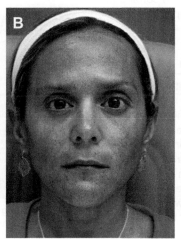
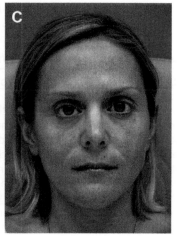

Fig. 3. Neurotoxin reduced lower face and masseteric hypertrophy. At the same time, deficient midface and temples were compensated with a biostimulant agent. (*A*) Before treatments. (*B*) After neurotoxin treatment (30 units). (*C*) After 3 PLLA sessions.

Table 1
FDA-approved injectable implants

	Technology	Product	Cross-Linking (%)	Hyaluronic Acid Concentration (mg/mL)
Hyaluronic acid	Hylacross	Juvederm Ultra	6	24
		Juvederm Ultra Plus	8	24
	Vycross	Volbella	–	15
		Vollure	–	17.5
		Voluma	<5	20
	NASHA	Restylane L	1	20
		Restylane Lyft	1	20
		Restylane Silk	1	20
	XpresHAn	Restylane Refyne	6	20
		Restylane Kysse	7	20
		Restylane Defyne	8	20
	Cohesive polydensified matrix	Belotero Balance	Variable	22.5
	Thixofix	Revanesse Versa	10	25
	Resilient hyaluronic acid	RHA 2	1.9–4.0	23
		RHA 3	1.9–4.0	23
		RHA 4	1.9–4.0	23
Biostimulant agents	PLLA	Sculptra	N/A	N/A
	Calcium hydroxyapatite	Radiesse	N/A	N/A

PLLA has the benefit of producing subtle results that are favored by many patients.[11,14] It is indicated for patients who desire global facial voluminization.[11]

Filler Material Selection

In general, HA fillers with high density, cross-linking, and viscosity are used for deeper volumization in areas such as the midcheek and malar regions.[1] In contrast, products that are softer and less dense are better suited for superficial injections in areas such as the lips (**Fig. 4**).[1]

Periorbital Area and Tear Trough

HA fillers are suitable for the periorbital area in part because they are reversible with hyaluronidase and temporary.[15] Fillers used in the tear trough and periorbital areas should be made of smaller particles, have less HA concentration, and contain less hydrophilic propensity. Hydrophilic fillers attract water, which can result in a degree of swelling that is undesirable in these regions.[11] Therefore, the use of fillers made with Hylacross technology is not recommended for the periorbital area and tear trough.[16] Fillers with a lower water binding capacity are less likely to result in swelling or bluish discoloration under the eyes.[5] The use of low-viscosity HA is considered safe, whereas

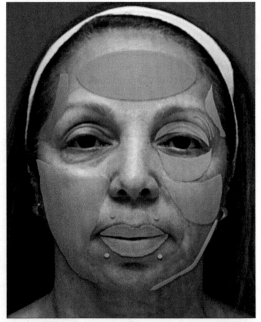

Fig. 4. Mapping of potential fillers for each facial zone. Pink: low HA concentration or HA with spreading capability. Purple: biostimulant agents, PLLA and calcium hydroxyapatite. Blue: high HA concentration, high lifting capability. Orange: low HA concentration or lower water-binding capacity.

injection of high-viscosity HA is not recommended for the tear trough.[17]

HA fillers made with NASHA, Vycross of low HA concentration, and cohesive polydensified matrix technologies are recommended for use in the tear trough and lower eyelid region.[5] NASHA fillers are most commonly used for periorbital volume augmentation.[18] HA fillers with a cohesive poly-densified technology have the lowest G' and allow for greater injection precision.[10,19] They are well-suited for injection of superficial regions of the face, as well as atrophic scars.[10,20] Because the skin of the tear trough is very thin, small amounts of filler are injected, and additional sessions are performed at another time if necessary.[5]

Temporal Fossa

Both HA fillers and biostimulant agents can be used for temporal fossa augmentation. The choice of dermal filler used for temporal fossa augmentation depends on whether treatment is superficial or deep. Lower G' products are preferred for superficial treatment of the temporal hollow, whereas products with a high G' and cohesivity are used for the injection of deep areas.[16] The placement of dermal fillers likewise depends on the dermal filler that is used.[16] HA fillers should be placed in either the subcutaneous plane or the plane between the superficial and deep temporal fascia.[16] When biostimulant agents and HAs with a high G' are used for augmentation of the temporal fossa, they should be placed deep to the temporalis muscle.[16] If placed within the muscle, their particles may migrate or lump, leading to undesirable results.[16]

HA fillers made with NASHA technology can be used for superficial volume augmentation in the temporal fossa owing to their small particle size and hydrophilic properties.[16] The filler should be injected into the subdermal space at the level of the superficial temporal fascia.[16] Viscous fillers with a larger particle size can be used in the temporal area, because it is thicker than surrounding areas such as the eyelids.[18] PLLA and calcium hydroxyapatite biostimulant agents are suitable for deep temporal fossa augmentation.[16]

Upper Eyelid

Moderately concentrated HA fillers, such as those made with NASHA, Vycross of low HA concentration, XpresHAn with low cross-linking, and cohesive polydensified matrix technologies, are recommended for use in the upper eyelid region.[21] These HA fillers are ideal for use in the thin upper eyelid region, because use of less concentrated fillers may result in diffusion of the product, whereas more viscous fillers can result in a lumpy appearance.[21] Use of the lift, inject, and massage technique is recommended when using HA fillers made with NASHA technology for postoperative upper eyelid hollows.[16] This maneuver elevates the brow adjacent to the hollow above the orbital rim. The HA injected is molded on the rim to diffuse through the tissue planes and smoothly fill the deficit. The biochemical characteristics of the NASHA product allow the injector to achieve a 3-dimensional lift, successfully restoring orbital volume loss secondary to aging or excessive fat removal during upper eyelid blepharoplasty.[16,18,22,23]

MIDFACE

Fillers with a high HA concentration and G' are recommended for deep injection at the midface.[10] These properties give fillers a high lifting capability that results in a desired plump appearance in this area.[10] HA fillers made with Vycross (20 mg/mL HA concentration) technology are indicated for augmentation in the cheek region.[10] These products can create a long-lasting lift while maintaining a low swelling capacity.[10] They are malleable, reversible, and can be injected into the subcutaneous and supraperiosteal levels.[24] Specifically, HA fillers with Vycross technology can be used for the lateral, anterior, and medial cheek areas.[2] HA fillers with Vycross and NASHA technologies are recommended for the lid–cheek junction.[2] Additionally, NASHA fillers with large particle size can be used for the midface region.

NEGATIVE VECTOR PATIENT

Youthfulness and facial attractiveness are usually correlated with a smooth transition between the periorbital zone and adjacent anatomic areas, such as the midface, temples, and brow complex.[21] The negative vector patient lacks support for the globe and orbit from the midface–bony maxilla or soft tissue (**Fig. 5**).[25] This lack of support leads to lower lid and cheek descent, undereye bags, and scleral show, giving the patient an aged appearance.[26,27] For the negative vector patient, infraorbital concavity demands convexity. HA fillers are an effective treatment option for correcting the negative vector.[28,29] This treatment modality is less invasive than methods such as fat repositioning and alloplastic implants; additionally, it can be reversed with hyaluronidase if necessary.[30–32]

The landing platforms for the negative vector patient are the bony tear trough and the maxillary face lateral to the infraorbital artery. A 2-pronged approach can be used, placing HA injections at

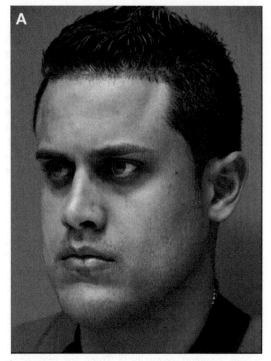
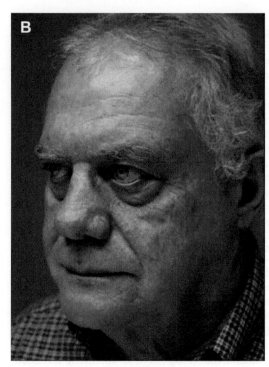

Fig. 5. Negative vector patient. (*A*) Young negative vector patient. (*B*) Older negative vector patient.

these locations. HA injection in these regions is safe, effective, and associated with high patient satisfaction.[30,33] HA is a suitable product for the tear trough because it tends to distribute evenly within the injected region and possesses adequate desired implant characteristics: it is malleable, smooth, and has a homogenous composition.[30] A patient with a weak maxilla resulting in negative vector and lower eyelid fat prolapse may be buttressed with deep biostimulant material (PLLA or calcium hydroxyapatite gel) deposited at the maxilla and orbital retaining ligament (**Figs. 6** and **7**). After a few treatment sessions, significant

improvement in appearance can be achieved without the use of surgical procedures (Video 1).

SHALLOW ORBIT PATIENT

A shallow orbit patient has a decreased depth of the orbits associated with prominent ocular globes (**Fig. 8**).[34] Neuroimaging can be used to confirm projection of the globes outside the orbital rim and rule out the presence of orbital or globe abnormalities. It is important to evaluate for conditions such as hyperthyroidism, because these patients may present with bilateral proptosis. Patients with a shallow orbit need support around the orbit,

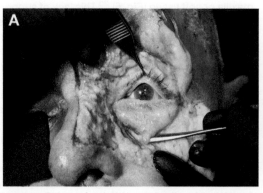
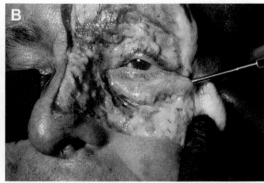

Fig. 6. Deep biostimulant material deposition. (*A*) At the maxilla. (*B*) At the tear trough ligament and orbital retaining ligament.

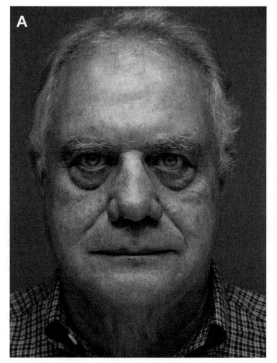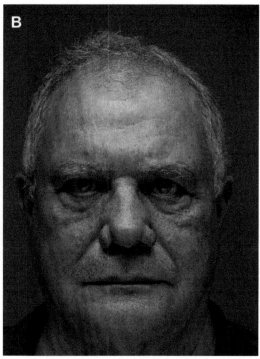

Fig. 7. Negative vector patient before and after treatment with deep biostimulant agent. (*A*) Before treatment. (*B*) After 3 PLLA sessions.

especially at the junction of the lower eyelid and midface. The preferred course of action in these patients is with nonsurgical correction using HA injections. The use of a smaller filler volume is recommended in these cases, and additional treatment sessions can be performed to obtain the desired results.[30]

NASHA and HAs made with cohesive polydensified matrix technology can be placed at the tear trough, resulting in subtle yet effective changes in appearance that can positively impact the patient's self-image. In the patient with a shallow orbit, the benefits of injecting both the midface and infraorbital areas should always be considered. Some experts recommend that patients

with shallow orbit receive treatment in the prezygomatic space, pyriform aperture, and deep midfacial fat before the tear trough, because it leads to more natural results.[30,35] Treatment with single-point injection of HA fillers at midface in close proximity to the suborbicularis oculi fat has been found to be successful in achieving midface volume restoration.[36] Additionally, patients report improvement in appearance of the tear trough and eyebags (Video 2).[36]

DEEP SET EYES PATIENT

The patient with deep set eyes has eyes that rest deeper into the skull and give the illusion of a

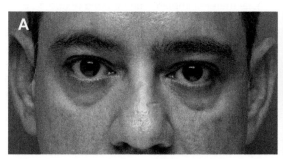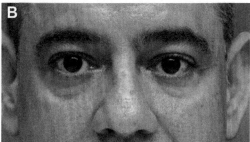

Fig. 8. Shallow orbit patient. (*A*) Before treatment. (*B*) After 1 mL of HA.

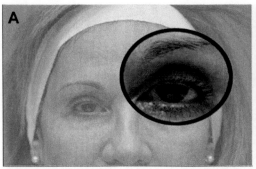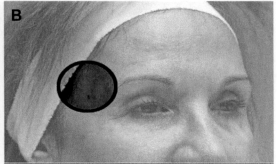

Fig. 9. Patient with deep set eyes. Inject the temple to dissimulate a "prominent roof" because injecting the upper eyelid will make the eye look smaller. (A) Deep upper eyelid sulcus. (B) Temporal fossa depression.

very prominent brow bone (**Fig. 9**). To dissimulate a prominent roof, the patient can be injected in the temple, because injecting the upper eyelid will make the eye look smaller. To conceal the bony brow prominence, the HA injection should be placed deep at the temporal fossa, about 1 cm above the temporal fusion line and 1 cm lateral (**Fig. 10**, Video 3).

PEANUT FACE

The term peanut face refers to a face that lacks temporal lateral volume (**Fig. 11**). It can be

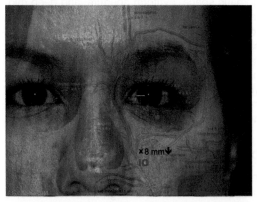

Fig. 10. Location of main vessels around the eye. The best way to locate the main vessels around the eye is to use your patient's pupil as your guiding compass. For instance, to find the foramen (or cleft where the bundle of supraorbital nerves and vessels emerges) use the iris' medial limbus and the orbit's superior margin. The neurovascular structures of the infraorbital foramen are aligned between the iris' medial limbus and the pupil at approximately 8 mm to 1 cm from the lower orbital rim. Remember that the supratrochlear artery is located approximately 1 cm medial to the supraorbital artery. All these structures emerge from deep within these foraminas. Hence, to ensure safety in injections, depth must definitely be taken into account.

reframed with biostimulant agents such as PLLA and calcium hydroxyapatite, and the goal is to make the facial shape as oval as possible. PLLA is used to stimulate collagen production in areas such as the temples, leading to volume restoration.[13,14] Filling the temporal region creates a smooth transition between the forehead and cheek, resulting in a more balanced appearance.[37]

Biostimulant agents and dermal fillers have been used to improve age-related volume loss in the temporal fossa and are also effective in counteracting the lack of temporal volume seen in patients with a peanut face. There are 2 schools of thought regarding temporal fossa augmentation.[37,38] Moradi and colleagues[37] (2011) injected dermal fillers in the subcutaneous space superficial to or just deep to the superficial temporal fascia. The needle is inserted perpendicular to the skin, and subsequent injections are administered in a fanned pattern.[37,38] Juhász Marmur[38] (2015) use a 3-injection approach: the first injection is placed in the center of the deepest concavity at the temporal fossa, followed by an injection superior or posterior to the first, and last, the third injection is administered in the lateral forehead. The purpose of the last 2 injections is to correct remaining defects, which leads to a smooth contour.[38]

Depending on the particular level of experience and skill, deep injections or the more taxing superficial material implant can be used (Video 4). Both approaches have their strengths and limitations, which the clinician must carefully evaluate. The temporal region contains vessels that anastomose with the ophthalmic artery, and intra-arterial injection of dermal fillers could result in embolization leading to blindness.[38–41] Deep injection below muscle prioritizes safety, because the deep central temporal fossa does not contain important vessels making embolization of filler unlikely during dermal filler injection.[38] The superficial technique is more cost efficient. Deep temple and

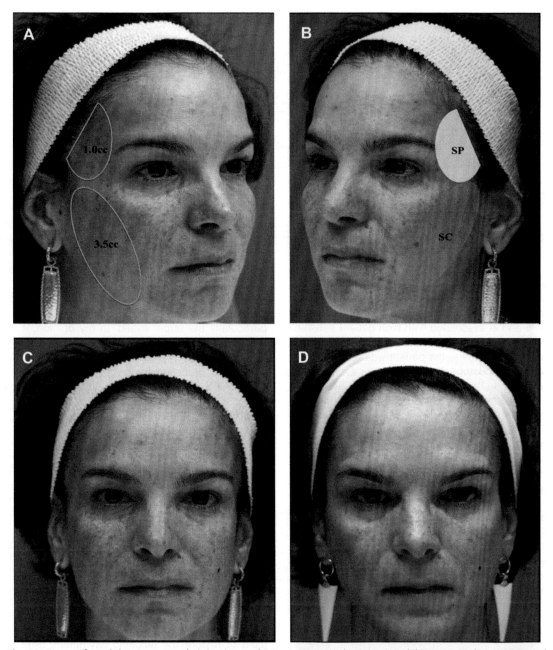

Fig. 11. Peanut face. (*A*) A 1-mL temple injection and 3.5 mL preauricular injection. (*B*) Deep temple injection and superficial preauricular injection. (*C*) Before treatment injection. (*D*) After 2 treatments of 1 vial per session.

superficial preauricular injections were used in a patient with peanut face, which achieved the goal of rounding out the facial contour (**Fig. 11**).

IATROGENICALLY ALTERED ANATOMY

By and large, oculoplastic surgeons have embraced the concept of volume preservation.

Regrettably, this approach has not been adopted yet as the gold standard in periocular surgery. This is particularly true of the upper eyelid region; although upper blepharoplasty results in the removal of undesired excess skin, over time, depletion of volume in this region can result in a hollow superior sulcus.[21] A loss of volume at the superior sulcus, then, can occur secondary to

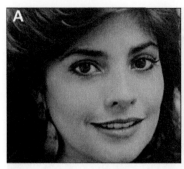
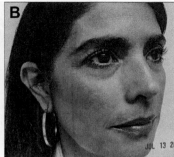
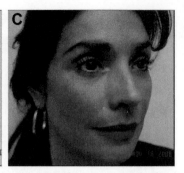

Fig. 12. Patient with postoperative deep upper eyelid sulcus. (*A*) At 32 years old. (*B*) Before surgery. (*C*) After 4 eyelid surgery.

upper blepharoplasty or aging, and it tends to give patients a tired and older appearance.[21]

HA fillers can be used to restore upper eyelid volume in patients with an iatrogenically induced deep upper eyelid sulcus.[21] This procedure is performed in the office setting with minimal recovery time and is associated with high patient satisfaction.[21] After undergoing an endoscopic brow lift and eyelid surgery, the patient was unhappy with a resulting postoperative deep upper eyelid sulcus (**Fig. 12**). In her youth, she had upper eyelid and brow volume that was later surgically removed. A postoperative deep upper eyelid sulcus can be corrected by filling the upper eyelids and eyebrows. Retro-orbicularis oculi fat (ROOF) injections can be used in such cases to both dissimulate the postoperative high crease and volume subtraction.

ROOF (eyebrow) injections can be used to enhance youthful convexity in younger patients. The other indications for filling this area are volume loss secondary to involutional changes or deflation associated with aging, as well as iatrogenic volume depletion. ROOF injections can be made either superficially in the subdermal region or

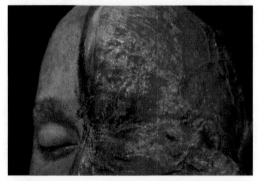

Fig. 13. Of concern on upper eyelid filler placement are the 2 major vascular structures near this region: the supraorbital (SO) and supratrochlear (ST) arteries.

deep in the supraperiosteum using stronger products. Injections must be made lateral to the supraorbital and supratrochlear arteries, which are adjacent to the medial upper eyelid area (**Fig. 13**).

Cannula injection is this author's preferred approach technique at the periocular zones, particularly the upper eyelid. In my opinion, it is safer and results in less bruising. The plane of injection is within the suborbicularis muscle and anterior to vascular structures (Video 5). In this way, HA fillers can restore periocular volume.

TRAUMA PATIENT

The trauma patient presents a challenge when the surgical reconstructive process reaches a plateau. Facial trauma can result in loss of integrity of soft tissues, an important component of an individual's facial features that must be restored to obtain an adequate cosmetic result.[42] We can step in with injectables to complete restoration. Successful use of dermal fillers to treat facial chronic post-traumatic scars has been reported, resulting in no complications and a favorable aesthetic outcome.[43] Our results demonstrate how biostimulant agents allow us to go the extra mile for a patient who has undergone multiple reconstructive surgeries. Filler and neurotoxin injections were used to restore the resulting asymmetry after a motor vehicle accident (**Fig. 14**). The following examples are trauma patients after gunshot wounds to their faces on their filler reconstructive phase. The patient had severe facial scarring and cheek descent after extensive facial reconstruction (see **Fig. 14**). A biostimulant agent was injected primarily on the midface zone, leading to soft tissue lift without the need for additional surgeries (**Fig. 15**). After a gunshot wound in her right eye and maxillary zone, this patient experienced periocular complex trauma that resulted in loss of the ocular globe, as well as deep superior sulcus and maxillary depressed fractures (**Fig. 16**). The

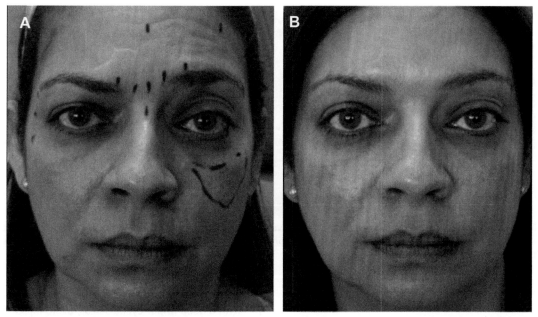

Fig. 14. Motor vehicle trauma patient after neurotoxin and filler injections. (*A*) Before neurotoxin (2.5 U) and HA filler on the midface. (*B*) After treatment.

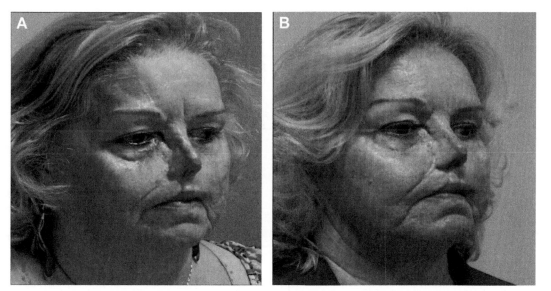

Fig. 15. Patient with a gunshot wound on her filler reconstructive phase. Biostimulant agents were injected on the midface to create a soft tissue lift. (*A*) Before treatment. (*B*) After 3 session with 3 vials of PLLA.

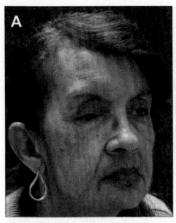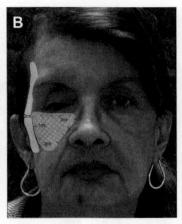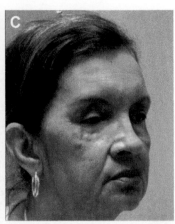

Fig. 16. Biostimulant agent PLLA was used to restore volume loss in the maxilla and temporal area in a patient with gunshot wound in the right eye and maxillary zone. (*A*) Before treatment. (*B*) After 3 sessions with 3 vials PLLA on the right side. (*C*) After treatment.

biostimulant agent PLLA was injected in the maxillary and temporal regions to restore volume loss in these areas.

SUMMARY

The beauty and challenge of oculofacial surgery is to achieve the perfect balance between function and cosmesis in every surgical approach or treatment. With the advent of injectable implants that are effective and specific for different facial zones, we have expanded our scope of work to masterfully complete facial restoration in patients with diverse signature features (Shamban 2019[3]). This review of cases treated with injectables are a testament that less invasive facial restoration plays a role in our work.

CLINICS CARE POINTS

- The cosmetic patient assessment must include visualization of the face on frontal, lateral, and oblique profile in resting and dynamic positions. Symmetry should be considered as an objective and the periocular zone a focal point on facial rejuvenation.

- HA fillers are preferred for the periocular zone because they can be easily dissolved with hyaluronidase.

- For the patients with a negative vector and those with a shallow orbit, consider a dual approach; tear trough and midface concomitant filler injections.

- The patient with deep set eyes may present with a deep upper eyelid sulcus; avoid injecting at the upper eyelid because it will make the eyes look smaller.

- The so-called peanut face patient lacks temporolateral volume. The goal of injectables is to make the facial frame as oval as possible.

- The iatrogenically volume depleted periocular zone after eyelid/eyebrow surgery can be restored with injectable implants on the lower, upper eyelids, and eyebrow (ROOF).

- When the surgical reconstructive process of a trauma patient hits a plateau, you can step in with injectables to complete restoration.

SUPPLEMENTARY DATA

Supplementary data related to this article can be found online at https://doi.org/10.1016/j.fsc.2021.01.003.

REFERENCES

1. Monheit GD. Nonsurgical facial rejuvenation. Facial Plast Surg 2014;30(4):462–7.
2. De Maio M, Swift A, Signorini M, et al. Facial assessment and injection guide for botulinum toxin and injectable hyaluronic acid fillers: focus on the upper face. Plast Reconstr Surg 2017;140(2):265e–76e.
3. Shamban A. The signature feature™: a new concept in beauty. J Cosmet Dermatol 2019;18(3):692–9.
4. Dayan S. Subliminally exposed: shocking truths about your hidden desires in mating, dating and communicating. Use cautiously. New York: Morgan James Publishing; 2013.

5. Hoenig J, Hoenig D. Minimally invasive periorbital rejuvenation. Facial Plast Surg 2013;29(4):295–309.

6. Rohrich RJ, Bartlett EL, Dayan E. Practical Approach and Safety of Hyaluronic Acid Fillers. Plast Reconstr Surg Glob Open 2019;7(6):e2172.

7. Micheels P, Sarazin D, Tran C, et al. Effect of different crosslinking technologies on hyaluronic acid behavior: a visual and microscopic study of seven hyaluronic acid gels. J Drugs Dermatol 2016;15(5):600–6.

8. Fagien S, Bertucci V, von Grote E, et al. Rheologic and physicochemical properties used to differentiate injectable hyaluronic acid filler products. Plast Reconstr Surg 2019;143(4):707e–20e.

9. Gutowski KA. FDA filler update: Revanesse Versa. Available at: https://drgutowski.com/wp-content/uploads/2020/01/292751.pdf. Accessed January 2, 2020.

10. Mansouri Y, Goldenberg G. Update on hyaluronic acid fillers for facial rejuvenation. Cutis 2015;96:85–9.

11. Dayan SH, Brennan TE, Arkins JP. Filler augmentation. In: Myint SA, editor. Nonsurgical peri-orbital rejuvenation. New York: Springer US; 2014. p. 75–87. https://doi.org/10.1007/978-1-4614-8388-5_6.

12. Lorenc Z, Fagien S, Flynn T, et al. Review of key Belotero balance safety and efficacy trials. Plast Reconstr Surg 2013;132(4 Suppl 2):33S–40S.

13. Beer K. Dermal Fillers and Combinations of Fillers for Facial Rejuvenation. Dermatol Clin 2009;27(4):427–32.

14. Fitzgerald R, Vleggaar D. Facial volume restoration of the aging face with poly-l-lactic acid. Dermatol Ther 2011;24(1):2–27.

15. Hwang CJ. Periorbital injectables: understanding and avoiding complications. J Cutan Aesthet Surg 2016;9(2):73–9.

16. Sykes JM, Cotofana S, Trevidic P, et al. Upper face: clinical anatomy and regional approaches with injectable fillers. Plast Reconstr Surg 2015;136(5):204S–18S.

17. Sharad J. Dermal fillers for the treatment of tear trough deformity: a review of anatomy, treatment techniques, and their outcomes. J Cutan Aesthet Surg 2012;5(4):229–38.

18. Morley AMS, Malhotra R. Non-surgical volume enhancement with fillers in the orbit and periorbital tissues: cosmetic and functional considerations. In: Guthoff RF, Katowitz JA, editors. Oculoplastics and orbit. Heidelberg (Germany): Springer; 2010. p. 211–29. https://doi.org/10.1007/978-3-540-85542-2_15.

19. Hevia O, Cohen BG, Howell DJ. Safety and efficacy of a cohesive polydensified matrix hyaluronic acid for the correction of infraorbital hollow: an observational study with results at 40 weeks. J Drugs Dermatol 2014;13(9):1030–6.

20. Lorenc Z, Fagien S, Flynn T, et al. Clinical application and assessment of Belotero: a roundtable discussion. Plast Reconstr Surg 2013;132(4 Suppl. 2):69S–76S.

21. Hartstein ME. Update on the treatment of the skeletonized upper eyelid. Adv Cosmet Surg 2019;2(1):135–42.

22. Broder KW, Cohen SR. An overview of permanent and semipermanent fillers. Plast Reconstr Surg 2006;118(3 Suppl):7S–14S.

23. Morley AMS, Taban M, Malhotra R, et al. Use of hyaluronic acid gel for upper eyelid filling and contouring. Ophthal Plast Reconstr Surg 2009;25(6):440–4.

24. Cotofana S, Schenck TL, Trevidic P, et al. Midface: clinical anatomy and regional approaches with injectable fillers. Plast Reconstr Surg 2015;136(5):219S–34S.

25. Non-Surgical Rejuvenation of the Periorbital Area. PRIME Journal. Available at: https://www.prime-journal.com/non-surgical-rejuvenation-of-the-periorbital-area/. Accessed May 9, 2020.

26. Frey ST. New diagnostic tenet of the esthetic midface for clinical assessment of anterior malar projection. Angle Orthod 2013;83(5):790–4.

27. Yaremchuk MJ. Infraorbital rim augmentation. Plast Reconstr Surg 2001;107(6):1585–92.

28. Zamani M, Thyagarajan S, Olver JM. Functional use of hyaluronic acid gel in lower eyelid retraction. Arch Ophthalmol 2008;126(8):1157–9.

29. Tan P, Kwong TQ, Malhotra R. Non-aesthetic indications for periocular hyaluronic acid filler treatment: a review. Br J Ophthalmol 2018;102(6):725–35.

30. Sharad J. Treatment of the tear trough and infraorbital hollow with hyaluronic acid fillers using both needle and cannula. Dermatol Ther 2020;33(3):e13353.

31. Goldberg RA. Transconjunctival orbital fat repositioning: transposition of orbital fat pedicles into a subperiosteal pocket. Plast Reconstr Surg 2000;105(2):743–51.

32. Flowers RS. Tear trough implants for correction of tear trough deformity. Clin Plast Surg 1993;20(2):403–15.

33. Carruthers A, Carruthers J. Non-animal-based hyaluronic acid fillers: scientific and technical considerations. Plast Reconstr Surg 2007;120(6 Suppl):33S–40S.

34. Hallinan JTPD, Pillay P, Koh LHL, et al. Eye globe abnormalities on MR and CT in adults: an anatomical approach. Korean J Radiol 2016;17(5):664–73.

35. Fitzgerald R, Carqueville J, Yang PT. An approach to structural facial rejuvenation with fillers in women. Int J Womens Dermatol 2019;5(1):52–67.

36. Liang C-P, Thong H-Y. A guide to cheek augmentation: single-point deep injection of hyaluronic acid filler at midface in close proximity to medial suborbicularis oculi fat (SOOF) area. J Cosmet Dermatol Sci Appl 2016;06(01):1–8.

37. Moradi A, Shirazi A, Perez V. A guide to temporal fossa augmentation with small gel particle

hyaluronic acid dermal filler. J Drugs Dermatol 2011; 10(6):673–6.

38. Juhász MLW, Marmur ES. Temporal fossa defects: techniques for injecting hyaluronic acid filler and complications after hyaluronic acid filler injection. J Cosmet Dermatol 2015;14(3):254–9.

39. Funt D, Pavicic T. Dermal fillers in aesthetics: an overview of adverse events and treatment approaches. Clin Cosmet Investig Dermatol 2013;6: 295–316.

40. Moradi A, Shirazi A, Moradi J. A 12-month, prospective, evaluator-blinded study of small gel particle hyaluronic acid filler in the correction of temporal fossa volume loss. J Drugs Dermatol 2013;12(4):470–5.

41. Tangsirichaipong A. Blindness after facial contour augmentation with injectable silicone. J Med Assoc Thail 2009;92:S85–7.

42. Wentrup-Byrne E, Grøndahl L, Chandler-Temple A. Replacement materials for facial reconstruction at the soft tissue-bone interface. In: Sharma CP, editor. Biointegration of Medical implant materials: science and Design. Cambridge, UK: Woodhead Publishing Limited; 2010. p. 51–85. https://doi.org/10.1533/9781845699802.1.51.

43. Hussain SN, Goodman GJ, Rahman E. Treatment of a traumatic atrophic depressed scar with hyaluronic acid fillers: a case report. Clin Cosmet Investig Dermatol 2017;10:285–7.

Complications of Periocular Dermal Fillers

Yao Wang, MD[a,b], Guy Massry, MD[a,b,c], John B. Holds, MD[d,e],*

KEYWORDS

- Hyaluronic acid gel • Dermal filler complication • Tyndall effect • Tear trough

KEY POINTS

- Dermal fillers, predominantly hyaluronic acid gels (HAGs), have great utility in treating aging changes of the periocular area.
- Dermal fillers vary in their results and suitability in the periocular area, with generally predictable results and complication rates.
- Clinical results and complications are related specifically to biochemical and rheologic characteristics of the product selected, the specific patient, and how the filler is injected.
- Hyaluronidase injection is an essential element in the treatment of most HAG dermal filler complications. Complications of other fillers are not treatable in this fashion.
- Blindness and neurovascular embolization complications after dermal filler injection is a special topic addressed separately in Catherine J. Hwang and colleagues' article, "Blindness After Filler Injection: Mechanism and Treatment," in this issue.

 Video content accompanies this article at http://www.facialplastic.theclinics.com.

OVERVIEW

Periocular aging is characterized by thinning of the tissues encircling the orbit, apparent sagging and redundancy of upper eyelid skin, and pseudoherniation of lower eyelid fat.[1] Surgical approaches may address all these factors, but the use of cosmetic dermal fillers, primarily hyaluronic acid gels (HAGs), is a popular approach to address volume deficit in these aging tissues. More than 1.5 million people undergo facial injection with a synthetic dermal filler yearly in the United States. These products have good utility and an excellent safety profile, even in the periocular area, although undesirable outcomes can occur.[2,3]

The most commonly used dermal fillers are synthetic HAG fillers, with a smaller representation of collagen, calcium hydroxylapatite gel, poly-L-lactic acid, and polymethylmethacrylate beads.[4] Autogenous fat also is employed surgically,[5] which is a different topic, and liquid silicone and other unapproved, imported, or withdrawn products are employed by some injectors.

The use of HAG and other fillers in the midface and upper face is associated with several risks, most commonly undercorrection or overcorrection of the soft tissue deficit or the placement of or migration of the filler into an inappropriate location (**Fig. 1**).[6–8] Use in the lower eyelid commonly is associated with the Tyndall effect,[7] whose origin is debated.[9]

Additional adverse outcomes include the most feared—vascular or embolization events—or may relate to placement issues, nodules and migration,

[a] Beverly Hills Ophthalmic Plastic and Reconstructive Surgery, 150 North Robertson Boulevard #314, Beverly Hills, CA 90211, USA; [b] Department of Plastic Surgery, Division of Oculoplastic Surgery, Cedars Sinai Medical Center, Los Angeles, CA, USA; [c] Department of Ophthalmology, Division of Oculoplastic Surgery, Keck School of Medicine, University of Southern California, Los Angeles, CA, USA; [d] Saint Louis University School of Medicine, St Louis, MO, USA; [e] Ophthalmic Plastic and Cosmetic Surgery, Inc., St Louis, MO, USA
* Corresponding author. Ophthalmic Plastic and Cosmetic Surgery Inc., 12990 Manchester Road #102, St. Louis, MO 63131, USA.
E-mail address: jholds@gmail.com

Facial Plast Surg Clin N Am 29 (2021) 349–357
https://doi.org/10.1016/j.fsc.2021.02.001
1064-7406/21/© 2021 Elsevier Inc. All rights reserved.

allergy or hypersensitivity to the product, acute or late chronic infection, granuloma formation, or other chronic edema.

Appropriate patient history and selection, preparation, procedural and product decision making, and aftercare, as needed, result in optimal results. Hyaluronidase injection is a vital tool in managing and reversing most adverse effects of HAG filler treatment, with other approaches needed in the treatment of other complications and classes of fillers.

GENERAL COMMENTS ON DERMAL FILLER COMPLICATIONS
Patient-Related Issues

Inappropriate patient selection often is the starting point in a complication. In that regard, it is the injecting physician's role to screen the patient and determine whether the patient is a suitable candidate for the desired treatment. Patients with inappropriate motivation, obvious active social or psychiatric issues, and body dysmorphic syndrome should be rejected, because it is the injector's role to select the patient and treatment, not vice versa.[3]

A thorough history of skin conditions, allergies, systemic diseases, current medications, and previous procedures is essential. Acne, rosacea, and other infectious or inflammatory skin conditions all compromise the epithelial skin barrier and may promote inflammatory and infectious or biofilm reactions to dermal fillers. A history of cold sore or herpetic outbreaks may mandate pretreatment and post-treatment antiviral prophylaxis.

Patients with active autoimmune disease, including rheumatologic and thyroid disease, must be delayed or rejected. The procedural checklist should include temporal distancing from dental cleaning and procedures, immunizations, other medical and surgical procedures, blood thinners, and treatments or activities that disrupt the epithelial barrier (longer delay for thin or compromised skin). Three patients with a history of HAG filler treatment were noted in the Moderna COVID-19 vaccine trial to have a localized inflammatory reaction at the site of injection.[10] These reactions were self-limited but certainly concerning. Contacting patients a week before treatments to review these checklist items is wise.

Product-Related Issues

There are vital general physical property–related differences between dermal filler products that intuitively provide some guide to their use. There also are properties discovered in the use of products that, in the realm of clinical consensus or expert injector advice, are recommended. In that regard, in the periocular area, the ability to reverse the effects of HAG fillers with hyaluronidase is a vital factor in the selection of those products for most periocular treatments. HAG fillers are hygroscopic in nature, with a variable tendency to pull water into them after injection. Undercorrection of defects generally is desirable, and various products have variable amounts of cross-linking, free or short-chain HAG, and HAG concentration that affect their suitability in the periocular area (and other areas). Related rheologic characteristics include viscosity, G′ (elastic modulus), and G or tan delta (viscous modulus).[11] These properties are crucial in determining the appropriate depth and site for the placement of a specific product.

Procedure/Injector-Related Issues

Like all cosmetic injectable products, the results achieved with dermal fillers in the periocular area

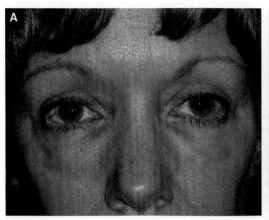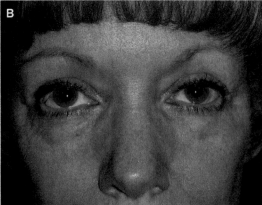

Fig. 1. (A) Woman with Tyndall effect in the lower eyelid 2 years after HAG filler injection elsewhere. (B) Ten minutes after 50 U of hyaluronidase injected subcutaneously into each lower lid.

ultimately largely are up to the treating practitioner's product selection and placement. Depth, volume, rate of flow, and device used for placement all are injector related. Good placement does not compensate for an inappropriate product selection, and vice versa. Injectable filler products are licensed as implants, and that is a good way to always think of them. The common preconception of many patients and, unfortunately, many injectors, that dermal fillers are injected and completely or largely dissipate, or dissolve over 6 months to 12 months, is false. HAG may persist with some breakdown, migration, and change in effect that goes on for a decade or more (**Fig. 2**). A thorough knowledge of facial anatomy as well as a history of an individual patient's previous treatments is essential for injectors.[12] Layering of various products intentionally or unintentionally occurs in many patients over time and has intentional and unintentional effects.

SPECIFIC COMPLICATIONS
Allergic/Hypersensitivity—Allergy Versus Late Onset

The severity of the allergic reaction is paramount (**Box 1** has a detailed list of soft tissue filler complications). Antihistamines may be effective if the reaction is mast cell–mediated. Oral steroids at doses and duration of treatment determined by the timing and severity of reaction are mainstays for allergic swelling and hypersensitivity not responsive to antihistamines. Delayed hypersensitivity reactions may require oral steroid or other treatment.[7,8]

Nodules/Granulomas/Inflammation/Infection

Noninflammatory nodules encountered early after hyaluronic acid (HAG) treatment may resolve with time and with judicious application of

hyaluronidase. Inflammatory nodules must be assessed and followed to determine if they are due to infection. Some inflammation is common early after treatment with some fillers, but persistence, increasing pain, or erythema or fluctuance should prompt antibiotic therapy (generally, a macrolide and/or tetracycline derivative along with a topical antibiotic, such as mupirocin) and drainage of fluctuance.[7] Treatment may require a biopsy with aerobic and anaerobic culture, holding the cultures for 14 days to 21 days. Dermal fillers form microglobules in the tissue that can support chronic biofilm infections, so chronic inflammatory reactions always must be presumed to be infectious until proved otherwise. Resolution of such infections likely requires a 4-week to 6-week course of antibiotics and multiple hyaluronidase injections to eliminate HAG fillers to the extent possible.

Box 1
Classification of soft tissue filler complications by onset of adverse event
Early reactions
Vascular infarction/soft tissue necrosis
Inflammatory reactions (acute/chronic)
Infection
Allergic reactions/hypersensitivity
Injection-related events
Pain
Ecchymosis
Erythema
Bruising
Bleeding
Inappropriate/superficial placement
Distant spread
Late reactions
Inflammatory reactions (acute/chronic)
Infection
Granuloma (typically chronic)
Differential diagnosis
Nodules
Dyspigmentation
Displacement of hyaluronic acid (HAG) filler material
Reproduced with permission from Signorini M et al., Global Aesthetics Consensus Group. Global Aesthetics Consensus: Avoidance and Management of Complications from Hyaluronic Acid Fillers-Evidence- and Opinion-Based Review and Consensus Recommendations. Plast Reconstr Surg. 2016 Jun;137(6):961e-71e.

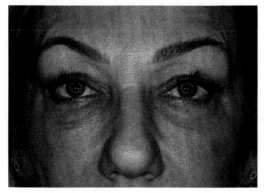

Fig. 2. Chronic HAG filler in patient 10 years after single treatment elsewhere.

The use of hydroxylapatite gel, poly-L-lactic acid, or polymethylmethacrylate beads in mobile structures, such as the lip, or over thin tissues, such as the tear trough, may result in visible nodules. Hydroxylapatite gel and poly-L-lactic dissipate over some time if the changes are not too severe. Polymethylmethacrylate beads do not resorb, and chronic nodules generally are surgically excised (**Fig. 3**),[13] although the injection of triamcinolone and 5-fluorouracil is reported in the treatment.[14] Inflammatory reaction to the collagen-containing vehicle of polymethylmethacrylate beads as well as poly-L-lactic acid may respond to injected steroid, and the injection of saline followed by vigorous massage has been performed with poly-L-lactic acid to break up clumps of possibly poorly mixed product causing nodules.[7] 5-Fluorouracil also has been injected to help soften scar tissue surrounding the implant.

Vascular Events

Vascular embolization with distal vascular occlusion and local necrosis is possible in almost any site, but the risk largely is technique related and occurs most commonly over the glabella and nasion. The use of 25-gauge or larger blunt cannulas for injection appears to diminish the risk of arterial embolization.[15] Immediate skin blanching occurs in an arterial distribution with arterial injection, and venous occlusion may occur due to excessive infiltration in a small area.

Rapid recognition and treatment are essential in the treatment of occlusive events.[7,12] Stopping injection, aspiration, massage, warm compresses, and hyaluronidase injection in significant doses (150–300 U) are performed, with consideration of the application of 2% nitroglycerine paste.[16] Patients are followed closely with local care to areas of skin necrosis to optimize outcome.

Embolization with visual loss or other neurologic complication is addressed in detail in Catherine J. Hwang and colleagues' article, "Blindness After Filler Injection: Mechanism and Treatment," in this issue.

COMMENTS ON THE TREATMENT OF THE TEAR TROUGH AREA
Undercorrection

Patients often have filler suggested or request filler injection of the tear trough in situations in which HAG filler injection is not appropriate to this area. Patients with marked tear trough depressions in this area who anticipate outstanding results are sure setups for disappointment. **Fig. 4** shows such a patient who experienced dissatisfaction with their tear trough treatment after 2 syringes (2 mL) of HAG filler. Additionally, product selection is paramount in this area, with the Hylacross fillers (Juvéderm Ultra and Juvéderm Ultra Plus, Allergan Aesthetics) particularly problematic and unsuitable to apply in the tear trough area (**Figs. 5** and **6**).[6] The authors see patients who desire correction and in whom more than 1 syringe of filler clearly is needed to achieve the desired result. The authors' preferred product in this area is Restylane-L (Galderma, Ft. Worth, TX, USA), and they rarely inject more than 1 mL to 1.5 mL of this HAG into the tear trough on the initial treatment. This and Restylane Silk (Galderma) generally are considered the most suitable products for this area by the most injectors based on physical properties, in particularly G′, and their track record in the tear trough. In the authors' hands, the incidence of lumps, Tyndall effect, or inadequate clinical effect has been greater when larger amounts are injected, and in most suitable patients the authors begin with part or all of 1 syringe (1 mL) (**Fig. 7**). The authors

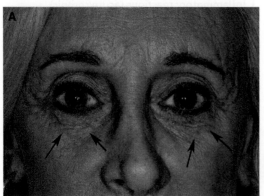 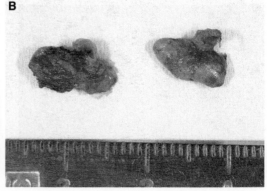

Fig. 3. Lower lid lumps from (*A*) attempted treatment of tear trough a year prior elsewhere with polymethylmethacrylate beads. Arrows at prominent lumps filler/scar. (*B*) Excised filler with encapsulating scar tissue.

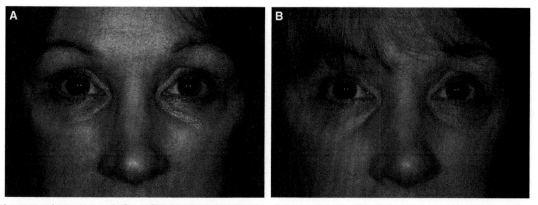

Fig. 4. Inadequate result from filler treatment elsewhere in a patient who is a better surgical than HAG filler candidate for surgery: (*A*) pretreatment and (*B*) post-treatment.

additionally prefer an upward-fanning technique utilizing a 25-gauge cannula technique in treating the tear trough to maintain the product in a deep plane and avoid embolic or other complications (Video 1). The clinician must have a perspective on what is achievable and know when to tell a patient to stop if an adequate result is not possible.

Overcorrection

A variety of untoward overcorrection consequences occur in the periocular area related to

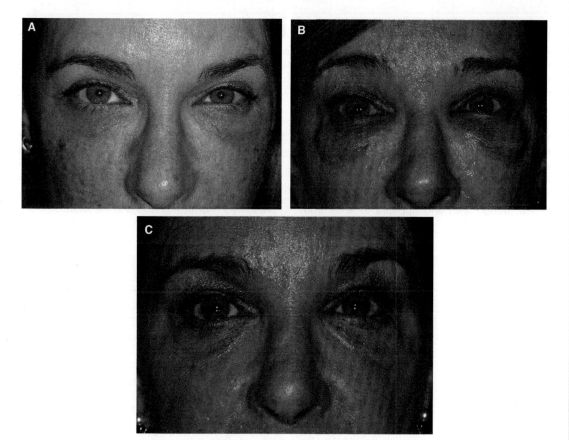

Fig. 5. Patient with skin discoloration and chronic edema after treatment of tear trough elsewhere with 2 mL Juvéderm Ultra (*A*) 6 years before treatment; (*B*) on presentation 6 months after treatment elsewhere; and (*C*) 18 months later after 750 U (total, 4 sessions) of hyaluronidase subcutaneously into the lower lids.

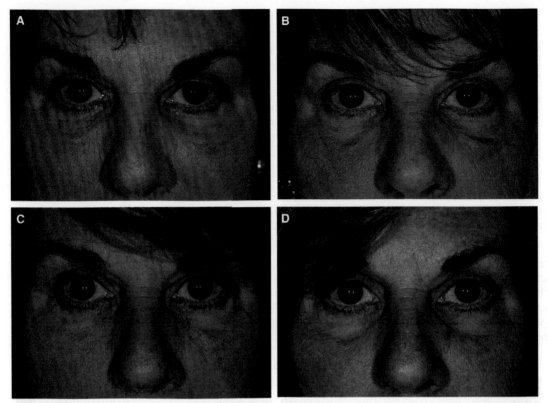

Fig. 6. Patient who received 1 mL of Juvéderm Voluma to each tear trough elsewhere 6 months prior: (A) on presentation; (B) after 75 U of hyaluronidase to each tear trough area (150 U total); (C) 2 weeks later after an additional 150 U; and (D) after a final 150 U (225 U total to tear trough each side). The patient preferred the prominent tear trough to the filler result.

the filler selection; method of administration, including volume, depth, persistence, and inflammation; and ecchymosis induced by the injection. The Tyndall effect, characterized by a bluish discoloration of the treated area, is a common in the tear trough area and appears to arise from the subcutaneous or intramuscular injection or migration of filler.[8] There is some debate as to whether the bluish color is a true Tyndall effect.[9] Overcorrection may occur immediately at placement or months or years later due to migration or presumed chemical changes in the filler.

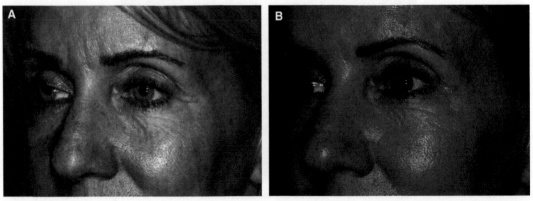

Fig. 7. Patient with good result after tear trough treatment with HAG filler (A) before treatment (B) after HAG injected into tear trough.

Product Issues—Author's Observations

Note that the first author has no financial interest in any company marketing a filler product, except for a small long-term investment in Revance Therapeutics (Revance Therapeutics, Nashville, TN, USA), and has not served as a consultant or taken an honorarium for any company marketing filler products for more than 10 years. Recommendations are based solely on personal experience, discussions with experienced colleagues, and published literature.

Migration of filler may occur months to many years after injection. The authors' perspective on this has significantly evolved over time. There are treatment issues due to inappropriate placement of products. Different products have different characteristics on initial placement and as they age in position. The authors have seen a wide variety of fillers used in the tear trough, including polymethylmethacrylate beads (Bellafill, Merz Aesthetics, Raleigh, NC, USA), hydroxylapatite gel (Radiesse, Merz Aesthetics, Raleigh, NC, USA), and every HAG filler in common use in the United States. The authors have seen significant aesthetic complications with virtually every product and note the following observations regarding the periorbital use of fillers in the tear trough area:

1. Polymethylmethacrylate bead (Bellafill) complications are severe and persistent. Visible filler requires covering the (hopefully deeply positioned) beads with HAG filler to camouflage it or surgical removal of the beads along with their capsule of fibrous encapsulation. Massage, needling, and injections with 5-fluorouracil and/or triamcinolone are described in the treatment of nodules resulting from this product, although these approaches work only early in the course[13,14] (see **Fig. 3**).
2. Hydroxylapatite gel (Radiesse) is noted to be contraindicated in the tear trough by many investigators. Bernardini and coworkers[17] have demonstrated its use favorably in the tear trough, although the authors have not used his technique.
3. HAGs all are prone to the development of an overfilled result, with or without the bluish appearance of the Tyndall effect (see **Figs. 1** and **2**). The authors have examined patients in whom the most recent treatment with a HAG filler was 12 years prior, and the Tyndall effect was first noted 10 years after that, two years prior to presentation. The common presumption and treatment paradigm that these products "go away" in 6-12 months is entirely false and must be rejected and updated.

Unfortunately most patients and injectors operate under these false assumptions.

4. The Allergan Pharmaceutical Hylacross family of HAG fillers (Juvéderm Ultra and Ultra Plus) are quite hydrophilic and appear to be especially unsuitable products in the tear trough area. Kami Parsa, MD (personal communication, 2019) has presented results of patients he has treated for aesthetically undesirable results with numerous HAG fillers, including these products. There was 1 patient who required more than 30 hyaluronidase injections to resolve subcutaneous edema associated with a Hylacross filler. Often the skin is stretched and altered by the chronic edema, and aesthetic reconstruction is difficult. The authors have seen several patients with this complication and confirm this observation (see **Fig. 5**A,B).
5. The Restylane family of fillers appears most appropriate for use in the tear trough, with the original Restylane or Restylane-L preferred by the most injectors due to its favorable properties, including high G. Restylane Silk shares similar properties and is preferred by some injectors. Advantages and properties noted in Restylane include the following:
   a. Appropriate physical properties of flow, viscosity, high G, and moderate hydrophilicity
   b. Low and slow apparent diffusion through tissues with appropriate placement
   c. Low risk of autoimmune reaction or nodule formation
   d. Readily and rapidly removed with low to moderate doses of hyaluronidase (60–100 U/mL) in cases of migration or over-effect
6. The Vycross family of fillers (Allergan Pharmaceuticals) similarly is prone to migration and Tyndall effect. Although not as hydrophilic as the Hylacross family of fillers, these products (Juvéderm Volbella, Juvéderm Vollure, and Juvéderm Voluma) are more resistant to and harder to remove with hyaluronidase injection than the Restylane (Galderma) family of fillers. As the heaviest of this family with the most persistence, Voluma appears to be the hardest to remove with hyaluronidase injection, with most patients requiring hyaluronidase doses greater than 200 U per 1 mL of filler for adequate resolution of overcorrections (see **Fig. 6**).
7. Suspicion of prior filler placement or migration from the cheek or midface is important in the assessment of patients. Some aesthetic patients are notoriously poor in providing history, especially in regard to spa treatments often not administered by a physician. This is

compounded when a treatment may have been many years ago and the problem has been noted recently. A therapeutic trial of hyaluronidase injection is advised whenever there is any suspicion of possible HAG filler migration in the tear trough area. Edematous festoons often have the bluish appearance of a Tyndall effect and are worsened by HAG filler migration. Filler migration always must be suspected in acquired dysmorphia!

8. Patients presenting for lower eyelid evaluation in which dysmorphia related to HAG filler treatment is suspected require careful counseling and planning of any intervention, including hyaluronidase treatment. As bad as the swollen blue lower eyelids may look to a surgeon, it is the aesthetic the patient has lived with for some time, and the real upset may begin when the filler is dissolved and the tear trough change, lower lid bag, and skin laxity reassert themselves. These consequences must be explained to the patient, and, if the plan is to pursue surgery after hyaluronidase treatment, it should be scheduled in the near future before proceeding. The surgeon may wish to leave enough time interval for at least 1 more round of hyaluronidase before the surgery date arrives. It is a bad idea to dissolve filler extensively at the time of surgery if the patient no longer is aware of their native anatomy. It is better for them to have a few days to absorb that picture before blepharoplasty surgery. In some cases, the patient may insist on additional filler treatment to the tear trough, which may be reasonable as an interim treatment or if the surgeon can achieve a more favorable result.

The authors' experience with patients presenting with dysmorphic filler is that a majority wish to pursue lower blepharoplasty and proceed with surgery after hyaluronidase treatment of the filler that they are aware is present (30%) or have filler unknown to them camouflaging their native anatomy and desire surgery, with hyaluronidase treatment performed preoperatively to unmask their native anatomy (30%). Approximately 75% of patients receive more than 1 hyaluronidase treatment. Skippen and colleagues[18] report a series in which 92% of patients received a single hyaluronidase treatment; only 10% of patients proceeded with lower blepharoplasty after hyaluronidase treatment; and 80% of patients were treated again with HAG fillers after hyaluronidase treatment. Those investigators are an expert group whose capabilities are not questioned, but they appear to have a different patient type, practice pattern, and appropriate approaches to therapy.

9. The authors' preferred technique for tear trough treatment (see Video 1) generally is as follows:
   a. Upward fanning technique using a 25-gauge cannula advanced superiorly from a needle stab incision 3 cm below the orbital rim in line with the pupil
   b. Initial infraorbital block with 0.3% lidocaine with epinephrine 1:600,000.
   c. With the cannula deep on the periosteum and the side port up, small aliquots (0.02–0.03 mL) of Restylane-L are placed in the tear trough. As treatment proceeds, subtle tear trough elevation is apparent, arcing across the tear trough with multiple advancements.
   d. Aiming for a modest undercorrection of the tear trough defect, because there is some swelling of the HAG after treatment, and overcorrection is undesirable.
   e. A separate lateral treatment pocket may be undertaken for the temporal hollow, but careful treatment with small aliquots across the area is needed, and again undercorrection is advisable.
   f. Some icing, short-term avoidance of blood thinners, and limited massage and activity for a day are advisable. Bruising generally is minimal with a 25-gauge cannula technique.
10. Tear trough patients are followed-up at 1 week to 2 weeks, with additional treatment or touch-up as desired. The authors use half-inch 29-gauge to 30-gauge standard hypodermic needles for limited touch-up treatments.

SUMMARY

Dermal fillers, in particular HAG fillers, are used in the treatment of aging changes in the periocular area, especially the tear trough. Filler treatment requires in-depth knowledge of specific issues relating to product performance and administration as well as knowledge of safety protocols and recognition and treatment of complications.

There are different approaches to treatment of the tear trough, with the authors favoring an approach from below, with a 25-gauge blunt cannula injecting Restylane-L as the preferred HAG. Prior filler treatment must be suspected in patients presenting for aesthetic evaluation, and the possibility of migration with a dysmorphic appearance and/or Tyndall effect appearance in the tear trough always is kept in mind. Treatment with hyaluronidase injection generally is effective in this area, although the aesthetic change may be drastic and a follow-up plan must be discussed with the patient before proceeding with this therapy.

CLINICS CARE POINTS

- Proper patient selection, product selection, and placement are paramount in achieving ideal results with dermal fillers.

- HAG fillers persist long term, even if the desired clinical effect dissipates, creating the frequently encountered Tyndall effect in the tear trough area.

- Inflammation in areas of filler injection must be treated as infectious in nature until proved otherwise.

- Hyaluronidase injection is a vital tool in treating many complications and overcorrection using HAG fillers

- Before hyaluronidase injection of the tear trough area, patient counseling must occur, discussing the patients' options and planning if the patient finds recurrence of the tear trough to be aesthetically undesirable.

- An upward fanning injection technique with Restylane-L and a 25-gauge cannula is recommended by the authors in treating the tear trough area.

DISCLOSURE

Dr J.B. Holds is a shareholder of Revance Therapeutics, Newark, CA, USA, and received book royalties from Springer. Dr G. Massry received royalties from Elsevier, Springer, Quality Medical Publishers, and Osmotica Pharmaceuticals.

SUPPLEMENTARY DATA

Supplementary data related to this article can be found online at https://doi.org/10.1016/j.fsc.2021.02.001.

REFERENCES

1. Stutman RL, Codner MA. Tear trough deformity: review of anatomy and treatment options. Aesthet Surg J 2012;32(4):426–40.

2. Injectable fillers guide. Available at: https://www.americanboardcosmeticsurgery.org/procedure-learning-center/non-surgical/injectable-fillers-guide/. Accessed January 1, 2021.

3. Heydenrych I, Kapoor KM, De Boulle K, et al. A 10-point plan for avoiding hyaluronic acid dermal filler-related complications during facial aesthetic procedures and algorithms for management. Clin Cosmet Investig Dermatol 2018;11:603–11.

4. FDA-Approved Dermal Fillers. Available at: https://www.fda.gov/medical-devices/aesthetic-cosmetic-devices/fda-approved-dermal-fillers. Accessed January 1, 2021.

5. Maamari RN, Massry GG, Holds JB. Complications associated with fat grafting to the lower eyelid. Facial Plast Surg Clin North Am 2019;27(4):435–41.

6. Zoumalan CI. Managing periocular filler-related syndrome prior to lower blepharoplasty. Aesthet Plast Surg 2019;43(1):115–22.

7. Sclafani AP, Fagien S. Treatment of injectable soft tissue filler complications. Dermatol Surg 2009;35(Suppl 2):1672–80.

8. Ozturk CN, Li Y, Tung R, et al. Complications following injection of soft-tissue fillers. Aesthet Surg J 2013;33:862–77.

9. Rootman DB, Lin JL, Goldberg R. Does the Tyndall effect describe the blue hue periodically observed in subdermal hyaluronic acid gel placement? Ophthalmic Plast Reconstr Surg 2014;30(6):524–7.

10. Rice SM, Ferree SD, Atanaskova Mesinkovska N, et al. The Art of Prevention: COVID-19 vaccine preparedness for the dermatologist. Int J Womens Dermatol 2021. https://doi.org/10.1016/j.ijwd.2021.01.007.

11. Sundaram H, Cassuto D. Biophysical characteristics of hyaluronic acid soft-tissue fillers and their relevance to aesthetic applications. Plast Reconstr Surg 2013;132(4 Suppl 2):5S–21S. Erratum in: Plast Reconstr Surg. 2013;132(5):1378.

12. Signorini M, Liew S, Sundaram H, et al. Global aesthetics consensus group. global aesthetics consensus: avoidance and management of complications from hyaluronic acid fillers-evidence- and opinion-based review and consensus recommendations. Plast Reconstr Surg 2016;137(6):961e–71e.

13. Park TH, Seo SW, Kim JK, et al. Clinical experience with polymethylmethacrylate microsphere filler complications. Aesthet Plast Surg 2012;36(2):421–6.

14. Ibrahim O, Dover JS. Delayed-onset nodules after polymethyl methacrylate injections. Dermatol Surg 2018;44(9):1236–8.

15. DeLorenzi C. Complications of injectable fillers, part 2: vascular complications. Aesthet Surg J 2014;34(4):584–600.

16. Dayan SH, Arkins JP, Mathison CC. Management of impending necrosis associated with soft tissue filler injections. J Drugs Dermatol 2011;10(9):1007–12.

17. Bernardini FP, Cetinkaya A, Devoto MH, et al. Calcium hydroxyl-apatite (Radiesse) for the correction of periorbital hollows, dark circles, and lower eyelid bags. Ophthalmic Plast Reconstr Surg 2014;30(1):34–9.

18. Skippen B, Baldelli I, Hartstein M, et al. Rehabilitation of the dysmorphic lower eyelid from hyaluronic acid filler: what to do after a good periocular treatment goes bad. Aesthet Surg J 2020;40(2):197–205.

Blindness After Filler Injection
Mechanism and Treatment

Catherine J. Hwang, MD*, Brian H. Chon, MD, Julian D. Perry, MD

KEYWORDS

- Filler complications • Filler ischemic complications • Filler blindness • Filler-induced blindness
- Filler orbital ischemia • Blindness and filler • Hyaluronic acid gel filler • Dermal filler complications

KEY POINTS

- Blindness and orbital ischemia can occur with dermal filler injections. The mechanism of action is thought to be inadvertent intraarterial injection of filler product causing ischemia.
- Injectors should be aware of the risk of blindness and visual compromise/orbital ischemia and discuss this small but potential risk with patients before filler injection and obtain informed consent.
- There is no proven treatment to reverse filler-induced blindness to date.
- Some injectors suggest the use of retrobulbar hyaluronidase for filler-induced blindness; however, it has its own risks and is unproved to date.

OVERVIEW

Fillers are commonly thought of as a straightforward and safe treatment and continue to be a popular nonsurgical facial rejuvenation treatment option. According to the American Society for Aesthetic Plastic Surgery, an estimated 870,000 filler injection procedures were performed in the United States in 2018.[1] Dermal fillers come from a variety of materials including hyaluronic acid, calcium hydroxyapatite, and poly-L-lactic acid (PLLA), with more than 30 dermal fillers approved by the Food and Drug Administration.[2] Hyaluronic acid gel fillers are the most popular dermal filler due to safety and side-effect profile, reversibility, variety of formulations, and applications. However, hyaluronic acid gel fillers still have associated complications. Although most of these complications are mild and reversible, rare but reported complications include tissue ischemia, skin necrosis, and permanent blindness. To reduce the likelihood of these complications, implementing "Global Filler Safety" is essential, which includes understanding the facial anatomy, proper patient and filler product selection, and proper placement of filler in a safe anatomic location. As with any other procedure, an informed consent should include a thorough discussion with the patient about the risks and potential complications.[3]

Although the incidence of filler-induced blindness is unknown, increasingly more cases of visual compromise are expected to be seen with the growing use of fillers. Beleznay and colleagues found 146 total reported cases of sudden vision loss secondary to filler injections, with 98 cases found between 1906 and 2015[4] and another 48 cases between 2015 and 2018.[5] The actual cases of filler-induced blindness are likely underreported, as we do not have a good way to capture all cases.

Injectors, staff, and patients should be aware of this known complication. Even with the appropriate understanding and implementation of filler injections, blindness can happen. Signs and symptoms associated with visual compromise include immediate loss of vision, double vision, pain, ophthalmoplegia, droopy eyelids (ptosis),

Unrestricted grant award from Research to Prevent Blindness to the Department of Ophthalmology at Cole Eye Institute (RPB1508DM).
Oculofacial Plastic Surgery, Department of Ophthalmology, Cole Eye Institute, Cleveland Clinic Foundation, 9500 Euclid Avenue, Cleveland, OH 44195, USA
* Corresponding author.
E-mail address: hwangc2@ccf.org

Facial Plast Surg Clin N Am 29 (2021) 359–367
https://doi.org/10.1016/j.fsc.2021.02.002
1064-7406/21/© 2021 Elsevier Inc. All rights reserved.

headache, soft tissue ischemia, and stroke symptoms due to cerebral infarcts.[4,6–11] The highest risk areas or "danger zones" for visual compromise from filler injection are the glabella, nasal area, nasolabial fold, and temple.[4,11,12]

This article focuses on the mechanism of filler-associated blindness, possible treatments, and future directions.

MECHANISM OF VISUAL COMPROMISE DUE TO DERMAL FILLERS

The primary mechanism of filler-induced blindness is due to direct intraarterial filler injection, leading to embolization of filler material via vascular pathways to the ophthalmic artery.

Filler injected at pressures that overcome arterial pressure and friction forces due to viscous flow can lead to ophthalmic artery embolization. With enough pressure, the filler material moves initially in a retrograde path, then after reduction of injection pressure, filler material moves in an anterograde direction with blood flow, resulting in a shower of emboli anteriorly, including into the ophthalmic artery circulation.

The main branches of the ophthalmic artery include the supratrochlear, supraorbital, dorsal nasal, lacrimal, ethmoidal, palpebral, muscular, posterior ciliary, and central retinal arteries. The facial artery may anastomose with the ophthalmic artery via the angular artery. In a cadaver study, the supratrochlear, supraorbital, and dorsal nasal artery directly connected to the ophthalmic artery in all cadavers, and the angular artery anastomosed to the ophthalmic artery in 54% (**Fig. 1**)[13]—this corresponds with the common "danger zones" for visual compromise or blindness. Although these arteries may present more direct routes to the ophthalmic artery, there are many other anastomoses from the arteries of the face with the ophthalmic artery, so nearly any area of the face is at some risk of vision-threatening complications.[4]

The degree of visual compromise depends on the level of obstruction within the ophthalmic artery and is likely related to the filler particle size. The approximate diameter of the ophthalmic artery is 2 mm and the central retina artery is 160 μm.[14,15] If the filler product is larger than the vessel, ischemia downstream will result.

All major types of filler materials can result in visual compromise, and particle size likely has an impact on arterial occlusion. Autologous fillers, such as fat, vary in particle size. Hyaluronic acid particle sizes are 400 μm for Restylane (Galderma, Ft. Worth, TX) and 750 to 1000 μm for Perlane (Galderma, Ft. Worth, TX). Juvederm (Allergan, Irvine, CA) products are not passed through sizing screens during processing and are instead "cohesive molecules" of cross-linked hyaluronic acid. Radiesse (BioForm Medical, San Mateo, CA) is a CaHA with particle size between 25 and 45 μm. Sculptra (Dermik Laboratories, Berwyn, PA) is a PLLA filler with particles ranging from 1 to 63 μm. Artefill (Suneva Medical, San Diego, CA) is a polymethyl-methacrylate microsphere (PMMA) filler with particles of 30 to 50 μm.[16] In the Beleznay and colleagues 2015 review[4] of filler-induced vision loss cases from 1906 to 2015, the most common filler causing vision loss was autologous fat (47.9%), followed by hyaluronic acid (23.5%). In their follow-up study in 2019, of cases between 2015 and 2019, hyaluronic acid was now the most common filler type (81.3%) associated with vision loss, followed by CaHA, and only one case of autologous fat injection,[5] which likely represents the increased popularity of hyaluronic acid filler use but could also be related to the size of the filler material, with PLLA and PMMA smaller than the diameter of the central retinal artery (160 μm).

In filler-associated vision loss, the most common type of obstruction is ophthalmic artery occlusion, followed by central retinal artery occlusion (CRAO) and branch retinal artery occlusion.[11] Ophthalmic artery occlusion causes not only CRAO but also occlusion of the downstream vessels (ciliary arteries) and can result in ptosis, ophthalmoplegia, and anterior segment ischemia (**Table 1**). Ophthalmoplegia and anterior segment ischemia may improve after ophthalmic artery occlusion; however, CRAO will not likely improve.[6]

Of note, in cases of filler-induced blindness, filler embolization likely involves many arterial areas, beyond the ophthalmic artery. In the cadaver head perfusion model by Cho and colleagues, after injection of the supratrochlear artery, filler was also seen in the dorsal nasal and supraorbital artery in addition to the ophthalmic artery,[17] which is consistent with findings of skin necrosis in patients with filler-related vision loss.[18] Filler may embolize not only to the ophthalmic artery but also to other arteries such as the supratrochlear, supraorbital, dorsal nasal, and angular arteries.

PREVENTION OF FILLER-INDUCED BLINDNESS

Although there is no method or technique that will reliably prevent vision loss, risk-modifying strategies may reduce the likelihood of filler-induced vision loss.

Before injecting dermal fillers, it is important to have a baseline level of understanding of the relevant facial vascular anatomy and proper placement of the filler material. Although any area of the face has a potential risk of ophthalmic artery

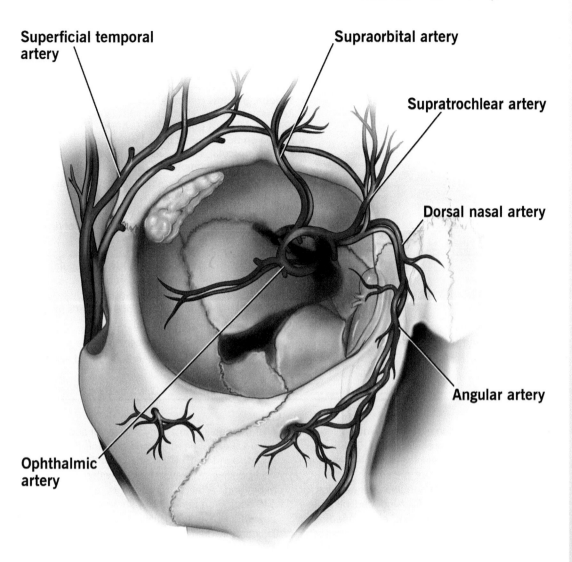

Superficial temporal artery

Supraorbital artery

Supratrochlear artery

Dorsal nasal artery

Angular artery

Ophthalmic artery

Fig. 1. Illustration of the right orbit demonstrates anastomoses between the internal (ophthalmic and tributaries) and external carotid arteries (superficial temporal, angular, and tributaries) (Reprinted with permission, Cleveland Clinic Center for Medical Art & Photography ©2021. All Rights Reserved.)

embolization, the common "danger zones" for vascular compromise include the glabella, nasal area, nasolabial folds, forehead, and temple **(Fig. 2)**.[4,11,12]

The possibility of loss of vision associated with fillers should be discussed with patients before injection and before informed consent is obtained.[3] Signs of filler-induced visual compromise include vision loss, sharp pain, ophthalmoplegia, ptosis, central nervous system (CNS) complications, and nausea/vomiting.[5] Pain may be variably present and can be masked by lidocaine, which comes in most of the filler products or by previously administered topical anesthetic agents or nerve blocks. If signs of filler-induced blindness are noticed, the filler injection should be immediately stopped,

and practitioners should be prepared to manage complications.[19]

Filler injectors should avoid high pressures and volumes on injection. In a study using a cadaver head perfusion model, the average injection pressure needed to embolize the ophthalmic artery by cannulating and injecting hyaluronic acid filler in the supratrochlear artery was 166.7 mm Hg.[17] The investigators noted that during injection "it is easy for the injector to exert the pressure well above 200 mm Hg within 2 to 3 seconds" and concluded that this provides support to the clinical recommendation to avoid high injection pressures during filler injections.

In addition, while injecting fillers, small aliquots should be used per pass. One cadaver study

Table 1
Signs and symptoms resulting from arterial occlusion

Artery	Signs/Symptoms if Occluded
Ophthalmic artery	• Sudden, painless complete unilateral vision loss • Retinal whitening, cherry red spot (+/−) • Relative afferent pupil defect (RAPD) • Effects on downstream branches (eg, dorsal nasal, retinal, muscular, ciliary, lacrimal, supraorbital, supratrochlear, ethmoidal)
Central retinal artery	• Sudden, painless complete unilateral vision loss • Retinal whitening, cherry red spot • Relative afferent pupil defect (RAPD)
Branch retinal artery	• Sudden, painless, partial unilateral vision loss (loss of peripheral field) • Visual acuity (VA) variable • Segmental retinal whitening (follows a vascular pattern)
Muscular arteries	• Ophthalmoplegia (extraocular muscles) • Ptosis (levator palpebrae superioris, Muller's muscle)
Dorsal nasal artery	• Nasal ischemia, possible necrosis
Supraorbital and supratrochlear arteries	• Forehead ischemia, possible necrosis
Ciliary arteries	• Long ciliary: ciliary body ischemia (reduced aqueous humor production, low IOP)
Lacrimal artery	• Lacrimal gland function, dry eye syndrome

showed the entire volume of the supratrochlear artery from glabella to orbital apex is 0.085 mL.[20] Therefore, small volumes, for example, less than 0.1 mL, should be used per pass.

Some have proposed cannulas over needles for filler injections; however, filler-induced blindness can result from injections using either needles or cannulas. In a review of 48 cases of blindness after filler injections from 2015 to 2018, in only 33% (16 of 48) were needle or cannula use documented, with 10 cases with needles and 6 with cannulas, with cannula diameters ranging from 27G to 23G.[5] The force needed to penetrate an arterial wall increases with both larger diameter cannulas and needles. For 27G needles and cannulas, the force needed to penetrate an artery is similar. For larger diameters (22G and 25G), cannulas require greater force to penetrate arterial walls than needles.[21] No clinical studies have shown cannulas are safer than needles or that they reduce the risk of arterial perforation.[22]

Reflux of the filler syringe is a commonly recommended technique to evaluate for intraarterial placement of the needle or cannula. In a study of 17 filler products (mostly hyaluronic acid, 1 PLLA, and 2 CaHA products), the syringe and needles provided in the filler package only showed a positive reflux in 53% of fillers, although larger bore needles did lead to positive aspirations in all

filler materials.[23] In a similar study of aspiration using a variety of needle types and soft tissue fillers, it was found that 112 of 340 aspiration tests (33%) had positive aspiration results within 1 second of aspiration. After 10 seconds of aspiration, 128/140 aspiration tests (38%) showed false-negative aspiration results.[24] Unlike aspiration tests when injecting fluids, filler materials have different rheological properties that make aspiration a less reliable test to confirm intraarterial placement of the needle or cannula.

Recommended injection techniques should be used, such as injecting small volumes per pass of the needle, continuously moving the tip of the needle or cannula during injection and using a low injection pressure, small aliquots of filler material, and possibly aspiration before injection; however, this has high false-negative results. Other recommendations to prevent intraarterial embolization of filler products include using local vasoconstrictors (eg, epinephrine) to constrict the blood vessels and limit entry, limiting the total volume of filler used, and occlusive pressure in the area of the supraorbital notch (**Box 1**).[25,26]

TREATMENTS FOR FILLER-INDUCED BLINDNESS

Unfortunately, to date, there are no proven treatments to reverse filler-induced blindness. Vision

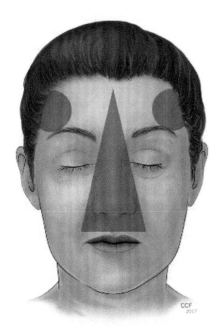

Fig. 2. Danger zones causing blindness for filler injections. The locations at highest risk for filler-associated vision loss include a central triangular area (glabella, nasal area, and nasolabial fold) and bilateral temples. (Reprinted with permission, Cleveland Clinic Center for Medical Art & Photography ©2021. All Rights Reserved.)

Box 1
Recommended injection techniques (clinics care points)

1. Understand periorbital anatomy.

2. Inject small volumes per pass and less than 0.1 mL in any one area.

3. Keep moving the tip of the injection needle/ cannula.

4. Attempt aspiration before injection; however, sometimes because of the length of the needle or nature of the filler product, it may not produce a flashback.

5. Use low injection pressure, do not force injection, especially in areas of previous scarring, injection, or surgery.

6. Consider the use of blunt cannulas, but remember they do not eliminate risk.

7. Smaller needles and cannulas may be more likely to penetrate vascular walls.

8. Always know where the tip of the needle or cannula is in 3-dimensional space, including depth (can use nondominant hand to protect globe and feel tip of cannula before injection)

9. Consider local anesthesia with epinephrine to vasoconstrict blood vessels; however, blanching may delay the recognition of ischemic complications.

---

recovery is time sensitive, and it is thought that the retinal circulation needs to be restored within 90 minutes of onset to prevent permanent vision loss.[27] If visual compromise or blindness develops after injection of fillers, the patient should be referred immediately to an ophthalmologist, preferably a retina specialist. Before initiating treatment, it is important to confirm the degree of vision loss (check visual acuity or at least determine light perception or no light perception) and evaluate the pupillary reaction for a relative afferent pupillary defect. It is important to evaluate for other signs of ischemia in the skin, orbit, and CNS. Proptosis (bulging of eye), extraocular motility, ptosis (droopy eyelid), and redness of the eye can be also present with filler-induced visual compromise.

Even with early recognition and prompt referral and evaluation, visual compromise associated with filler injection is often irreversible due to the terminal effects on the retina. The other signs such as ptosis and ophthalmoplegia will recover over time due to the rich blood supply and ability of muscles to regain function.[10]

Treatment options for filler-induced blindness resulting in blindness and CRAO include traditional treatments for CRAO to try and dislodge emboli: lowering intraocular pressure (IOP) with ocular massage, IOP-lowering eye drops, systemic medications such as acetazolamide and mannitol, and possibly anterior chamber paracentesis.[28] Although none of these treatments have been shown to reverse CRAO, most are relatively low risk and can be attempted in filler-induced blindness.

HYALURONIDASE

High-dose hyaluronidase is the only proven treatment of the reversal of soft tissue ischemia associated with inadvertent intraarterial injection of hyaluronic acid gel fillers. Hyaluronidase has been suggested as a treatment option for filler-related blindness, but this remains unproved. Hyaluronidase is an enzyme that depolymerizes hyaluronic acid by degrading glycoside bonds and may be used to reverse the effects of hyaluronic acid filler material. Hyaluronidase is derived from a variety of formulations: purified bovine testicular hyaluronidase (Amphadase, Hydase), purified ovine testicular hyaluronidase (Vitrase), and recombinant human DNA (Hylenex). Hyaluronidase products are standardized so that 1 International Unit (IU) is equivalent in hydrolysis of hyaluronic acid, regardless of the source of formulation.[29] The effectiveness of hyaluronidase depends on many factors, including the amount of filler needed to be reversed, surface area of hyaluronic acid for interaction with hyaluronidase, temperature, and pH.[29]

Hyaluronidase may take several hours to hydrolyze hyaluronic acid filler. Using 150 IU of hyaluronidase can hydrolyze 0.1 cc of hyaluronic acid in approximately 4 hours.[29] By depolymerizing hyaluronic acid filler materials, hyaluronidase may reverse ischemic complications. Different hyaluronic acid fillers respond at different rates, given different formulations, concentrations, and crosslinking properties. In one study, hyaluronidase in the form of Vitrase and Hylenex were used in vitro: Restylane showed the most degradation, followed by Juvederm, then Belotero (most resistant to degradation).[30] In general, more hyaluronidase is required for larger volumes of filler, and higher concentrations of hyaluronidase dissolves filler faster.

Hyaluronidase for filler-associated blindness potentially can be administered as an intraarterial, intravitreal, intravenous (IV), or retrobulbar injection. Although there are reported cases of improvement in vision with retrobulbar and intraarterial hyaluronidase injections, this has not been proved and is not consistently effective.[31]

Intraarterial hyaluronidase given near the ophthalmic artery, via the supratrochlear, supraorbital arteries, or with interventional radiology, could potentially dissolve hyaluronic acid filler causing filler-induced blindness.[32,33] Given the small time window for efficacy of hyaluronidase, intraarterial injections with interventional radiology are highly unlikely to be coordinated within a short time window, as this requires transfer to a hospital, administration of anesthesia, and establishing femoral artery access. Although supraorbital and supratrochlear arteries are close to the skin surface, this route relies on hyaluronidase being injected into the artery and following the path of least resistance, which may not be toward the filler material embolus. Two case reports[34,35] have shown that supraorbital and/or supratrochlear injections helped symptoms, although visual acuity and pressures were not checked. In addition, direct cutdown and cannulation of the supraorbital and/or supratrochlear artery has been proposed; however this requires surgical exposure, knowledge of the anatomy, and surgical expertise.

Intravitreal hyaluronidase potentially could provide a more direct access of hyaluronidase to the retinal and choroidal vessels, as it could diffuse across these vessels. Intravitreal hyaluronidase has been reported in the use of vitreous hemorrhage in diabetic retinopathy, showing no serious safety issues.[36] In addition, there are risks associated with retinal injections such as cataract formation or acceleration, raised IOP, retinal tears or detachments, and endophthalmitis. The authors, in their unpublished rabbit study data (Catherine J. Hwang, unpublished data, 2016), have not found reversal with intravitreal injections alone and needs to be administered by a skilled eye specialist.

IV hyaluronidase may be promising, as it could be administered in the office or emergency room setting by peripheral vein. In a rabbit model, Chiang and colleagues[37] showed improvement in ophthalmic and retinal artery perfusion with hyaluronidase and urokinase when given IV within 30 minutes, although large doses were required (5000 IU/kg). Urokinase is thought to help by dissolving any arterial thrombosis in the area of occlusion. IV hyaluronidase may be a promising route, as it could be administered quickly, has been shown to be safe in large doses, and can be administered by peripheral venous access.[38,39] However, this large dose of IV hyaluronidase in a 50 kg human (250,000 IU) may be cost prohibitive.

Retrobulbar hyaluronidase is another route of administration for filler-induced vision loss. Retrobulbar hyaluronidase theoretically works given its ability diffuse through arterial walls into intraarterial hyaluronic acid filler material.[40] Hyaluronidase, however, has not been found to penetrate the optic nerve sheath in in-vitro studies of human optic nerves.[41] In one rabbit study, retrobulbar hyaluronidase administered at 30 minutes using 1000 IU of hyaluronidase failed to reverse or restore filler-associated vision loss.[42] In a separate rabbit study, there seemed to be an improvement with 3000 IU retrobulbar hyaluronidase injection 5 to 10 minutes after filler retinal artery occlusion. However, in this study there were no pretreatment electroretinograms to verify abnormal function before retrobulbar hyaluronidase, so it is unknown if the eyes were truly occluded pretreatment and the hyaluronidase was given remarkably rapidly.[43] In the literature, the volume of retrobulbar hyaluronidase used for filler-induced blindness ranges from 120 IU up to 6000 IU.[31] Although there have been a few cases reported with successful use of retrobulbar hyaluronidase, there was no vision checked before treatment, questioning the reported visual improvement after treatment.

Given there are no proved treatments of filler-induced blindness, retrobulbar hyaluronidase is a frequently attempted treatment option but does have risks including retrobulbar hemorrhage and inadvertent globe perforation. In addition, less than 7 cc of hyaluronidase must be used, as higher volumes risks increased orbital pressure and optic disc edema.[44] Retrobulbar hyaluronidase, if administered, should be given by a trained professional, and the patient should understand that the treatment may not reverse the visual loss, can have some other risks, but could help with orbital pain.

FUTURE DIRECTIONS AND STUDIES

An ideal filler would be without complications, fully reversible, and could age with the individual. Unfortunately, an ideal treatment of visual compromise and blindness remains to be determined. Further research efforts are needed to find a treatment or possible prevention protocol. The ideal filler would be one that does not lead to complications, particularly the devastating complication of vision loss, and would have a reliable treatment if a complication were to occur.

Further studies may evaluate various routes of hyaluronidase administration (intraarterial, IV, intravitreal, and retrobulbar) by themselves or in combination as well as possible other adjunctive medications such as thrombolytics, corticosteroids, and vasodilators. The authors look forward to the day when they have a proved treatment of filler-induced blindness.

SUMMARY

Dermal fillers remain popular treatments for facial rejuvenation. Although relatively safe and effective, complications can occur, including visual compromise and blindness. Before any filler injection, careful planning and informed consent including vision loss and blindness should be discussed with the patient. In addition, injectors, staff, and patients should all be aware of and educated of potential complications, be able to identify filler complications, and promptly initiate treatment. For filler-induced vision loss, there are no proved treatments to date. Various rescue methods can be attempted such as those used for CRAO (ocular massage, lowering IOP, rebreathing into a bag) and potentially hyaluronidase. Hyaluronidase can be administered in various routes to attempt to reverse filler-induced blindness but unfortunately none have been proved to be effective. Regardless, hyaluronidase should always be available at all times when injecting hyaluronic acid fillers, as it is the only proved treatment to reverse filler-induced skin ischemia.

DISCLOSURE

The authors have nothing to disclose.

REFERENCES

1. 2018 Cosmetic (Aesthetic) Surgery National Data Bank Statistics. The American Society for Aesthetic Plastic Surgery. Available at: https://www.surgery.org/sites/default/files/ASAPS-Stats2018_0.pdf. Accessed Jan 2020.
2. Approved Dermal Fillers as of 11/26/2018. FDA. Available at: https://www.fda.gov/medical-devices/aesthetic-cosmetic-devices/fda-approved-dermal-fillers. Accessed January 2020.
3. Rayess HM, Svider PF, Hanba C, et al. A cross-sectional analysis of adverse events and litigation for injectable fillers. JAMA Facial Plast Surg 2018;20(3):207–14.
4. Beleznay K, Carruthers JD, Humphrey S, et al. Avoiding and Treating Blindness From Fillers: A Review of the World Literature. Dermatol Surg 2015;41(10):1097–117.
5. Beleznay K, Carruthers JDA, Humphrey S, et al. Update on avoiding and treating blindness from fillers: a recent review of the world literature. Aesthet Surg J 2019;39(6):662–74.
6. Yang HK, Lee Y, Woo SJ, et al. Natural course of ophthalmoplegia after iatrogenic ophthalmic artery occlusion caused by cosmetic filler injections. Plast Reconstr Surg 2019;144(1):28e–34e.
7. Yang Q, Lu B, Guo N, et al. Fatal cerebral infarction and ophthalmic artery occlusion after nasal augmentation with hyaluronic acid-a case report and review of literature. Aesthet Plast Surg 2020;44(2):543–8.
8. Tran AQ, Staropoli P, Rong AJ, et al. Filler-associated vision loss. Facial Plast Surg Clin North Am 2019;27(4):557–64.
9. Bae IH, Kim MS, Choi H, et al. Ischemic oculomotor nerve palsy due to hyaluronic acid filler injection. J Cosmet Dermatol 2018;17(6):1016–8.
10. Ramesh S, Fiaschetti D, Goldberg RA. Orbital and ocular ischemic syndrome with blindness after facial filler injection. Ophthalmic Plast Reconstr Surg 2018;34(4):e108–10.
11. Kapoor KM, Kapoor P, Heydenrych I, et al. Vision loss associated with hyaluronic acid fillers: a systematic review of literature. Aesthet Plast Surg 2019. https://doi.org/10.1007/s00266-019-01562-8.
12. Ortiz AE, Ahluwalia J, Song SS, et al. Analysis of U.S. Food and Drug Administration Data on Soft-Tissue Filler Complications. Dermatol Surg 2019. https://doi.org/10.1097/DSS.0000000000002208.

13. Wu S, Pan L, Wu H, et al. Anatomic study of ophthalmic artery embolism following cosmetic injection. J Craniofac Surg 2017;28(6):1578–81.

14. Hedges TR. Ophthalmic artery blood flow in humans. Br J Ophthalmol 2002;86(11):1197.

15. Dorner GT, Polska E, Garhöfer G, et al. Calculation of the diameter of the central retinal artery from noninvasive measurements in humans. Curr Eye Res 2002;25(6):341–5.

16. Attenello NH, Maas CS. Injectable fillers: review of material and properties. Facial Plast Surg 2015; 31(1):29–34.

17. Cho KH, Dalla Pozza E, Toth G, et al. Pathophysiology Study of Filler-Induced Blindness. Aesthet Surg J 2019;39(1):96–106.

18. Kim YK, Jung C, Woo SJ, et al. Cerebral Angiographic Findings of Cosmetic Facial Filler-related Ophthalmic and Retinal Artery Occlusion. J Korean Med Sci 2015;30(12):1847–55.

19. Goodman GJ, Magnusson MR, Callan P, et al. A consensus on minimizing the risk of hyaluronic acid embolic visual loss and suggestions for immediate bedside management. Aesthet Surg J 2019. https://doi.org/10.1093/asj/sjz312.

20. Khan TT, Colon-Acevedo B, Mettu P, et al. An anatomical analysis of the supratrochlear artery: considerations in facial filler injections and preventing vision loss. Aesthet Surg J 2017;37(2):203–8.

21. Pavicic T, Webb KL, Frank K, et al. Arterial wall penetration forces in needles versus cannulas. Plast Reconstr Surg 2019;143(3):504e–12e.

22. Yeh LC, Fabi SG, Welsh K. Arterial penetration with blunt-tipped cannulas using injectables: a false sense of safety? Dermatol Surg 2017;43(3): 464–7.

23. Casabona G. Blood aspiration test for cosmetic fillers to prevent accidental intravascular injection in the face. Dermatol Surg 2015;41(7):841–7.

24. Van Loghem JA, Fouché JJ, Thuis J. Sensitivity of aspiration as a safety test before injection of soft tissue fillers. J Cosmet Dermatol 2018;17(1):39–46.

25. Beleznay K, Humphrey S, Carruthers JD, et al. Vascular compromise from soft tissue augmentation: experience with 12 cases and recommendations for optimal outcomes. J Clin Aesthet Dermatol 2014; 7(9):37–43.

26. Carruthers JD, Fagien S, Rohrich RJ, et al. Blindness caused by cosmetic filler injection: a review of cause and therapy. Plast Reconstr Surg 2014;134(6): 1197–201.

27. Hayreh SS, Podhajsky PA, Zimmerman B. Nonarteritic anterior ischemic optic neuropathy: time of onset of visual loss. Am J Ophthalmol 1997;124(5):641–7.

28. Park KH, Kim YK, Woo SJ, et al. Iatrogenic occlusion of the ophthalmic artery after cosmetic facial filler injections: a national survey by the Korean Retina Society. JAMA Ophthalmol 2014;132(6):714–23.

29. DeLorenzi C. Discussion: Assessing Retrobulbar Hyaluronidase as a Treatment for Filler-Induced Blindness in a Cadaver Model. Plast Reconstr Surg 2019;144(2):321–4.

30. Rao V, Chi S, Woodward J. Reversing facial fillers: interactions between hyaluronidase and commercially available hyaluronic-acid based fillers. J Drugs Dermatol 2014;13(9):1053–6.

31. Paap MK, Milman T, Ugradar S, et al. Examining the role of retrobulbar hyaluronidase in reversing filler-induced blindness: a systematic review. Ophthalmic Plast Reconstr Surg 2019. https://doi.org/10.1097/IOP.0000000000001568.

32. Tansatit T, Apinuntrum P, Phetudom T. A cadaveric feasibility study of the intraorbital cannula injections of hyaluronidase for initial salvation of the ophthalmic artery occlusion. Aesthet Plast Surg 2015;39(2):252–61.

33. Surek CC, Said SA, Perry JD, et al. Retrobulbar Injection for Hyaluronic Acid Gel Filler-Induced Blindness: A Review of Efficacy and Technique. Aesthet Plast Surg 2019;43(4):1034–40.

34. Goodman GJ, Roberts S, Callan P. Experience and Management of Intravascular Injection with Facial Fillers: Results of a Multinational Survey of Experienced Injectors. Aesthet Plast Surg 2016;40(4): 549–55.

35. Thanasarnaksorn W, Cotofana S, Rudolph C, et al. Severe vision loss caused by cosmetic filler augmentation: Case series with review of cause and therapy. J Cosmet Dermatol 2018;17(5):712–8.

36. Kuppermann BD, Thomas EL, de Smet MD, et al. Safety results of two phase III trials of an intravitreous injection of highly purified ovine hyaluronidase (Vitrase) for the management of vitreous hemorrhage. Am J Ophthalmol 2005;140(4):585–97.

37. Chiang C, Zhou S, Chen C, et al. Intravenous Hyaluronidase with Urokinase as Treatment for Rabbit Retinal Artery Hyaluronic Acid Embolism. Plast Reconstr Surg 2016;138(6):1221–9.

38. Pillwein K, Fuiko R, Slavc I, et al. Hyaluronidase additional to standard chemotherapy improves outcome for children with malignant brain tumors. Cancer Lett 1998;131(1):101–8.

39. Hyaluronidase therapy for acute myocardial infarction: results of a randomized, blinded, multicenter trial. MILIS Study Group. Am J Cardiol 1986; 57(15):1236–43.

40. DeLorenzi C. Transarterial degradation of hyaluronic acid filler by hyaluronidase. Dermatol Surg 2014; 40(8):832–41.

41. Paap MK, Milman T, Ugradar S, et al. Assessing Retrobulbar Hyaluronidase as a Treatment for Filler-Induced

Blindness in a Cadaver Model. Plast Reconstr Surg 2019;144(2):315–20.

42. Hwang CJ, Mustak H, Gupta AA, et al. Role of Retrobulbar Hyaluronidase in Filler-Associated Blindness: Evaluation of Fundus Perfusion and Electroretinogram Readings in an Animal Model. Ophthalmic Plast Reconstr Surg 2019;35(1):33–7.

43. Lee W, Oh W, Ko HS, et al. Effectiveness of retrobulbar hyaluronidase injection in an iatrogenic blindness rabbit model using hyaluronic acid filler injection. Plast Reconstr Surg 2019;144(1):137–43.

44. Akar Y, Apaydin KC, Ozel A. Acute orbital effects of retrobulbar injection on optic nerve head topography. Br J Ophthalmol 2004;88(12):1573–6.

Moving?

Make sure your subscription moves with you!

To notify us of your new address, find your **Clinics Account Number** (located on your mailing label above your name), and contact customer service at:

Email: journalscustomerservice-usa@elsevier.com

800-654-2452 (subscribers in the U.S. & Canada)
314-447-8871 (subscribers outside of the U.S. & Canada)

Fax number: 314-447-8029

Elsevier Health Sciences Division
Subscription Customer Service
3251 Riverport Lane
Maryland Heights, MO 63043

Printed and bound by CPI Group (UK) Ltd, Croydon, CR0 4YY

08/05/2025

01864692-0006